Sport and Exercise Medicine

The complete guide for all candidates studying and working in the field of sport and exercise medicine, including higher specialist training and post graduate examinations. This revision guide covers all key elements of the UK National Curriculum in Sport and Exercise Medicine. Key features to facilitate learning include:

- A pictorial summary at the start of each chapter
- 'Clinical consideration' sections that show how knowledge can be applied to working clinical practice
- MCQ questions for each chapter, including answers

MFSEM examination candidates, MSc students in sport and exercise medicine, sport and exercise medicine specialist trainee doctors, physiotherapists and general practitioners with an extended role in musculoskeletal or sport and exercise medicine will all benefit from this new text.

MasterPass Series

For more information about this series please visit: www.routledge.com/MasterPass/book-series/ CRCMASPASS

Sport and Exercise Medicine

An Essential Guide

Edited by

Dr David Eastwood MBBS MSc (SEM) MFSEM (UK)
MRCGP DipMskMed

Locala, MSK department, Princess Royal Health Centre, Huddersfield, UK
Newcastle United Football Club, Newcastle-Upon-Tyne, UK
Leeds School of Medicine, University of Leeds, Leeds, UK

Dr Dane Vishnubala MBBS PGCME DipSEM (UK)
MRCGP MSc (SEM) FFSEM FHEA

Faculty of Biological Sciences, University of Leeds, Leeds, UK
Hull York Medical School, York
Yorkshire Sports Medicine Clinic and YSM Academy, York, UK

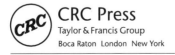

CRC Press
Taylor & Francis Group
Boca Raton London New York

CRC Press is an imprint of the
Taylor & Francis Group, an **informa** business

First edition published 2023
by CRC Press
6000 Broken Sound Parkway NW, Suite 300, Boca Raton, FL 33487–2742

and by CRC Press
4 Park Square, Milton Park, Abingdon, Oxon, OX14 4RN

CRC Press is an imprint of Taylor & Francis Group, LLC

© 2023 Taylor & Francis Group, LLC

ISBN: 978-1-032-01772-3 (hbk)
ISBN: 978-1-032-01762-4 (pbk)
ISBN: 978-1-003-17997-9 (ebk)

DOI: 10.1201/9781003179979

Typeset in ITC Legacy Serif
by Apex CoVantage, LLC

For Claire and Mari, constant sources of support and love,
and in memory of my grandad, who still inspires me every day.
David Eastwood

To my family: Katie, Rían, Fiadh, Arani and Arthy who support, encourage and inspire me everyday.
To JP for all the guidance, support and advice over the years.
Dane Vishnubala

Contents

Foreword

It is a privilege to be invited to write the foreword for David Eastwood and Dane Vishnubala's essential guide for sport and exercise medicine.

Accelerated by the awarding of the 2012 Olympics to London, sport and exercise medicine in the United Kingdom (UK) has made enormous progress since the turn of the century. It is now a fully accredited, well recognised and much sought after full medical specialty with an extensive training programme and a challenging final examination.

It is with that final examination in mind that David and Dane, with the help of a large number of extraordinarily knowledgeable co-authors, have produced this excellent book which will be an invaluable resource for both those taking the exam and others merely wanting a concise sport and exercise medicine resource.

As someone who has laboured through writing a few books over the years, I have a good appreciation of the work that goes into a volume such as this and as such I offer my heartiest congratulations to David and Dane, and their colleagues. The book will undoubtedly be a valuable contribution to the field of sport and exercise medicine.

Peter Brukner OAM, FACSEP
Professor of Sports Medicine,
La Trobe University, Melbourne, Australia
Co-author, *Clinical Sports Medicine* textbook

As sport and exercise medicine becomes more established across the world as a medical speciality, it is only fitting that the breadth of the subject is recognised by formal examination in various guises.

This compendium covers a wide, and far-reaching exploration of the syllabus of the UK higher specialist training program but is equally suited for those studying sport and exercise medicine in other territories and in other contexts, not just examination preparation. The subject summaries are comprehensive and yet concise giving the reader an aide memoire alongside robust and challenging questions of the type seen in examination. Each expanded answer to these questions gives the reader the opportunity to target further in-depth revision if required and will prove invaluable in examination preparation.

The text is also invaluable to those involved in teaching as both a guide to trainee expectation but also as a means of assessing progress against the curriculum from undergraduate to postgraduate level.

One striking feature is the breadth of new sport and exercise medicine consultants in the authorship, giving real world experience and currency to this excellent text which I highly recommend.

Dr Andrew Franklyn-Miller MBBS PhD
MRCGP FFSEM
Chief Medical Officer GB and England Hockey
Former Director of Sports Medicine,
Sports Surgery Clinic, Dublin, Ireland

Preface

As former candidates of the Faculty of Sport and Exercise Medicine examinations, as well as former MSc SEM students ourselves, we were both surprised and frustrated at the lack of texts on the market for sport and exercise medicine examinations. As such, we felt there was a perfect opportunity to develop a guide for those in a similar position. We wanted to produce something concise that can aid knowledge and revision, and we feel that this is a unique guide, ideal for those studying sport and exercise medicine, sitting examinations or working in various clinical settings where sport or exercise play a role.

Sport and exercise medicine is a developing specialty. Recent years have seen an increase in the number of institutions offering diplomas and MSc degrees in sport and exercise medicine. The Faculty of Sport and Exercise Medicine (FSEM) membership examination is now open to doctors from different specialty backgrounds, which has not always been the case.

Surprisingly, there is little sport and exercise medicine content taught at undergraduate level. Therefore, knowing examined material in this discipline can be challenging; and we hope we have addressed this need. The book is divided into chapters based on the brand new 2021 sport and exercise medicine curriculum, with a chapter dedicated to each curriculum component.

Each chapter contains:

- *An infographic overview:* This includes some key learning points from the chapter content that may appeal to the more visual learner.
- *Clinical considerations:* These are tips throughout the text with thoughts on how to apply knowledge to clinical situations.
- *Multiple choice questions:* At the end of each chapter we have included some questions to test knowledge and understanding.

This book aims to target a wide range of readers studying postgraduate sport and exercise medicine, including doctors, physiotherapists, allied health care professionals and students.

We thank the many authors and reviewers who have contributed to this text, many of whom are experts in their field or who have recently completed examinations and postgraduate qualifications in this subject. We have allocated authorship with the first author having made the most significant contribution to the chapter and the last author providing a senior review.

It is important to note that we have included key references and suggested further reading, rather than extensive referencing. We hope that this text can also act as a platform to further resources in the reader's learning journey.

Dave and Dane

About the Editors

Dr David Eastwood. MBBS MSc (SEM) MFSEM (UK) MRCGP DipMSKMed. David is a general practitioner and sport and exercise medicine physician. He currently works within the National Health Service (NHS) in general practice and at Locala Health and Wellbeing musculoskeletal medicine clinic. He has wide ranging experience working in professional sport, including football, rugby league and international multisport events, and is currently working with the first team at Newcastle United football club. He enjoys teaching and is a physical activity clinical champion for the Office for Health Improvement and Disparities (OHID). He is a director of Medisense, an innovative medical education organisation, and a visiting lecturer at Leeds University.

Dr Dane Vishnubala. MBBS MRCGP PGCME MSc (SEM) DipSEM (UK) FFSEM FHEA. Dane is a consultant physician in sport and exercise medicine and the education lead for the British association of sport and exercise medicine (BASEM). He is currently the clinical lead of the MSc in sport and exercise medicine at the University of Leeds and the training programme Director for SEM higher specialist training in Yorkshire and Humber. He is the lead doctor for the Office for Health Improvement and Disparities (OHID) peer to peer physical activity education programme.

He is the founder of CORE Fitness Education, a fitness training provider, and Medinotes, a medical notes system for SEM.

Clinically, Dane works for the Ministry of Defence (MOD) and for Yorkshire Sports Medicine Clinic. He is currently the Chief Medical Officer for Basketball England and the Welsh Football senior womens team doctor.

Contributors

Brook Adams
Consultant Radiologist
York Teaching Hospitals NHS Foundation Trust
York UK

Pippa Bennett
Consultant in Sport and Exercise Medicine
English Institute of Sport (EIS)
Peterborough, UK

Simon Boyle
Consultant Orthopaedic Surgeon
York and Scarborough Teaching Hospitals NHS
Foundation Trust
York, UK
Yorkshire Sports Medicine Clinic and YSM Academy
York, UK

James W. Burger
Psychiatry Registrar
University of Cape Town
Cape Town, South Africa

Victoria Campbell
GP and Sport Doctor
UK Ministry of Defence
Glasgow, UK

Sean Carmody
GP and Sport Doctor
Crystal Palace Football Club
London, UK

Natalie Cheyne
Orthopaedic Senior Clinical Fellow
Manchester University NHS Foundation Trust
Manchester, UK

Richard Collins
Consultant in Sport and Exercise Medicine
English Institute of Sport, Milton Keynes, UK
School of Biomedical Sciences, Faculty of Biological
Sciences, University of Leeds, Leeds, UK

Michael Cooke
Consultant in Emergency Medicine
Bradford Teaching Hospitals NHS
Foundation Trust
Bradford, UK

Robert Cooper
Consultant Cardiologist
Liverpool Heart and Chest Hospital NHS
Foundation Trust
Liverpool, UK

Rishi Dhand
GP and Sport Doctor
Leeds United Football Club
Leeds, UK

Linda Evans
GP Registrar and Sport Doctor
Leeds Teaching Hospitals NHS Trust
Leeds, UK

Daniel Fitzpatrick
Sport and Exercise Medicine Registrar
Imperial College Healthcare NHS Trust
London, UK

Ian Gatt
Upper Limb Technical Consultant
English Institute of Sport (EIS)
Sheffield, UK

Nick Grantham
Performance Specialist and Coach
Newcastle United Football Club
Newcastle upon Tyne, UK

Steffan Griffin
GP Registrar and Sport Doctor
Imperial College Healthcare NHS Trust
London, UK

Roshan Gunasekera
Sport and Exercise Medicine Registrar
Sheffield Teaching Hospitals NHS Foundation Trust
Sheffield, UK

James Hamilton
Consultant Radiologist
York and Scarborough Teaching Hospitals NHS
Foundation Trust
York, UK
Yorkshire Sports Medicine Clinic and YSM Academy,
York, UK
School of Biomedical Sciences, Faculty of Biological
Sciences, University of Leeds, Leeds, UK

Sarah Hattee
Senior Physiotherapist
Yorkshire Rugby, Leeds, UK
Yorkshire Sports Medicine Clinic, York, UK

Anthony Hoban
GP and Sport Doctor
Shamrock Rovers Football Club and Football
Association of Ireland
Dublin, UK

Andrew Howse
Specialist Sport and MSK Physiotherapist
Bristol Physio, Bristol, UK
Basketball England, Manchester, UK

James Hull
Consultant Respiratory Physician
Royal Brompton Hospital, Guy's and St Thomas'
NHS Foundation Trust
London, UK

Allan Johnston
Consultant Psychiatrist
English Institute of Sport (EIS)
Sheffield, UK

Kush Joshi
Consultant in Sport and Exercise Medicine
Homerton University Hospital Foundation Trust
London, UK

Saurav Kataria
GP Registrar and Sport Doctor
Bradford Teaching Hospitals NHS Foundation Trust
Bradford, UK

Nicky Keay
Sports and Dance Endocrinologist
University College London
London, UK

Thomas Leggett
GP and Sport Doctor
Loomer Medical
Staffordshire, UK

Raymond Leung
Consultant in Sport and Exercise Medicine
Homerton University Hospital NHS Foundation Trust
London, UK

Emma Jane Lunan
Consultant in Sport and Exercise Medicine
Marnock Medical Group
Kilmarnock, UK

Katie Marino
Academic GP Registrar
Keele University
Keele, UK

Jude McDowell
Specialist Musculoskeletal Physiotherapist
York and Scarborough Teaching Hospitals NHS
Foundation Trust
York, UK
Yorkshire Sports Medicine Clinic, York, UK

Luke McMenamin
Anaesthetic Registrar
Leeds Teaching Hospitals NHS Trust
Leeds, UK

Andrew Duncan Murray
Consultant in Sport and Exercise Medicine
University of Edinburgh
Edinburgh, UK

James Noake
Consultant in Sport and Exercise Medicine
Pure Sports Medicine
London, UK

John Noonan
Performance Coach
Noonan Performance Ltd
Cheshire, UK

Camilla Nykjaer
Academic Lead MSc SEM and PG Cert MSK
Medicine
School of Biomedical Sciences, Faculty of
Biological Sciences, University of Leeds, Leeds, UK

Patrick O'Halloran
Sport and Exercise Medicine Registrar
University Hospitals Birmingham NHS Foundation
Trust Marker Diagnostics UK Ltd
Birmingham, UK

Carles Pedret
Sport Medicine and Sport Orthopaedic Doctor
Clínica Diagonal, Esplugues de Llobregat
Barcelona, Spain

Jonathan Power
Consultant in Sport and Exercise Medicine
School of Biomedical Sciences, Faculty of
Biological Sciences, University of Leeds
Leeds, UK
Yorkshire Sports Medicine Clinic and YSM Academy
York, UK
Liverpool Football Club, Liverpool, UK

Andy Pringle
Professor in Physical Activity and Health
Intervention
University of Derby
Derby, UK

Anoop Raghavan
GP and Sport Doctor
York and Scarborough Teaching Hospitals NHS
Foundation Trust
York, UK

Hamish Reid
Consultant in Sport and Exercise Medicine
Moving Medicine, Faculty of Sport and Exercise
Medicine, Edinburgh, UK

Ashley Ridout
Sport and Exercise Medicine Registrar
Oxford University Hospitals NHS Foundation Trust
Oxford, UK

Rebecca Robinson
Consultant in Sport and Exercise Medicine
Sheffield Teaching Hopitals NHS Foundation Trust
Sheffield, UK

Peter Rosenfeld
Consultant Orthopaedic Surgeon
Imperial College Healthcare NHS Trust
London, UK

Claire Ryan
Radiology Registrar
Leeds Teaching Hospitals Trust
Leeds, UK

David Salman
Academic Clinical Fellow in Primary Care
Imperial College London
London, UK

Andrew Shafik
GP Registrar and Sport Doctor
Millwall Football Club
London, UK

K Pumi Senaratne
Consultant in Sport and Exercise Medicine
Nottingham University Hospitals NHS Trust
Nottingham, UK

Suzy Speirs
Consultant Podiatric Surgeon
Central London Community NHS Healthcare
Trust
London, UK

Luke Taylor
Senior Lecturer in Sport and Coaching Sciences
Oxford Brookes University
Oxford, UK

Gui Tran
Consultant Rheumatologist
Harrogate and District NHS Foundation
Trust
Harrogate, UK

Patrick Tung
Consultant in Emergency Medicine
Mid Yorkshire Hospitals NHS Trust
Dewsbury, UK

Justin Varney
Consultant in Public Health Medicine
Birmingham City Council
Birmingham, UK

Amit Verma
Consultant in Sport and Exercise Medicine
Liverpool Football Club and Connect Health
Liverpool, UK

Anita Vishnubala
GP and A&E Doctor
Kings College Hospital NHS Foundation Trust
London, UK

Steven Whatmough
Sport and Exercise Medicine Registrar
St James's University Hospital
Leeds, UK

David Whittaker
Sport and Exercise Medicine Registrar
University College London Hospitals NHS Trust
London, UK

Mark Williams
Senior Lecturer
Department of Sport, Health and Wellbeing
Writtle University College
Chelmsford, UK

Craig Zalecki
Consultant in Sport and Exercise Medicine
School of Biomedical Sciences, Faculty of Biological
Sciences, University of Leeds, Leeds, UK
Yorkshire Sports Medicine Clinic, York, UK

Basic Science 1

David Eastwood, Mark Williams, Nick Grantham, John Noonan and David Salman

BACKGROUND

A person's physiological response to exercise depends on a number of factors, including: the type of exercise, the age, gender, genetic makeup and body composition of the person, as well as environmental conditions (e.g. geographical area, climate and social factors). This chapter aims to outline some of the mechanisms and homeostatic responses involved in exercise.

ANATOMY

Bone

Bone is a rigid tissue that constitutes the skeleton. Its metabolism (known as remodelling) is a continuous cycle of growth and resorption that is influenced by hormones, osteoclastic and osteoblastic activity. Bone also plays a metabolic role in managing the balance of calcium and phosphate in the body (Figure 1.2).

The key components of bone metabolism include:

- *Bone matrix:* this is mostly made of the mineral hydroxyapatite (calcium phosphate) as well as organic material that is mostly type 1 collagen.
- *Osteoclasts:* these multinucleated cells attach to bone and commence resorption of the matrix by using enzymes and hydrogen ions.
- *Osteoblasts:* deposit new collagen and minerals in the spaces created by osteoclasts.
- *Osteocytes:* these are the most common cell type and exist within the bone matrix. They transmit signals to other osteocytes to indicate bone stress as a result of mechanical forces.

Various hormones can impact bone remodelling and calcium metabolism:

- *Parathyroid hormone (PTH):* this hormone is secreted by parathyroid gland chief cells. It raises blood calcium levels by increasing osteoclast activity. Conversely, high levels of plasma calcium bind to the parathyroid gland and inhibit PTH production. PTH also acts on the kidneys by upregulating ion channels, increasing the reabsorption of calcium into the blood and releasing calcitriol.
- *Calcitonin:* this is released from thyroid C cells in response to high calcium levels. It binds to osteoclasts to inhibit resorption and acts on the kidney to cause calcium clearance in the urine.
- *Vitamin D:* sourced from either ingestion or synthesised from a cholesterol precursor, its presence increases the amount of calcium absorbed in the intestine. It is metabolised to its major circulating form, Calcidiol (25(OH)D), in the liver, and then to its hormonal form, Calcitriol (1,25(OH)2D), in the kidney.

Exercise is generally considered beneficial to bone and can be an effective management option for osteoporosis or bone loss. The most significant osteogenic response is gained from high-impact, high exercise-specific intensity activity, whereas sports with low-impact forces—such as cycling—do not typically provide much benefit. An acute bout of exercise increases bone resorption and, initially, increases osteoclastic activity. As adaptation occurs, osteoblasts up-regulate bone formation. Bone is extremely responsive to nutrient intake and good bone health needs adequate energy availability.

DOI: 10.1201/9781003179979-1

BASIC SCIENCE

Exercise Capacity

- Borg scale (rating of perceived exertion, RPE) 6–20
- Lactate threshold
  - blood lactate ≥ 4mmol/L
  - velocity indicates endurance performance
- VO_2 max Q $(CaO_2\text{-}CvO_2)$
  - RER (Respiratory Exchange Ratio) > 1.15
  - RPE >17
  - Heart rate within 10bpm of maximum
  - Plateau ≤ 150ml O_2/min

Nutrition

Daily calorie intake should be calculated using:
  - basal metabolic rate
  - age
  - sex
  - physical activity levels

Male 2500+ calories
Female 2000+ calories

Carbohydrates 2–12g/kg/day

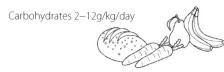

Protein 0.8–1.5g/kg/day

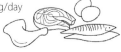

Fat 0.5–1.5g/kg/day

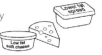

Tissue

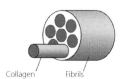

Myofibril
Fascicle
Fibre

Muscle
- Type 1a - ↑ mitochondria
  ↑ oxidative
- Type 2a - ↑ oxidative
  ↑ glycolytic capacity
- Type 2x/2b - ↓ oxidative
  ↑ glycolytic capacity

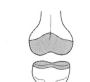

Collagen microfibrils
Fibrils

Ligament
- Fibroblasts
- Collagen (type I)
- Water
- Elastin
- Lipids
- Proteoglycans

Cartilage
- Water
- Collagen (type II)
- Proteoglycans
- Chondrocytes

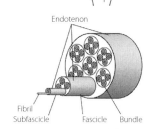

Endotenon
Fibril
Subfascicle
Fascicle
Bundle

Tendon
- Water
- Collagen (type I)

Energy Systems and Yield

1) ATP-PCr   ATP - 1

2) Anaerobic glycolysis   ATP - 2

3) Oxidative phosphorylation   ATP - Carbohydrates: 36-39
                                  Fat: > 100

Figure 1.1 Pictorial chapter overview.

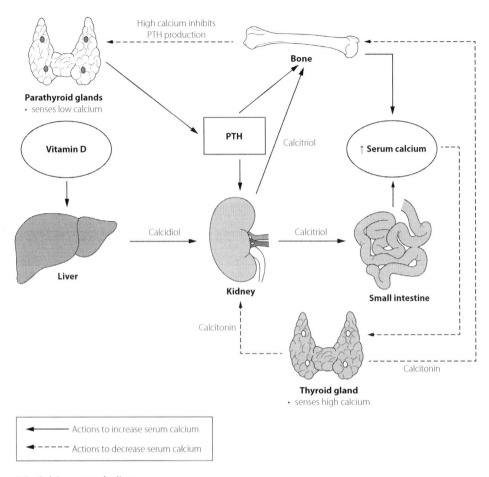

Figure 1.2 Calcium metabolism.

Tendon

This is the transitional tissue connecting bone and muscle. It transfers the mechanical energy, generated by muscle contraction, to the bone, thereby producing movement. Tendon primarily consists of water and type I collagen. These molecules group together to form fibrils, which group further to form fibres. A number of fibres are grouped into a subfascicle and a number of subfascicles into a fascicle. An endotenon is the connective tissue that encases collagen bundles including the fibres and fascicles, allowing them to glide amongst each other and providing further support. Tendons are highly structured, which permits great strength to sustain mechanical load.

Tendons are subject to many forms of injury, including tendinopathy. The pathophysiology of this injury is still debated, but tendons fail to repair, leading to

disorganised type I and III collagen fibres, capillary overgrowth and rounded fibroblasts unevenly distributed throughout the tissue. There is an increase in the ratio of type III to type I collagen, which has poorer biomechancial properties. Multiple intrinsic risk factors (including age and nutrition), as well as extrinsic risk factors (such as changes to mechanical load and poor training technique) may contribute.

Acute tendinous and musculotendinous injuries take longer to heal compared to myofascial injuries. Stages of tendon healing include haemostasis (platelets trigger the coagulation cascade over a period of around 15 minutes), inflammation (where fibroblasts produce type III collagen over around 7 days), proliferation (tissue modelling over approximately 7–21 days) and remodelling (type III collagen is replaced by type I collagen, which can take up to 18 months).

Ligament

This is the transitional tissue connecting bone to bone. Ligaments provide structural support, limit excessive movement and contribute to joint proprioception through mechanoreceptors and free nerve endings. The main constituents of ligaments are fibroblast cells, type I collagen, water, elastin, lipids and proteoglycans. Compared to tendons, ligaments generally contain less collagen and are less organised in their structure.

An injury to ligament can cause sprain or rupture. Sprains are often graded (grade I: stretching of the ligament with microscopic, but no macroscopic, tearing; grade II: partial tearing of the ligament and grade III: complete rupture). Management of these injuries will depend on the location, severity and the individual needs of the patient. For example, a young, high functioning athlete with an anterior cruciate ligament rupture may require surgical repair.

Stages of ligament healing include inflammation (an influx of inflammatory cells, neutrophils and the production of type III collagen, typically over 7 days), proliferation (where type III collagen is replaced by type I over approximately 7–21 days), remodelling and maturation (which can take up to 18 months). Extra-articular ligaments generally have a greater capacity to heal.

Articular Cartilage

Articular or hyaline cartilage acts to inhibit friction and distribute load between joints. There are other forms of cartilage including fibroelastic (or meniscal) cartilage and fibrocartilage, which is located in tendon and ligament bone insertions.

Articular cartilage is avascular and is sustained by bone and superficial synovial fluid. It comprises of water, collagen (mostly type II), proteoglycans and chondrocytes. The water content tends to decrease with normal ageing, but increases in osteoarthritis, due to increased tissue permeability.

Injury may cause an intra-articular fracture. Here, the healing response produces type I collagen and fibrocartilage, which is less resilient and may predispose to osteoarthritis. Osteoarthritis is a degenerative disease that is characterised by a progressive loss of articular cartilage. In this process, water content is increased, proteoglycans decrease and collagen becomes less organised. Ultimately, changes also occur to the joint capsule and bone.

Muscle

Muscle is soft tissue and is usually grouped into smooth, skeletal and cardiac muscle. Skeletal muscle is striated and constitutes between 30–40% of human body mass. When stimulated, muscle contracts to produce movement.

The functional contractile unit of muscle is the sarcomere—this is comprised of actin and myosin protein filaments. These filaments make up myofibrils, which are grouped into fibres. Endomysium encases fibres to form a fascicle, and these fascicles are surrounded by perimysium to group into muscle.

During muscle contraction, the binding sites on actin are exposed by calcium ions, and myosin binds, as well as binding to ATP—the necessary source of energy. This facilitates the cross-bridge stroke of myosin on actin, generating contraction of the sarcomere unit.

Skeletal muscle consists of different fibre types, dependent on the myosin heavy chain (MyHC) protein that they express: a slow-contracting type 1 fibre and a fast-contracting type 2, further classified into 2a, 2b and 2x.

Although 2b and 2x are sometimes used interchangeably, type 2b fibres are not expressed in large mammals (humans), but are in smaller mammals, such as mice.

- *Type 1 fibres ('slow-twitch fibres'):* These contain a high number of mitochondria and a rich blood supply. Subsequently, they are highly oxidative and have a low glycolytic capacity, meaning they fatigue less easily but generally generate lower forces. They are used in long duration contractile activities such as endurance sports.
- *Type 2a fibres ('fast-twitch oxidative fibres'):* these fibres are resistant to fatigue as they are highly oxidative but have high glycolytic capacity. There is a high number of mitochondria. They are used in activities such as repeated weightlifting, where continued effort is needed.
- *Type 2x fibres ('fast-twitch glycolytic fibres'):* these fibres are lowly oxidative and have high glycolytic capacity. They fatigue very easily and are used for high intensity exercise such as sprinting. Typically, there is a low number of mitochondria.

Neuromuscular Response to Exercise

When a muscle is recruited and used, it progressively adapts to load and fibres can hypertrophy. Exercise stresses the musculoskeletal system and microtrauma stimulates a repair process by cells, including myosatellite cells.

Different types of exercise training will stimulate the presence of different types of muscle fibres. The recruitment of muscle fibres is determined by the size principle, which states that motor units with smaller fibres are recruited first, followed by larger fibres as more force is required. Strength training causes high concentric and eccentric forces, which in turn, 'overloads' the muscle, causing protein synthesis, hypertrophy of muscle fibre and a preference to type II fibres.

Endurance training, such as long-distance running, increases the presence of mitochondria, which increases gas exchange availability and makes type I muscle fibres more abundant.

EXERCISE PHYSIOLOGY

Cellular Metabolism

Adenosine Triphosphate (ATP) is the energy source required for skeletal muscle. It consists of adenosine and three phosphate groups. Splitting the terminal phosphate bond on this molecule creates this energy. This takes place with the addition of water (hydrolysis) and the enzyme ATPase. As cells store a limited amount of this energy, re-synthesis is necessary. A phosphate group is added to ADP—a process called phosphorylation—to restore ATP.

$$ATP \rightarrow ADP + P + Energy$$

Energy Production Pathways

ATP-PCr

In addition to storing a small amount of free ATP, cells contain phosphocreatine (PCr). The enzyme creatine kinase acts on PCr to separate a phosphate molecule (P) from creatine. The energy released in this process can be used to add this free phosphate molecule to ADP to form ATP. This is a form of substrate-level metabolism. It does not require oxygen,

but supplies are limited, and the combination of free ATP and PCr can only sustain energy for up to 15 seconds in a full sprint. A high volume of fast-twitch muscle fibres with adequate creatinine, as well as tailored training, can influence the output of this energy system.

ANAEROBIC GLYCOLYSIS

This process relies on ATP production from the breakdown of glucose via a pathway involving glycolytic enzymes (Figure 1.3). Glucose comes from carbohydrate ingestion or glycogen stores. Glycogen is stored in the liver and muscle. When it is required, it is broken down into glucose 1-phosphate in hepatocytes and myocytes, before entering the glycolysis pathway. At the start of this process, glucose or glycogen is first converted into glucose-6-phosphate. This stage costs 1 ATP molecule when glucose is converted. A process of 10–12 reactions then takes place, resulting in pyruvic acid. There is a net gain of 2 ATP molecules for each glucose molecule. If this process begins with glycogen, there is a net gain of 3 ATP molecules.

Pyruvic acid can be reduced by lactate dehydrogenase to produce lactic acid. The lactic acid at the end of this process dissociates to produce a salt (lactate) and a hydrogen ion. These ions need to be buffered, otherwise the acidity will inhibit cellular activity. Lactate can be metabolised aerobically by other tissues. This energy system, alongside ATP-PCr, is the primary system for short, intense exercise, such as a 400 m sprint.

OXIDATIVE PHOSPHORYLATION

Prolonged exercise requires a greater amount of energy. This process occurs in cell organelles called mitochondria and is initiated more slowly (Figure 1.4). Oxidative production of ATP involves aerobic glycolysis, the Krebs cycle and the electron transport chain. In the same glycolytic process explained for anaerobic glycolysis above, the resultant pyruvic acid is converted to acetyl coenzyme A (Acetyl-CoA) in the presence of oxygen. Acetyl-CoA then enters the Krebs (or citric acid) cycle, a complex series of processes that directly forms 2 ATP molecules as well as carbon dioxide and hydrogen.

A hydrogen ion is produced in the Krebs cycle. During glycolysis, a hydrogen ion is also released when glucose is broken down into pyruvic acid. These

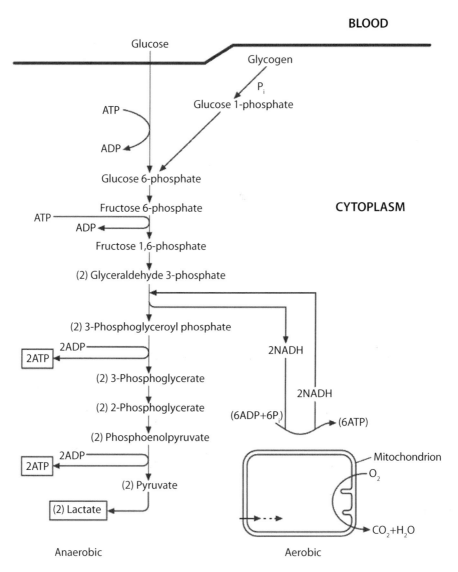

BLOOD

Glucose

Glycogen

P_i

Glucose 1-phosphate

ATP

ADP

Glucose 6-phosphate

Fructose 6-phosphate   **CYTOPLASM**

ATP

ADP

Fructose 1,6-phosphate

(2) Glyceraldehyde 3-phosphate

(2) 3-Phosphoglyceroyl phosphate

2ADP

2ATP   2NADH

(2) 3-Phosphoglycerate

2NADH

(2) 2-Phosphoglycerate

$(6ADP+6P_i)$ (6ATP)

(2) Phosphoenolpyruvate

2ADP

2ATP   Mitochondrion

(2) Pyruvate O_2

(2) Lactate

CO_2+H_2O

Anaerobic   Aerobic

Figure 1.3 Glycolysis and gluconeogenesis overview.

Source: Saghiv and Sagiv, 2020

ions are carried by coenzymes to the electron transport chain where they are divided into protons and electrons. The hydrogen ion combines with oxygen to form water, preventing acidity, and the electrons undergo further reactions to provide the energy needed to phosphorylate ADP. With one molecule of glucose, the maximal net gain is 38 molecules of ATP. With glycogen, the maximal net gain is 39 molecules

of ATP (one ATP molecule is used in converting glucose to glucose-6-phosphate before glycolysis begins).

When carbohydrate sources expire, this process can use fat as a fuel; whilst this is far slower, the energy yield is far greater. Because oxygen is required, factors such as cardiac and respiratory function, altitude or the abundance of 'slow-twitch' muscle fibres can influence its efficiency in athletes.

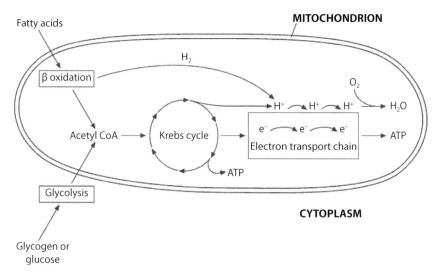

Figure 1.4 Aerobic processes.

Source: Saghiv and Sagiv, 2020

Table 1.1 Energy systems

Approximate Duration	Type	Fuel	Example
Up to 4 seconds	Anaerobic	ATP (muscle store)	Tennis serve
Up to 15 seconds	Anaerobic	ATP + PCr	Sprint
Up to 3 minutes	Anaerobic	ATP + PCr + muscle glycogen	Swim
Beyond 3 minutes	Anaerobic and aerobic	Muscle glycogen and lactic acid	Basketball match
Beyond 3 minutes	Aerobic	Muscle glycogen and free fatty acids	10 K run

Energy Systems During Exercise

Different sports will use different energy systems to different degrees (McArdle et al. 2015). Table 1.1 provides some examples.

EXERCISE NUTRITION

Energy intake must equal energy expenditure and an adequate diet is important to sustain this. It is key to maintain a diet that provides health benefits, maximises athletic performance and maintains an appropriate body composition.

Recommended calorie intake will vary depending on the amount of physical activity and basal metabolic rate (BMR), but should be around 2000 calories daily in women and 2500 in men.

BMR is the minimum amount of energy needed for the body's basic metabolic processes. It should be calculated in a thermoneutral environment when the body is not digesting food, and gives an estimation of energy costs before any physical activity or exercise.

Weight, height and sex are important variables when calculating BMR. The Harris-Benedict and Mifflin St Jeor equations are commonly used to calculate this. Daily calorie expenditure can then be determined by multiplying by a value representing the activity levels of an individual. If free fat mass (FFM) is available, then BMR can be predicted more accurately by the Katch-McArdle formula.

A combination of carbohydrates, protein and fat make up the majority of diet, and carbohydrates tend to be the main source of energy in exercise. For most people, a diet will consist of around 50% carbohydrate and 10-30% fat with the remainder being protein. For endurance athletes, carbohydrate intake may be substantially higher. Diet should depend on the energy requirements and exercise performed by the individual. Those participating in gymnastics, for example, where lean muscle mass is required, may require a diet with greater protein content. An endurance runner, however, may require greater levels of carbohydrate and fat.

Carbohydrate

Carbohydrates (CHO) are either monosaccharides, disaccharides or polysaccharides (such as glycogen), depending on the molecular chain length. Major dietary sources include fruit, grains, pasta, beans, vegetables and sweets. It is the main energy source. Recommended carbohydrate intake for exercising individuals can be anywhere between 2-12 g/kg/day depending on the energy requirements of the individual. Low intensity or skill-based activities may require 3-5 g/kg/day, team sport participants should aim for 5-7 g/kg/day and endurance athletes should consume anywhere up to 12 g/kg/day depending on energy requirements. Sometimes, carbohydrate loading is used by distance endurance athletes. Training exercise is tapered in the days prior to competition, whilst the percentage of dietary carbohydrate is increased, sometimes to as much as 70-80% of total calories consumed.

CLINICAL CONSIDERATIONS

Fatigue in an endurance athlete is often due to depleted muscle glycogen and low blood glucose levels. The point at which this is reached can be termed 'hitting the wall.' Before and during exercise, nutrition strategies should be considered to optimise fuel for competition. High glycaemic foods that are quickly oxidised can be useful, such as gels containing glucose or sucrose. For intense exercise

lasting greater than 30 minutes duration, up to 90 g/hour of carbohydrate can be consumed to avoid fuel depletion.

Protein

Proteins are molecules consisting of amino acid chains. Recommended protein intake for sedentary individuals is 0.8 g/kg/day. In exercising individuals, it should be closer to 1.0 g/kg/day and 1.5 g/kg/day for endurance athletes, or those striving to increase muscle mass or lose weight. Strength and power based athletes should consider at least 2.0 g/kg/day. Intake should be tailored to the individual, depending on weight and the frequency and intensity of exercise. Meat, fish, seafood, lentils, beans, tofu and dairy are common dietary sources.

Fat

Fats are organic compounds with limited water solubility. Most fat in the body is stored as triglyceride—three fatty acid molecules linked to a single glycerol molecule. It is a significant energy source, is a component in structures such as nerves and assists in the transport of fat-soluble vitamins. Milk, butter, oils and avocado are sources. Carbohydrates and proteins have an energy density of 4 kcal/g, whereas fats have a higher energy density of 9 kcal/g.

Vitamins

These are a group of compounds that the body needs in small amounts but are essential for tissue growth and metabolism. Fat-soluble vitamins include D, A, K and E. Water-soluble vitamins include vitamin C (ascorbic acid) and the B vitamins—thiamine (B1), riboflavin (B2), niacin (B3), pantothenic acid (B5), biotin (B7), folate (B9) and cobalamin (B12). With regards to sport, vitamins A and D are needed in bone development. Deficiency in B vitamins has been shown to impair performance, so having adequate dietary intake in athletes is essential. Vitamin B12 is needed in red blood cell production; a key part in gas exchange and oxidation. Thiamine is required in the transformation of pyruvic acid to Acetyl-CoA. Riboflavin is crucial for mitochondrial electron transport chain (ETC) function, in oxidative phosphorylation. Niacin helps make up Nicotinamide Adenine Dinucleotide Phosphate (NADP), a coenzyme in glycolysis.

Minerals

These are needed in cellular level processes. Macrominerals include calcium, magnesium, sodium, potassium and phosphorus. Microminerals include iron, copper, selenium and zinc.

Iron is a key component in haemoglobin and myoglobin, as well as being located in muscle, liver, spleen and bone marrow. Menstruation, poor diet and footstrike haemolysis in runners can lead to iron deficiency. Exercise, particularly endurance exercise, can also lead to dilutional anaemia, whereby plasma expansion is greater than red blood cell increase, leading to a falsely low haemoglobin level. Dietary iron can be found in leafy vegetables, red meat, beans, liver, nuts and fortified breakfast cereals. Men should consume around 9 mg of iron per day and menstruating females 15 mg per day.

Calcium is found in milk, cheese and leafy green vegetables. Most calcium is stored in bones and is necessary for their metabolism and growth. It is also integral to nerve pulse transmission and muscle contraction. Adults require 700 mg of calcium per day. If dietary intake is insufficient, this can lead to weakened bones, or osteopenia, which can then lead to osteoporosis and increased fracture risk.

Supplements

Debate exists as to whether dietary supplements provide ergogenic value to athletes, and most supplements do not have sufficient evidence to back their use if dietary intake is already appropriate and balanced. Caffeine ingestion has been shown to improve exercise performance with regard to muscle endurance, muscle strength, anaerobic power and anaerobic endurance. Caution should be taken with increased caffeine and energy drink consumption; there have been reported pro-arrhythmic effects due to the very high adrenergic activity developed during intense exercise.

Creatine is one of the most popular dietary ergogenic aids used within athletic populations today.

Supplementation has reliably shown increased intramuscular concentrations of creatine in the literature, although in practice, ergogenic benefit is more variable. Renal dysfunction and cramping has been reported with its use, suggesting individual responses should be monitored. Nonetheless, creatine is particularly useful to improve high-intensity exercise capacity, and other training adaptations, such as increased muscular strength, power and recovery from exercise.

Sodium bicarbonate ($NaHCO_3$) has been suggested to aid performance by reducing acidosis in exercise. The literature is mixed, with some studies reporting improvements in swimming and endurance running times; whereas other research suggests it may even impair performance, perhaps via its mechanism of neutralising gastric acid and causing gastrointestinal upset.

Hydration

Water is crucial in exercise. It helps regulate body temperature, maintains blood pressure and allows transportation at a cellular level. In terms of hydration, the general advice is to 'drink to thirst' and restore water loss that ensues due to sweating and insensible losses during exercise. Aerobic performance is impaired with dehydration. However, over-drinking can also lead to other problems such as dilutional hyponatraemia.

Energy Costs of Exercise

The body deals with the stress of exercise in a complex way. Exercise training increases antioxidant enzymes, which prevent excessive muscle damage from free radicals. Eccentric exercise has been shown to induce more delayed onset muscle soreness (DOMS) and muscle damage. Neutrophils infiltrate injured muscle tissue and release cytokines to trigger an inflammatory response. Following exercise-induced muscular damage, phagocytes break down cellular debris, before regeneration occurs after around 4 days. Satellite cells respond initially, before forming myoblasts (which develop into muscle), whilst a repair process occurs at cell membranes. Muscle will generally hypertrophy as a response to these processes.

MONITORING EXERCISE CAPACITY, TRAINING AND OVERTRAINING

Determining exercise capacity can be important in a number of settings (Kenney et al., 2020). In elite sport, it provides an evaluation of ability or a threshold that can be used in training and to improve performance. It can also help determine information that will guide exercise prescription in the general population, or examine the effectiveness of rehabilitation in altering exercise capacity.

Borg Scale

This is a subjective Rating of Perceived Exertion (RPE) that helps determine exercise intensity. It was initially developed on a 6–20 scale, with 6 equivalent to no exertion at all and 20 equivalent to maximal exertion. There is an association between the RPE number and heart rate, with heart rate being approximately 10 times the RPE number.

Metabolic Equivalent of Task (MET)

This is a unit that can be a useful gauge of physical activity intensity. 1 MET is considered the rate of energy expenditure or oxygen consumption at rest. This equals 3.5 mL of oxygen per kg of body weight per minute. MET permits a method of comparison of the intensity of physical activities. For example, walking slowly is 2 METs and swimming moderately hard is 8 METs.

Repetitions in Reserve (RIR)

This is a method used in resistance training to assess perceived exertion or exercise intensity. It is a measure of how many repetitions remain in a set before technical failure (or the inability to complete a repetition).

It is considered a more accurate method of determining near-limit loads for resistance training compared with traditional RPE scales and is relative to an individual's strength and ability.

Anaerobic (Lactate) Threshold

In anaerobic glycolysis, when lactate removal is slower than lactate production, it can accumulate. This occurs in intense exercise when aerobic metabolism in neighbouring tissues is unable to meet exercise demands. The point at which blood lactate appears to rise disproportionately above resting values is considered the lactate threshold. Another way of determining this point is when blood lactate concentration reaches 4 mmol/L.

The lactate threshold can be communicated as a percentage of maximal oxygen uptake at which it occurs. Usually, this is at around 55% of an untrained person's aerobic capacity (VO_2 max). It may also be expressed as the running velocity (kilometres/hour) at which the point is reached.

An anaerobically trained athlete is able to generate up to 30% more blood lactate compared to untrained individuals. Because blood lactate accumulation contributes to fatigue, a higher lactate threshold is a marker of better endurance performance.

Aerobic Capacity

In oxidative phosphorylation, the use of oxygen by cells is known as oxygen uptake (VO_2). This uptake rises rapidly at the start of exercise, but plateaus when supply meets demand. Maximal oxygen uptake (VO_2 max) is a measure of the maximum rate at which the body can extract oxygen, supply exercising tissue and aerobically resynthesise ATP.

In practice, it is when there is a plateau in oxygen consumption during a graded exercise test (GXT) or ramp test, beyond which no increase in effort can raise it. This usually involves a treadmill or cycle ergometer, whilst ventilation, oxygen and carbon dioxide concentration of the inhaled and expired air are recorded.

The respiratory exchange ratio (RER) is the comparison of the volume of carbon dioxide exhaled against the volume of oxygen consumed. This ratio should be >1.15 at VO_2 max. Other suggested criteria to help determine VO_2 max include heart rate within 10 bpm of age predicted maximum, a plateau of ≤ 150 mL O_2/min and perceived exhaustion (such as RPE >17 on the Borg scale).

$$VO_2 \text{ max} = Q(CaO_2 - CvO_2)$$

The Fick equation outlines that VO_2 max equals cardiac output (Q) multiplied by the amount of oxygen working muscles are able to take from the blood passing through them. CaO_2 = arterial oxygen and CvO_2 = venous oxygen content.

VO_2 max is an indicator of endurance performance. In the general population, it ranges from 20–90 mL/kg/min, with endurance trained athletes having the highest readings. VO_2 max can be difficult to achieve, particularly in non-athletic populations. In such cases, VO_2 peak can be recorded. This is when a plateau in VO_2 is not reached with increasing work rate. Provided the individual achieves over 80% of predicted work, a heart rate >80% of predicted maximum and a RER >1.15, it can be assumed that a maximal effort has been reached.

Other Factors

Both anaerobic threshold and aerobic capacity can be markers of performance; however other factors also contribute to success. These include tactical decisions, psychological differences and economy—an individual with a lower oxygen consumption (VO_2) for a given pace or load has a better economy.

As an example, running economy is complex and represents the combination of various metabolic, biomechanical, cardiorespiratory and neuromuscular characteristics during running. Favourable genetics are thought to play a role in determining economy, however many factors may be modifiable and include:

- Muscle fibre types
- Substrate utilisation
- Heart rate
- Core temperature
- Training volume and fatigue
- Biomechanics including running style/gait
- Body composition
- Muscle force production
- Stiffness (muscle-tendon compliance)

TRAINING

Training programmes should work on the principle of 'progressive overload.' This means that to continue to gain the benefits of training, the exercise or stimulation must be increased as the body adapts to the current level. If this is too low, then optimal performance will not be reached. When this principle is carried out too far, the body may not progress but instead decline. The volume of training can be increased either with the amount of work or the intensity.

Overreaching occurs when the body is intentionally overworked in order to adapt and improve. In functional overreaching, there is a short decrease in performance that can last days to weeks, before an expected increase in performance.

Overtraining is when overreaching results in a prolonged deterioration in performance (widely accepted as >2 months duration) alongside other symptoms. It is often a result of both physical and psychological causes. A decrease in performance may be associated with weight loss, gastrointestinal symptoms, insomnia, anxiety, depression or loss of motivation. Excessive training has also been shown to suppress normal immune function and can lead to vulnerability to infection. The primary treatment is rest. There is a close association between overtraining and Relative Energy Deficiency in Sport (RED-S), with both sharing hypothalamic-pituitary involvement, and overlapping symptoms.

BODY COMPOSITION

Body composition refers to the proportion of fat, muscle, bone and water that constitutes a person. Fat can be found in muscle tissue, subcutaneously or viscerally—around organs. Higher body fat distribution is associated with environmental factors including smoking, alcohol consumption and childhood obesity, as well as genetic factors. Increased upper body fat and visceral fat composition is associated with an increased risk of hyperlipidaemia, hypertension, type 2 diabetes amongst other health issues.

Obesity and Measuring

Body mass index (BMI) is a commonly used health tool for assessing health risk (Table 1.2). It is calculated

Table 1.2 Body Mass Index (BMI)

BMI	Weight status
<18.5	Underweight
18.5–24.9	Healthy weight
25–29.9	Overweight
30–34.9	Obesity 1
35–39.9	Obesity 2
≥ 40	Obesity 3

using weight in kg/[(Height in m)^2]. Having a BMI greater or equal to 30 is considered obese. The difficulty with this measurement, is that it does not differentiate between muscle and fat mass, and therefore, is not a reliable reference for individuals with high muscle mass—such as competitive athletes.

Other forms of assessing body composition include skinfold testing, hydrostatic weighing, Bioelectrical Impedance Analysis (BIA) and Dual Energy X-ray Absorptiometry (DEXA) scanning. Skinfold thickness may be inaccurate because it is user-dependent and may vary based on the skin calliper used. Various calculations can estimate fat percentage depending on the skin-fold thickness at sites including calf, triceps and the subscapularis regions. In BIA, an electrical current passes through the body and the voltage is measured. Having a lower impedance suggests more muscle content, as this contains more water. The hydration status of an individual can affect these results. DEXA scanning is considered the most accurate method. It can also give an accurate measurement of bone density, in addition to visceral fat. There is a small radiation dose, but less than conventional X-ray.

Exercise is recommended to achieve weight loss. The evidence that exercise contributes significantly to weight loss is not firmly established. The challenges of monitoring dietary intake, exercise intensity and exercise duration over a long period of time may contribute to limited research in this area. Moreover, physical activity has significant health benefits that are independent of weight loss, and these benefits make it a vital adjunct when considering general health, irrespective of weight.

A negative energy balance (i.e. exercising and losing more calories than those acquired by diet) results in weight loss over time through the loss of body fat and muscle mass. Fatigue from the loss of glycogen stores after intense exercise may affect performance and training. Therefore, intentional weight loss in athletes should be monitored carefully and dietary modifications may be more favourable.

MULTIPLE CHOICE QUESTION (MCQ) QUESTIONS

1. In bone metabolism, which one of the following hormones inhibits osteoclast activity?

   A. Thyroid hormone
   B. Parathyroid hormone
   C. Calcitonin
   D. Calcitriol
   E. Adrenocorticotropic hormone

2. You are giving dietary advice to an athletics team. Which numbers best describe the recommended average calorie intake in females and males?

   A. Females 2000, males 2500
   B. Females 2400, males 2800
   C. Females 2000, males 3000
   D. Females 2800, males 3000
   E. Females 2800, males 3500

3. Which one of the following is recognised as a limiting factor of the anaerobic (glycolytic) energy system?

   A. Lack of AMP
   B. Lack of lactic acid
   C. An accumulation of pyruvic acid
   D. Depletion of glycogen
   E. Lack of ATP

4. You are providing track-side medical cover at the Olympic games. The next event is a 200 m heat. Which energy system is predominantly used by competitors?

   A. PCr system
   B. Aerobic system (Oxidative Phosphorylation)
   C. Glycolytic system (Anaerobic glycolysis)
   D. Citric acid cycle
   E. ATP body stores

5. Whilst attending some exercise testing, the sport scientist tells you that Runner A has a better running economy than Runner B. Which of the following factors in Runner A is most likely to give them a better running economy?

   A. Increased leg stiffness
   B. Greater stride length
   C. Greater pace
   D. Greater VO$_2$ max
   E. Less type 2a muscle fibres

MULTIPLE CHOICE QUESTION (MCQ) ANSWERS

1. Answer C
    Calcitonin, a hormone produced by thyroid C-cells, inhibits osteoclast activity and opposes the action of Parathyroid hormone (B). Calcitriol (D) is a form of Vitamin D and can be used to treat hyperparathyroidism, whereas Adrenocorticotropic hormone (E) stimulates cortisol from the adrenal glands.

2. Answer A
    Although the average calorie intake in an active athletics team is likely to be much higher, the NHS recommended daily intake is 2000 calories in females and 2500 calories in males (A). The other answers describe various combinations that may be appropriate depending on multiple factors including frequency and intensity of exercise. Some powerlifters or gymnasts may require up to 6000 calories daily.

3. Answer D
    AMP can be converted to ADP and ATP, but a lack of it will not impair glycolysis, so A is incorrect. A lack of lactic acid (B) is incorrect. When there are high levels of lactic acid, it accumulates in muscle, lowers pH and can impair anaerobic respiration. Pyruvic acid is an intermediate in many metabolic pathways, so when it accumulates (C) it may be a) converted back to carbohydrates via gluconeogenesis; b) to fatty acids; c) enter the Krebs cycle or d) produce lactic acid. Although the anaerobic energy system requires ATP to function, ATP stores can be replenished quickly via a number of pathways including the PCr system. It directly relies on glycogen stores to be broken down into glucose, so once glycogen stores are depleted, the body cannot rely on this energy pathway to produce ATP. Therefore, D is the correct answer.

4. Answer C
    Although at the start of the event, ATP stores (E) and the PCr system (A) will contribute, the majority of energy in a 200 m sprint will be provided by the Glycolytic system (Anaerobic glycolysis), therefore C is correct.

5. Answer A
    Pace is not related to economy (the two runners could be running at the same pace with very different oxygen consumption) so C is incorrect. VO_2 max and running economy are thought to be determined independently, making D incorrect. B is incorrect as athletes are thought to use their optimal stride length. Overly long strides can be detrimental as misplaced strike position can cause friction, whereas overly short strides cause increased muscle work and energy loss. Type 2a muscle fibres are more oxidative, therefore less of them may decrease running economy (E). This leaves A as the correct answer. Leg stiffness is a measure of how well a runner recycles energy applied to the ground, and a greater stiffness can exploit stored elastic energy, improving economy.

REFERENCES AND FURTHER READING

The British Association for Sport and Exercise Sciences (BASES). 2023. *Learning Resources for Students.* Available from: https://www.bases.org.uk/spage-students-studying_and_learning_resources.html

Kenney, W.L., WIlmore, J.H and Costill, D.L. 2020. Physiology of Sport and Exercise. *Human Kinetics.* 7th Edition.

McArdle, W.D., Katch, F.I and Katch, V.L. 2015. Exercise Physiology: Nutrition, Energy and Human Perofrmance. *Wolters Kuwer.* 8th Edition. Philadelphia, USA.

Saghiv, M.S., Sagiv, M.S. (2020). *Basic Exercise Physiology: Clinical and Laboratory Perspectives.* 1st ed. Cham: Springer International Publishing: Imprint: Springer, pp. 15–16.

Gait and Biomechanics **2**

Thomas Leggett and Luke Taylor

BACKGROUND

Where mechanics is the study of forces and their subsequent effects, biomechanics applies this to the structure and function of biological systems. A sport and exercise medicine clinician should understand kinematics and kinetics to perform an assessment of movement and how it plays a role in performance and injury.

Simple mechanics can be measured with simple equipment—such as a fulcrum and a lever—which can be easily reproduced for study. Human biomechanics are complex. Levers (or joints) are never perfect; there is rarely one force acting in a single direction and anatomy differs between individuals. Modelling can be applied to different body systems so they can be analysed and assessed more closely. A simple biomechanical assessment, to an extent, is applying a model to a joint or structure. The more understanding and knowledge the assessor has, the more factors apply to that 'model.' For example, one could model a knee joint as a simple hinge. However, as the appreciation of anatomy deepens, more variables can be introduced to an assessment: other planes of movement, different forces, direction(s) of forces, the effect of adjacent soft tissue structures on the joint and external variables. Application of biomechanics can improve injury prevention, aid assessment, diagnosis, rehabilitation and improve physical performance.

MOVEMENT ANALYSIS

Understanding biomechanical variables is key to being able to assess an individual's specific movements. The main variables are external load (force applied), internal load (muscle forces), motion or movements that can occur and body structure (such as physical limits and tissue characteristics).

Kinematics and Kinetics

- Kinematics are the movements occurring in body segments, without reference to the forces applied.
- Kinetics are the reason these movements occur— i.e. the forces affecting the movements.

Kinematics

Kinematics is the study of movement—which is modelled as linear and angular movement. Linear movement occurs when the whole moving object follows a straight path, covering the same distance at constant speed. This is rarely applied to human movement, given the angular movement of joints. Even a 100 m run is an approximation of linear movement, as the individual components, e.g. the legs and arms, are rotating. Angular movement is rotational, such as the movement of a joint around a fixed axis.

Understanding certain variables is required to understand kinematics. The simple variables are: time, displacement, velocity, speed and acceleration.

- An object's displacement is its change in position, and has direction and magnitude. For example, a body moves two metres (magnitude) to the right (direction).

DOI: 10.1201/9781003179979-2

GAIT AND BIOMECHANICS

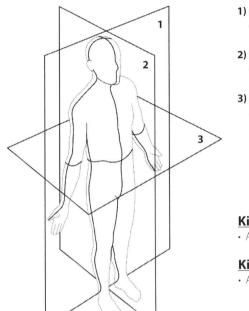

1) Coronal plane (frontal)
- Anterior and posterior portions

2) Sagittal plane (longitudinal)
- Left and right portions

3) Axial plane (horizontal)
- Superior and Inferior portions

Kinematics
• A description of movement

Kinetics
• A description of forces and how movement occurs

Walking gait cycle

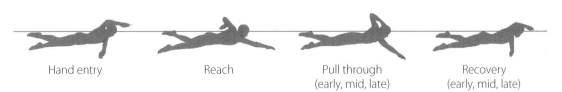

| Heel strike | Foot flat | Mid stance | | Heel off | Toe off | Mid stance | | Heel strike |

| Stance phase | | | | | Swing phase | | | |

Swim cycle

| Hand entry | Reach | Pull through (early, mid, late) | Recovery (early, mid, late) |

Figure 2.1 Pictorial chapter overview.

- Time is the interval over which a change has occurred.
- Speed is distance divided by time.
- Velocity is the displacement divided by time of travel. Velocity has direction, unlike speed. It is normally measured in metres per second (m/s).
- Acceleration is the change in velocity of a body per second, measured in metres per second^2. As velocity has direction, acceleration can be positive or negative—i.e. an increasing or decreasing variable. Simply: how fast the body is speeding up or slowing down.

Kinetics

Kinetics considers the forces that affect movement. The basis of kinetics is derived from Newton's laws of motion. Force is either a push or pull and has magnitude and direction. Due to this, it is a vector quantity (this means at least two forces are competing to achieve an outcome). For example, a person could exert a force on a ball in order to throw it in a certain direction.

Newton's first law of motion (law of inertia) states a body must remain at rest, or, if in motion, remain in motion at a constant velocity, unless acted on by an external force. For example, an ice-hockey player will move in the same direction, at the same speed unless there is an action from an external force.

Newton's second law of motion (law of acceleration) states that acceleration of a system is directly proportional to, and in the same direction, as the net external force acting on the system, and inversely proportional to the mass. If a footballer kicks a ball, it will move in the same direction of the force. The greater the force of the kick, the greater the speed the ball has.

Newton's third law of motion (law of reaction) states that whenever one body exerts a force on a second body, the first body experiences a force that is equal in magnitude and opposite in direction to the force that the first body exerts. In a sprinter, the action of feet pushing against starting blocks must be matched by an equal but opposite force of the blocks pushing back.

The understanding of kinematics and kinetics can impact our understanding of individuals and how they interact with the environment around them. This is particularly important in sport, where the execution of movement is crucial to performance.

Technological Aids—Biomechanical and Motion Assessment

A biomechanical assessment should form and enhance any clinical examination within sport and exercise medicine. The significance of 'normal' and altered biomechanics on sporting performance or injury is not straightforward; however, it can provide additional direction to your assessment and subsequent management of an injury or athlete.

Understanding alignment and normal anatomy is the initial step, before assessing single plane movements and then complex sport-specific movements. It is also important to acknowledge that there is no single perfect way to complete a task or action. Each individual has unique physical characteristics that will dictate a movement style (e.g. asymmetries, strength, height, weight). External factors such as the environment and sport equipment also contribute. Within each sport however, it is recognised that some movement patterns are more effective than others. For example, keeping legs and feet straight and submerged when swimming front crawl.

Biomechanics can be measured by observation, but this is a learnt skill. Initially, observations in standing and sitting can highlight underlying structure alignment. This is then observed during movement—initially a single plane movement; then, more complex, sports-specific movements, such as walking, running or throwing.

Observation and analysis can be enhanced with technology, which is based around wearable devices that measure joint displacement. Three-dimensional analysis is required to describe more complex movements. Force plates are mechanical sensing devices that measure ground reaction forces and can be useful in human movement analysis. These resources will not be available to every clinician, but can provide more in-depth data that can influence management. Video analysis using mobile or tablet applications can also provide similar data and may be more accessible.

CLINICAL CONSIDERATIONS

Below is an example of a brief lower limb biomechanical assessment:

1) Feet

- Assess the appearance of the hind, mid and forefoot in standing and whether there is obvious pes planus or pes cavus.

- Determine if the talar head is more prominent on one side.
- Look at the malleolar curves and their symmetry from behind.
- Look at whether the calcaneus is level with the floor from behind.
- Assess if the medial arch is present and uniform.
- Look whether the forefoot is seen equally on lateral and medial sides from behind. If only the lateral forefoot is visualised, this suggests pronation, whereas seeing only the medial forefoot suggests supination.

2) Knee

- Assess for tibiofemoral symmetry and determine if there is genu valgum or genu varum.

3) Pelvis

- See whether the pelvis is level and identify any obvious leg-length discrepancy. Trendelenberg testing can be used.

4) Dynamic movements

- Walking—Assess gait pattern to determine gross movement quality. An antalgic gait describes walking with a short stance phase and limp to avoid musculoskeletal pain.
- Bilateral leg squat and single leg squat (if able)—Assess the control of the trunk, pelvis, tibia and feet. If the knees do not remain aligned over the feet, the pelvis drops (leading to femoral adduction), or a shoulder drops (causing trunk asymmetry), this can suggest poor coordination and muscle imbalance. A single leg squat is a difficult skill for many people and faults are common but practising the movement and improving motor control will help. Strengthening of the Vastus medialis oblique (VMO) may help knee stability, addressing tight hip flexors and weak gluteal muscles may improve pelvic stability.

Influence of Posture

Posture and issues with posture have links to widespread pain. A poor posture can impact gait, which can alter ankle, knee, hip, shoulder and spine range of movement, inhibiting movement strategies. Posture is described as being adaptive or maladaptive. Adaptive is when a posture is adopted to achieve pain relief.

Maladaptive is when the person adopts a new posture, which causes pain. An example of this is slouching forward, leading to upper cervical extension and strain on facet joints, leading to pain.

Cervical postural syndrome presents as protruding chin and upper cervical lordosis. Additional consequences may be rounded shoulders, short and tight pectoral muscles, restricted shoulder movements and reduced thoracic extension. Pain is often worsened by prolonged static postures and movement alleviates pain.

In order to impact a movement strategy or posture, the root cause should always be considered. A weakness or tightness in one muscular group may have a subsequent effect on another. For example, tight hip flexors may cause increased pelvic anteversion, which may cause an increased lumbar lordosis, which may present with lower back pain.

Principles of Body Morphology

Body morphology refers to the body's shape or size and is unique to every individual. Broadly, morphology can be grouped into ectomorph, endomorph and mesomorph subtypes. Ectomorphs are long and lean with low levels of body fat and muscle. Endomorphs have higher levels of body fat and muscle. Mesomorphs are more middle ground—they often appear more 'athletic' with a balance of fat and muscle. A different body morphology will result in different forces acting in different ways around a body. For example, a taller athlete will need to generate a different force to flex their hip when compared to a shorter athlete. An athlete with more mass will experience more force through their ankles, knees, hips and spine on landing compared to a lighter athlete.

Additionally, an individual's bone structure will vary and needs to be assessed in any biomechanical assessment. For example, each person has an individual Q-angle of the hip, resulting in varying knee valgus/varus appearances. The Q-angle is formed between the quadriceps muscles and the patella tendon. It is the angle between a line from the Anterior superior iliac spine (ASIS) to the patella centre and the patella centre to the tibial tubercle. A normal angle is considered 12–20 degrees. Excessive angles can affect patella movement in the femoral groove, contributing to anterior knee pain and chondromalacia. Increased strength in the VMO and gluteal muscles can help mitigate an excessive angle.

GAIT CYCLE

Normal Walking

The normal gait cycle consists of heel strike, stance phase, toe off and then swing phase which leads to heel strike once more.

- *Heel strike:* initial contact of one foot with the ground (the start of the loading phase/shock absorption).
- Stance phase (body supported by one leg).
  - *Midstance:* centre of mass is directly above the ankle joint.
  - *Terminal stance:* flat foot to heel off. Centre of mass is moving forward over the forefoot (Shock absorption/loading biomechanics shifting toward propulsion forces).
- *Toe off—propulsion:* The midfoot locks into position creating a rigid lever, allowing propulsion.

Gait Analysis

A clinician should be able to recognise abnormal gait patterns. This is based on a good understanding of a normal gait cycle. An initial assessment can be a direct observation as part of an examination. Gait can be further analysed with video footage. Additionally, more sophisticated systems (such as a force plate) observe, measure and analyse multidimensional kinematic and kinetic data.

BIOMECHANICAL ANALYSIS OF SPORT-SPECIFIC TECHNIQUES AND FAULTY BIOMECHANICS, LEADING TO INJURY

When considering specific sporting movements, they can be broadly grouped into simple movement patterns:

- *Push-like patterns:* where a heavy load is being lifted away (e.g. weight lifting) or the distal segment is pushing against a resistance (e.g. cycling).
- *Pull-like patterns:* where a heavy load is brought closer (e.g. rowing).
- *Throw-like patterns:* developing a high-speed movement, which is then transferred to an object, like throwing or kicking a ball.

More complex movements aim to result in propulsion of the athlete, such as swimming or running.

Walking

Following heel strike, the foot pronates to increase contact with the ground. Toe-off occurs after the foot supinates. This phase relies on flexibility of the subtalar joint to allow for conversion of rotatory forces of the lower limb. A stiff subtalar joint will result in poorer dissipation of shock.

Excessive pronation (low arch) may contribute to biomechanical abnormalities elsewhere in the kinetic chain, leading to abnormal loading patterns on medial structures of the foot, ankle and knee.

Excessive supination (high arched) may contribute to iliotibial band syndrome. Foot alignment and degree of pronation or supination needs to be assessed; this includes the angle between the calcaneus and the Achilles tendon. Pelvic tilt may highlight a leg length discrepancy.

Running

During running, the gait cycle is maintained; however, stance phase tends to consist of midfoot or forefoot only, rather than heel strike. The cycle is around a third shorter and the velocity is much higher. As a result of this, the shock absorption forces are higher and, as a consequence, there is a predisposition to overload injuries.

In running, conservation of energy is vital. A biomechanical weakness or issue with the kinetic chain can result in poorer efficiency and a subsequent loss of energy and early fatigue. Poor foot biomechanics may result in issues higher up in the kinetic chain, which will result in earlier fatigue and poorer performance. Similarly, poor gluteal strength or endurance may become more apparent further into a run. When running, it is essential to stabilise the hip and pelvis.

The muscles are required to oppose the high forces generated during running.

There is some retrospective evidence to suggest a relationship between rearfoot strike technique and running-related injuries. Transitioning to a non-rear-foot strike pattern has also been reported to improve symptoms of patellofemoral pain (Alexander et al., 2021). Despite this, gait retraining can cause increased training loads, and therefore interventions should be considered on a case-by-case basis. Strength training has been shown to improve economy in runners and there may be other appropriate strategies.

Jumping

Jumping can be described as a ballistic or plyometric movement. The stretch shortening cycle can be used to illustrate the biomechanical features of a jump. The movement is initiated by an eccentric pre-stretch of the glutes, hamstrings, quadriceps and calves, as the hips and knees flex. There is then an amortization phase (brief isometric state) before a concentric shortening phase of these muscle groups (the 'explosive' jumping movement). On landing, deceleration in opposing muscles or other tissue structures, such as ligaments, takes place.

Coordination of arm movements during jumps is vital to achieving a maximum jump. Long and triple jumps involve a run-up and are more complex movements.

Kicking

Kicking is another ballistic movement. It consists of preparation, action and follow-through phases. The preparation phase is the player's approach or set-up to the ball. The action is the moment their foot strikes the ball and the follow through is once the ball has left the foot of the player.

The preparation phase allows the body to get into an advantageous position for the action phase. Being too far from the ball will put increased stresses on different structures. Each athlete will strive to work out their optimum positioning with respect to the ball. Initiating a strong core in this phase is vital for when they reach the action phase. If the core is not activated or weak, the forces being generated can lead to muscular or tendon injury. Commonly in football,

adolescents with underdeveloped core strength can get into a position to kick and overextend their hip before quickly flexing (kicking) resulting in a rectus femoris injury. Being in the correct position for the preparation phase allows the larger, stronger segments of the body to initiate movement. The preparation phase stretches the agonist muscles (hamstrings), increasing the storage of elastic energy. When maximum tension is developed, the movement can be executed.

The action phase is initiated by the large muscle groups and the movement is then continued by faster, smaller and more distal muscles, which allow speed to increase throughout the movement and apply force to the ball. The accuracy of this movement is increased through better muscle recruitment. The recovery phase involves controlled deceleration by the opposing (antagonist) muscle groups.

Throwing

Throwing arm pain is thought to be attributed to three major factors: insufficient physical competencies (elbow/shoulder strength and mobility), technique errors and excessive or inadequate workload. During a throw, the scapula must work alongside the humerus to maintain glenohumeral stability.

Throwing is typically divided into six components:

- Preparation phase
- Stride
- Arm cocking
- Acceleration
- Deceleration
- Follow through

The highest stresses to the upper limb occur during arm cocking, acceleration and deceleration. These phases are where the majority of injuries occur. During arm cocking, external rotation of the shoulder in abduction can lead to repetitive impingement of the under-surface of the supraspinatus tendon and the posterosuperior glenoid. The interaction of these structures, with high forces and repetition, can cause glenoid labrum lesions, internal impingement and anterior subluxation. If there is anterior instability of the shoulder, or poor scapular control, these forces are increased, as is subsequent injury risk.

Acceleration starts at maximal shoulder external rotation and finishes at ball release. As the arm accelerates forward, this puts tension on the long head of biceps. There is also some twisting of the tendon— these forces can result in tearing of the superior labrum, shoulder instability or long head of biceps tendinopathy.

During deceleration, the long head of biceps is working to prevent shear forces around the shoulder, but to also decelerate elbow extension and pronation, which can be another mechanism for superior labral anterior to posterior (SLAP) lesions and posterior cuff tendinopathies. This is regarded as the most harmful phase of throwing. Elbow pain in throwers is linked to valgus stress. The forces in throwing can exceed the tensile strength of the ulnar collateral ligament, leading to strains and tears.

Swimming

Swimming relies on the upper and lower limbs propelling the body through water. Roughly 90% of this propulsion comes from the upper limbs. The kinetics of this movement require the forward propulsive forces to overcome the drag of the water.

Freestyle (front-crawl) is the fastest and most commonly used stroke. It requires the swimmer to maintain as horizontal a position as possible. The latissimus dorsi, pectoralis major, subscapularis and serratus anterior muscles all play a key role in the freestyle stroke. The swimming cycle consists of reach, pull through (early, mid and late), end of pulling and recovery (early, mid and late).

- *Pull through:* adduction and internal rotation of the shoulder as the elbow flexes and then extends.
- *Recovery phase:* abduction and external rotation of the shoulder; followed by elbow flexion and then extension.

Shoulder pain in swimmers is common and can be a result of poor biomechanics and ineffective scapula control. Rotator cuff tendinopathy may arise from repetitive microtrauma and labral injury, or instability, is associated with an increased laxity in the swimming population.

Biomechanical faults may contribute to dynamic muscle imbalances. The following movement patterns in swimming may predispose to injury:

- Arms entering the water too far outside the line of the shoulder, or too close together, in butterfly stroke.
- A pull through with elbows in full extension, rather than an S-shaped pull through, in backstroke.
- A pull through that crosses the midline, or striving for too much length, in freestyle.
- Excessive elbow extension in breaststroke.

EQUIPMENT REQUIREMENTS AND CHOICES IN ATHLETIC PERFORMANCE

Different sports use equipment for different applications. Some are extensions of limbs: footwear, tennis racquet, golf club, hockey stick, etc. Some enhance speed of movement: bicycle or wheelchair. Some are protective: shin pads, shoulder pads, or protective helmets.

Regardless of the purpose or intended function of the equipment, there needs to be a balance between optimising sporting function, limiting or enhancing the athlete's biomechanical strain and obeying the rules of the sport.

Equipment will be sized and adjusted depending on the athletes age, size and biomechanics at that time. Macro-adjustments can be made initially. This roughly dictates the size of the equipment: shoe size, racquet size, bike frame size, etc. Then further micro-adjustments can be made: arch support, handle length, string tightness, saddle height, etc. It is vital to consider these small changes, as the athlete is likely to reproduce a sport specific movement thousands of times or more. This could include a foot-plant on running, a forehand swing in tennis, or a downward pedal stroke in cycling. If the equipment is appropriately fitted, not only can the athlete's action be more efficient, it reduces the risk of overuse injury. The adjustments need to be assessed in neutral, but also throughout sporting activity.

Orthotic Prescription

There are no definitive criteria or a 'one fits all' method to prescribing an orthotic. An orthotic is aimed to correct a biomechanical abnormality. Understanding the biomechanical issue is part of this, but having a firm grasp on the history is imperative. Appreciating the duration of the problem is the most appropriate way to correct it. A longstanding issue needs to be corrected gently to avoid a drastic correction and subsequent over-compensation of other structures. For example, an athlete who has had severe pes planus (flat feet) for many years needs a gradual increase in arch height. This is compared to other conditions where you can be more aggressive with orthotic changes.

The conventional aim is to achieve a neutral position of the subtalar joint; however, this does not consider movements during more complex sequences or the gait cycle. An orthotic prescription should not only aim to move the foot into a neutral position, but provide support through the desired range of motion. An orthotic for cycling cleats will have a different purpose to sprinting spikes.

Excessive supination is difficult to correct with orthotics and these individuals should be directed to buying shoes with maximum shock absorption.

Use of Splinting, Bracing and Taping Techniques

A good understanding of biomechanics is vital for the application of splinting, bracing and taping techniques. It is imperative to understand the anatomical structures, and their associated biomechanics, which you are attempting to support. These techniques can be applied for various reasons:

- Immobilisation
- Restriction of movement
- Support of soft tissue structure (joint capsule, ligament, muscle)
- Enhance proprioceptive feedback
- Compression of muscle-tendon units
- Protective padding

Although a taping technique might be used to completely immobilise a joint or structure whilst acceptable healing can occur, taping is commonly used in sport to protect or support a joint or structure, whilst allowing for participation to continue. Creating a support that is adequate in its role but is not too restrictive, requires an understanding of:

- Normal anatomy
- Normal biomechanics
- Underlying mechanism of injury
- Grading of injury
- Biomechanical requirements of sporting activity
- Properties of different taping/bracing materials
- Sport specific rules

MULTIPLE CHOICE QUESTION (MCQ) QUESTIONS

1. In the walking gait cycle, what is the approximate ratio of the stance to swing phase?

   A. 50:50
   B. 40:60
   C. 60:40
   D. 65:35
   E. 70:30

2. You are learning more about cycling biomechanics. You read that the power (or push) phase occurs between 12 o'clock to 6 o'clock during pedalling. The recovery (or draw) phase occurs between 6 o'clock to 12 o'clock. Which of the following muscles are NOT activated during the power phase?

   A. Gluteus maximus
   B. Lateral gastrocnemius
   C. Tibialis anterior
   D. Erector spinae
   E. Rectus femoris

3. You are providing medical cover at an archery competition. One of the competitors draws his bow. What is the name of the energy present, by virtue of the bowstring's position called?

   A. Elastic energy
   B. Potential energy
   C. Kinetic energy
   D. Stored energy
   E. Mass energy

4. Whilst providing medical assistance at a golfing tournament, you observe two players tee off. One player drives the ball a much greater distance than the other. They appeared to swing their club with a greater force. Which biomechanical principle is most applicable to this scenario?

   A. Newton's first law of motion
   B. Newton's second law of motion
   C. Newton's third law of motion
   D. The stretch-shortening cycle
   E. The kinetic link principle

5. As part of a biomechanical assessment on an athlete, you decide to assess shoulder internal and external rotation. Which plane do these movements mainly occur in?

   A. Sagittal (or longitudinal)
   B. Horizontal (or axial, or transverse)
   C. Frontal (or coronal)
   D. Superior
   E. Median

MULTIPLE CHOICE QUESTION (MCQ) ANSWERS

1. Answer C
   The stance phase occupies 60% of the gait cycle and starts with heel strike, finishing with toe off. During running, the swing phase is prolonged and constitutes 60% of the gait cycle (B).

2. Answer C
   From the top of the pedal stroke, the hip extensors are activated (A), followed by the knee extensors (E). The gastrocnemius' (B) main role is as a stabiliser, as are the abdominals and erector spinae (D) muscles. Tibialis anterior is a key commencer of the recovery phase by initiating dorsiflexion.

3. Answer B
   Potential energy is the energy possessed by a body for doing work (in this case the bowstring), by virtue of its position (pulled taut). Kinetic energy is the energy for doing work by virtue of its velocity of motion and mass (C).

4. Answer B
   Newton's second law of motion (Law of acceleration) states that acceleration is directly proportional to the net external force acting on the system. In this case, a greater acceleration drives the ball further.

5. Answer B
   The shoulder is a multiplanar joint. Forward to backward movements take place in the sagittal plane (A), lateral movement in the frontal plane (C) and internal/external rotation in the horizontal plane (B).

REFERENCES AND FURTHER READING

Alexander, J.L.N., Willy, R.W., Napier, C., et al. (2021). Infographic: Running myth: Switching to a non-rearfoot strike reduces injury risk and improves running economy. *British Journal of Sports Medicine*, 55, pp. 175–176.

Physiopedia. (2023). *Biomechanics in Sport*. Available from: https://www.physio-pedia.com/Biomechanics_In_Sport

The Biomechanics Initiative. (2023). *Virtual Content Collection*. Available from: https://thebiomechanics initiative.org/virtual-content/

Musculoskeletal Medicine Overview

Steffan Griffin, Roshan Gunasekera, David Eastwood and Dane Vishnubala

INTRODUCTION

The following chapters explore musculoskeletal (MSK) medicine. Each chapter explores key anatomy, examination method and core conditions (with the presentation, investigations and management covered). When it comes to MSK pathology, most clinicians will be familiar with the acronyms: 'RICE', 'POLICE' and 'PEACE and LOVE' (Dubois and Esculier, 2020), but how does knowing that help in the wider rehabilitation process? Whilst they may provide a structure for the acute management of MSK injuries, they fail to consider the broader and more holistic elements that affect patients' recovery. The following holistic and multi-disciplinary model can be tailored to anyone, from sedentary patients to elite athletes.

THE #DREAM APPROACH

The #DREAM acronym encapsulates some of the key domains that clinicians should consider when seeing patients with an MSK injury. Each MSK complaint will have its own specific '#DREAM', which, in practice, would be informed by scientific evidence, the experience of the practitioner and a multitude of patient-specific factors.

D: DIAGNOSIS

In all cases, a thorough history and clinical examination should take place, cognisant of red-flags or significant "not-to-be-missed" pathology. Gathering information is a highly skilled task, involving careful questioning, responding to patient cues and exploring the history critically. Examination should then be used to aid in reaching key differential diagnoses.

Regarding investigations, every practitioner should be able to robustly defend the clinical reasoning behind each request. To help with this, questions that may be helpful include:

- Are objective investigations needed? Is there a specific clinical question, the answer to which will influence clinical care?
- What could be the impact of an incidental finding not related to the presentation and how will this be explained to the patient?
- Is there a specific context to this injury? Is a definitive return-to-play (RTP) timeline needed (as is often the case in elite sport), and would investigations help inform that?

R: RISK FACTORS AND REHABILITATION

Risk-Factors: Though the patient may be seen after the injury has occurred, prevention is better than cure. This is a potential window to reduce the chances of recurrence; factor(s) contributing to the injury should be identified in order to reduce the likelihood of this happening again.

Rehabilitation: This should not refer to a one-off prescription of exercises. A biopsychosocial, multidisciplinary approach to patient management should be adopted to maximise the chance of a good outcome:

- Considering whether the patient wants to involve the wider support team (coaches, team-mates, parents etc.).
- Drawing a rehabilitation timeline and signposting to the stages. If there has been a delay in the

patient presenting for clinical care, establishing where they are on this timeline already, and ensuring that the patient understands the fluid nature and criteria to progress through the stages.

E: EDUCATION

Considering injury as an opportunity for patients to increase their health understanding and empowering them to take control of their rehabilitation process can be done by:

- Providing information relating to their condition in practical and relatable terms.
- Considering and acknowledging the patient's ideas, fears, expectations and goals, as well as their own personal and social situations. Provide reassurance where needed.
- Ensuring that the patient is happy with the role of pain during and after rehabilitation exercises.
- Providing resources that patients can refer to throughout their journey.

A: ANALGESIA AND 'ACCESSORIES'

Analgesia: There are numerous options. Clinicians should be familiar with the relevant anti-doping codes and the goal of the medication. Prescribing holistically and considering wider issues with chronic NSAID and opioid use is important.

'Accessories': These will depend on several factors (including cost, risks and evidence), but can be useful in many contexts (e.g. injection therapy). The patient should be made aware of their adjuvant role to the fundamentals of recovery, such as exercises and load management.

M: MAINTAIN PHYSICAL ACTIVITY LEVELS AND/OR FITNESS

Portraying the injury in a way that highlights what a patient can still do can have a positive influence.

The patient should remain physically active and optimise other lifestyle factors (e.g. diet, smoking, alcohol intake and sleep). Motivational Interviewing or a brief intervention can be utilised, if appropriate. For athletes, injury could be approached as an opportunity to improve in other areas (e.g. strength in other parts of the body, tactical awareness).

SUMMARY

The #DREAM model proposes a holistic and multi-disciplinary approach to MSK medicine and SEM care, and works well both clinically and as a revision aid.

The following chapters aim to improve and test musculoskeletal medicine knowledge. Learners are advised to seek a range of patients, in order to fulfil a checklist of the core conditions. A suggested approach:

- Critically review the notes.
- Practice MSK-focused history taking.
- Be aware of, and carry out, a variety of techniques to examine the MSK system.
- Be critical of the sensitivity and specificity of 'special tests' as well as their indications and limitations.
- Recognise the strengths and weaknesses of a variety of investigations
- Management strategies for MSK conditions is rapidly evolving. Finding mentors with whom to discuss cases, while maintaining engagement with current literature, is advised.

REFERENCES AND FURTHER READING

Dubois B, Esculier J. Soft-tissue injuries simply need PEACE and LOVE. British Journal of Sports Medicine 2020;54:72–73.

Griffin, S., Gundasekera, R., et al. 2021. Proposing a #DREAM approach to Musculoskeletal medicine. BJSM Blog.

Proposing a #DREAM approach to musculoskeletal medicine

What should all clinicians consider when seeing patients with musculoskeletal complaints?

Griffin, Gunasekera et al., BJSM blog 2021

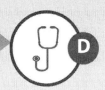

Diagnosis

Are there red-flags present? Would clinical investigations add diagnostic value and affect the treatment provided/eventual outcome? How would you explain 'incidental findings' to the patient? Treat the patient in front of you, not the report.

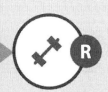

Risk Factors & Rehab

Can you work out what factor(s) contributed to the injury in the first place and reduce the likelihood of this happening again?

Draw a rehab continuum with clear progression criteria, and adopt a holistic interdisciplinary approach to patient recovery that utilises various skill-sets and backgrounds.

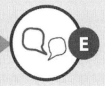

Education

Provide information in practical and understandable 'chunks'. Can you get the patient to repeat back to you what they understand after your explanation? Consider and acknowledge the patient's ideas, fears, expectations and goals. Provide reassurance where needed.

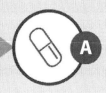

Analgesia & 'Accessories'

Ensure you are in line with the relevant anti-doping codes when prescribing, and be aware of wider issues with chronic NSAID/opioid use.

Use 'accessories' such as injection therapies, supplements & shockwave only for specific reasons and explain their roles clearly. Don't chase the 1% 'marginal gain' if you haven't nailed the basics first.

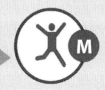

Maintain Physical Activity Levels ± Fitness

Re-frame the injury in a way that highlights what the patient *can* still do. Highlight the importance of being/remaining physically active & optimise other lifestyle factors (*e.g. diet, smoking, alcohol intake and sleep*). For athletes, highlight that this injury is an opportunity to improve in other areas (e.g. tactically).

Shoulder and Elbow 3

Victoria Campbell and Simon Boyle

INTRODUCTION

The shoulder is one of the most complex joints in the body, connecting the humerus, scapula and clavicle. It is made up of four joints, comprising the sternoclavicular, acromioclavicular, glenohumeral and scapulothoracic joints (Figures 3.2–3.4).

The central articulation of the shoulder is the glenohumeral joint. This is a highly mobile ball and socket joint, which allows the hand to be placed in space and also to undertake sporting activities. Glenohumeral joint stability is conferred by both passive and active stabilisers. The passive stabilisers include the concave shape of the glenoid and its articular cartilage, which is further deepened by the labrum peripherally. Attached to the labrum are the glenohumeral ligaments and capsule that serves to restrict excessive translation of the humeral head in specific arm positions. Active stabilisation is delivered by the rotator cuff muscles, which act to centre the humeral head in the glenoid, as well as enabling glenohumeral joint movement. There are several bursae surrounding the joint to help reduce friction.

There are a number of different muscles that work together to provide both stability and movement of the shoulder. The superficial muscles include pectoralis major in the anterior aspect of the shoulder and latissimus dorsi and trapezius in the posterior aspect of the shoulder. The deltoid muscle provides the characteristic contour of the shoulder and is the largest muscle of the shoulder.

The deep muscles include pectoralis minor and subclavius in the anterior aspect. Posteriorly, the periscapular muscles include levator scapulae, rhomboid major/minor and teres major. The rotator cuff muscles are engaged in concavity-compression as well as being responsible for elevating/abducting the arm and the rotational movements of the shoulder. The four rotator cuff muscles are supraspinatus, subscapularis, infraspinatus and teres minor.

ELBOW

The elbow joint is a synovial joint made up of three bones: the humerus, the radius and the ulna. These give rise to two joints that give the elbow its hinge-like properties: the humeroulnar joint and humeroradial joint. The proximal ulnar and radius articulate giving the proximal radioulnar joint, which permits rotational movement of the forearm and hand. The elbow joint complex is enveloped by a joint capsule that is strengthened by the radial collateral ligament laterally and ulnar collateral ligament medially. There are also a number of bursae present helping to reduce friction between the moving joints (Figures 3.4–3.6).

EXAMINATION OF THE SHOULDER

Inspection

- Standing
- Inspect both shoulders. The shape and position of each shoulder should be relatively similar. Inspect the position of the scapula and observe scapulothoracic movement from behind during repeated forward flexion of the shoulder for any winging. Look for wasting of the deltoid or of the rotator cuff in the supra/infraspinous fossa.

DOI: 10.1201/9781003179979-3

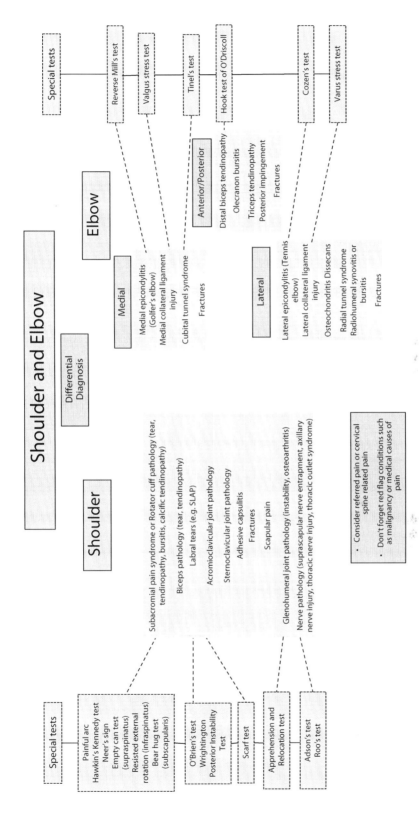

Figure 3.1 Differential diagnosis chart.

Rotator Cuff Muscles

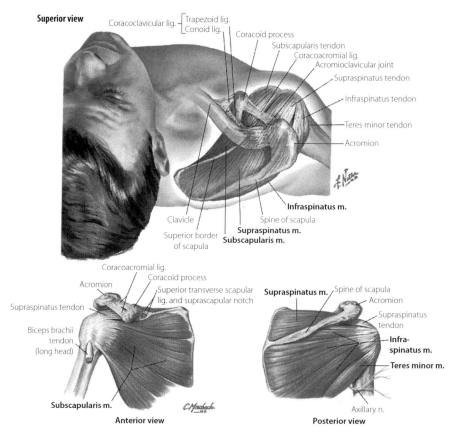

Figure 3.2 Muscles of the shoulder.

Source: Cleland et al. (2016). *Netter's Orthopaedic Clinical Examination: An Evidence-Based Approach.* 3rd ed. Philadelphia: Elsevier. With permission.

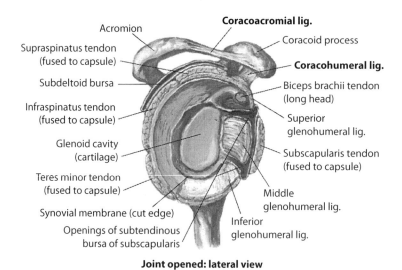

Figure 3.3 View of the glenohumeral joint.

Source: Cleland et al. (2016). *Netter's Orthopaedic Clinical Examination: An Evidence-Based Approach.* 3rd ed. Philadelphia: Elsevier. With permission.

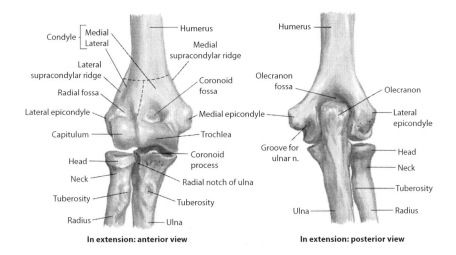

Figure 3.4 Bones of the elbow joint.

Source: Cleland et al. (2016). *Netter's Orthopaedic Clinical Examination: An Evidence-Based Approach.* 3rd ed. Philadelphia: Elsevier. With permission.

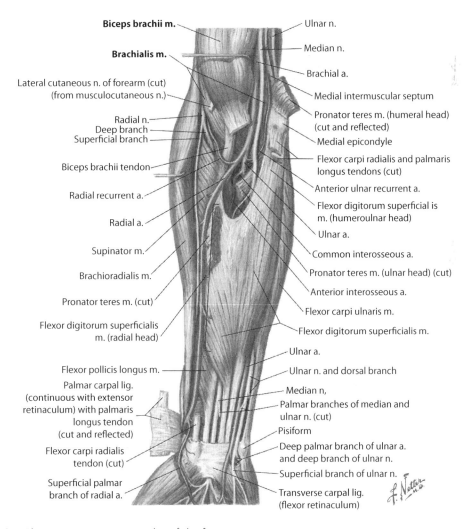

Figure 3.5 Flexor compartment muscles of the forearm.

Source: Cleland et al. (2016). *Netter's Orthopaedic Clinical Examination: An Evidence Based-Approach.* 3rd ed. Philadelphia: Elsevier. With permission.

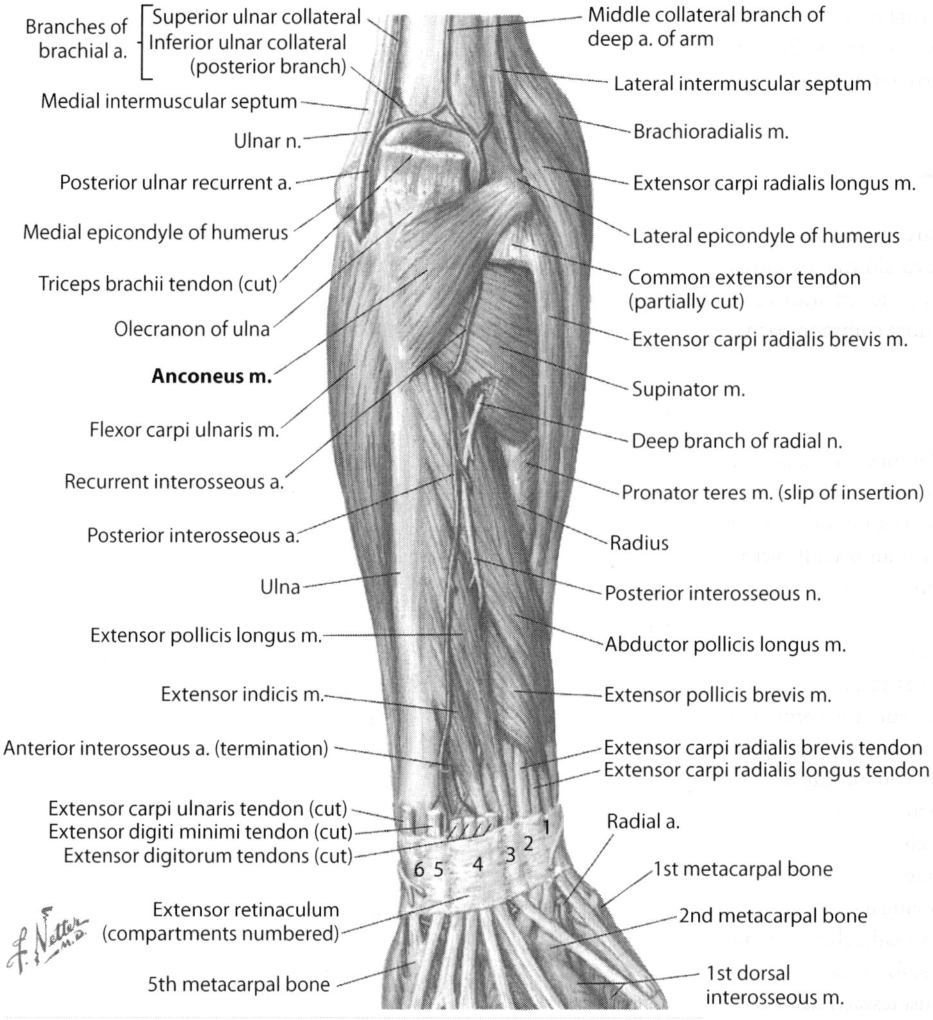

Figure 3.6 Extensor compartment muscles of the forearm.

Source: Cleland et al. (2016). *Netter's Orthopaedic Clinical Examination: An Evidence-Based Approach.* 3rd ed. Philadelphia: Elsevier. With permission.

Screening Tests

- Examine the cervical spine to exclude a more proximal neural pathology as a cause for shoulder/arm symptoms.

Palpation

- Sternoclavicular joint
- Clavicle

- Acromioclavicular joint (ACJ)
- Rotator cuff muscle insertions/tuberosities
- Long head of biceps tendon

Movement

ACTIVE AND PASSIVE

- Forward flexion/extension
- Abduction in scapular plane (30 degrees anterior to coronal plane)

- External rotation with elbows at side (ER$_1$) and 90 degrees of abduction (ER$_2$)
- Internal Rotation (spinal level)

Special Tests

There are numerous special tests that can be performed to aid the diagnosis of shoulder pathologies. This list is not exhaustive but may help identify some of the more common pathologies seen.

ROTATOR CUFF TESTS

Shoulder movements are compound and it is impossible to specifically isolate any single muscle with a clinical test. Taking this into account, the following tests help form an overall picture of the integrity/pathology of the individual rotator cuff muscles.

- Empty Can test (in the scapular plane—with 90 degrees abduction and the arm 30 degrees forward from the coronal plane) to test for supraspinatus pathology. Pain or weakness against resistance can indicate a positive test.
- Resisted external rotation (with the arm adducted and elbow flexed to 90 degrees) to test for infraspinatus and teres minor pathology.
- Bear Hug test (with the palm of the affected side on the opposite shoulder and the elbow held horizontal) to test for subscapularis pathology. Pain or weakness against resisted elevation can indicate a positive test.

SUBACROMIAL PAIN/IMPINGEMENT TESTS

These tests are used to bring the subacromial structures (rotator cuff and bursa) into contact with the acromion and the coracoacromial ligament. This can reproduce the 'impingement' pain the patient experiences during the active act of abduction.

- Neer's sign to test for subacromial pathology. Pain between 60 and 120 degrees of abduction with internal rotations in the scapular plane indicates a positive test.
- Neer's test for subacromial pathology. If the pain from the test above is improved/abolished after the administration of a local anaesthetic injection into the subacromial space, this is known as a positive Neer's test.

- Hawkins Kennedy test for subacromial pathology. Pain with internal rotations whilst the shoulder and elbow are in 90 degrees of flexion indicates a positive test.
- These tests may yield positive results in the presence of other pathologies e.g. labral lesions, ACJ arthritis, calcific tendinopathy, etc.

ACROMIOCLAVICULAR JOINT TESTS

- Scarf test for acromioclavicular joint pain.

LABRAL AND INSTABILITY TESTS

- Apprehension and Relocation test for identifying anterior capsulo-labral pathology. If pain or apprehension are experienced with passive external rotation in supine, this may indicate an underlying anterior capsulo-labral injury. If pain or apprehension improves with application of a posterior directed force on the shoulder, this is a positive Relocation test.
- O'Brien's test for identifying Superior Labral Anterior/Posterior lesions (SLAP). This is a resisted test with the shoulder in 90 degrees of flexion, 15 degrees of adduction and internal rotation (thumbs down) followed by a repeat test with palms facing upwards and shoulders in a neutral position. The test is considered positive if the pain produced on the first test is relieved by the neutral position of the second test.
- Wrightington Posterior Instability Test (WPIT) for posterior instability/labral lesions. The test is considered positive if there is weakness in maintaining the horizontal position or posterior joint pain with a modified O'Brien's test.

EXAMINATION OF THE ELBOW

Inspection

- Standing
- Look for any swelling, bruising, deformity, asymmetry, muscle atrophy, rheumatoid or gouty nodules, olecranon bursa
- Look at the appearance of the biceps for a Popeye sign (LHB rupture) or proximal migration (distal biceps rupture)

- Observe the carrying angle of elbow—usually 10 degrees in men and 13 degrees in women

Palpation

- *Lateral side of elbow:* tenderness at or just distal to the lateral epicondyle may indicate ECRB tendinosis/tennis elbow
- *Medial side of elbow:* palpate over the bony prominences and medial epicondyle. Tenderness over the medial epicondyle may indicate medial epicondylitis/golfer's elbow.
- Olecranon
- Radial Head
- *Ulnar nerve/cubital tunnel:* palpation for tenderness/Tinel's test and stability in flexion/extension

Movements

- Active and Passive Testing:
  - Elbow flexion and extension
  - Forearm pronation and supination—performed with the elbows flexed to 90 degrees and asking the patient to rotate the hand to make the palms face up/down
  - Wrist flexion and extension
- Resisted Testing
  - Elbow flexion and extension
  - Forearm pronation and supination
  - Wrist flexion and extension

Special Tests

TENDINOPATHIES

Tennis Elbow

- Cozen's Test (resisted wrist extension with the forearm pronated and wrist extended/radially deviated) for lateral epicondylitis.

Golfer's Elbow

- Reverse Mill's (passive forearm supination, wrist extension and then elbow extension) for medial epicondylitis.

Distal Biceps Tendinopathy

- Hook Test of O'Driscoll. When pain is elicited with a finger hooking the biceps tendon from lateral to medial, this is indicative of distal biceps tendinopathy. Where the tendon is absent then this indicates a distal biceps rupture.

Ulnar Nerve

- Tinel's Test on the ulnar nerve as it sits in the cubital tunnel/ulnar groove for ulnar neuropathy. The nerve can also be assessed for stability and signs of dislocation in flexion and extension.

Elbow Ligaments

- Valgus stress test (in approximately 30 degrees of elbow flexion and the humerus in full external rotation) to assess the integrity of the Ulnar Collateral Ligament.
- Varus stress test (in approximately 30 degrees of elbow flexion and the humerus internally rotated) to assess the integrity of the Lateral Collateral Ligament.

SHOULDER

Subacromial Pain Syndrome

Subacromial pain syndrome (SAPS) refers to pain generated from one of the structures within the subacromial space. The most common cause is intrinsic, which is related to overuse, muscle imbalance or cuff degeneration. This leads to abnormal contact of the rotator cuff on the coracoacromial arch. Extrinsic causes result from pathological structures abnormally pressing on the rotator cuff and bursa such as subacromial spurs, coracoacromial ligament hypertrophy, etc. SAPS accounts for between 40–65% of all presentations of shoulder pain.

- *Presentation:* Patients tend to present between 35 and 60 with an insidious onset of shoulder pain in the absence of trauma. They will describe discomfort with movements, in particular, through a mid-arc of abduction (70–120 degrees—painful arc). Sleep may be disturbed.

- *Examination:* There is no single test which is diagnostic of SAPS but using a combination of Neers/Hawkins Kennedy tests will help aid in diagnosis. It is important in younger patients (<35) to consider instability/microinstability as the cause for subacromial pain.
- *Investigations:* X-rays can be useful to look for pathologies such as subacromial spurs or calcific tendinopathy. Ultrasound has shown to be effective in identifying bursitis as well as dynamic impingement or rotator cuff tears. MRI and MRA scans are rarely needed unless intra-articular pathology is considered. Overall, SAPS is a clinical diagnosis and imaging may be normal.
- *Management:* Management of subacromial pain syndrome will depend on several factors including age, level of activity and the underlying pathological process responsible for the pain. Most cases should be initially managed conservatively. Conservative measures include activity modification, analgesia and structured kinetic chain physiotherapy. This includes working on core strength, scapular retraction and posterior chain/cuff balancing. Corticosteroid injections can be helpful in some cases if pain is an issue and can help in achieving more useful physiotherapy rehabilitation. They can be particularly useful in painful pathology such as bursitis or calcific tendinopathy. Ultrasound-guided barbotage is effective for calcific tendinopathy. As a last resort, surgery can be used to remove extrinsic causes of impingement such as acromial spurs, ACJ spurs or excision of calcific deposits. Patients who have a good response to a subacromial injection are most likely to see a benefit from surgery.

Adhesive Capsulitis

Adhesive capsulitis (also known as frozen shoulder), predominantly affects adults aged 40–60 and more commonly affects women. It can be associated with systemic disease such as thyroid disease and diabetes. The shoulder joint capsule is normally an elastic structure that permits the large range of motion we require from the shoulder. Environmental and genetic factors can lead to stiffening and contraction of the capsule, which initially results in pain followed by a gradual loss of range of motion and function.

- *Presentation:* Adhesive capsulitis tends to present in three stages. Freezing, frozen and thawing. The freezing stage can last between 3 and 9 months in which the patient's main complaint is of pain and evolving stiffness. As they progress into the frozen phase, the pain improves but range of motion continues to be reduced (12 to 24 months). Following this, the shoulder begins to 'thaw' and there is gradual restoration of motion and function as pain and stiffness eases (9 to 12 months). Usually, there is gradual onset of pain with gradual reduction in range of motion. Patients will describe difficulty with everyday tasks such as dressing or brushing their hair and they may have difficulty sleeping. Severe pain is characteristically described with sudden or unexpected movements.
- Examination findings may vary depending on what stage a patient is experiencing. A loss of passive external rotation is a typical finding with a frozen shoulder.
- *Investigations:* Investigations aren't routinely required for this condition as it is a clinical diagnosis. An X-ray is useful in excluding arthritis and other painful pathologies. If there is a history of trauma or previous cancers then an MRI may be requested to rule out other pathologies such as cuff tears or metastases.
- *Management:* Adhesive capsulitis is often a self-limiting condition and can take approximately 12–24 months to resolve. Physiotherapy has been shown to have some benefit in improving range of motion and preventing stiffness but it is important to avoid painful stretching. Corticosteroid injections can be considered if pain is significant however these are short lived and do not generally improve range of movement. Hydrodilatation injections involve injecting a larger volume of saline, local anaesthetic and steroid into the glenohumeral joint capsule. This serves to provide pain relief but also plastic deformation of the capsule and occasionally capsular rupture to improve range of movement. This is generally performed by radiologists under image guidance. For those patients recalcitrant to this treatment, surgery can be considered in the form of an arthroscopic capsular release. All treatment modalities should be followed by structured physiotherapy and well managed analgesia to obtain the best outcome.

Glenohumeral Instability

Dislocations/instability of the glenohumeral joint are most commonly traumatic and 95% occur in the anterior direction. The bones, muscles and capsulo-labral structures around the shoulder act to stabilise the joint and disruption of any of these can lead to recurrent instability. Atraumatic instability can occur as a result of previous trauma, hyperlaxity and muscle patterning issues.

- *Presentation:* Traumatic glenohumeral joint instability can be anterior, posterior or multidirectional and the presentation may depend on the direction of instability. The majority of patients will recall a history of a frank dislocation followed by episodes of the shoulder feeling unstable or loose. In sports, dislocations usually occur in a collision event such as a tackle or as a result of a fall or diving catch.
- *Investigations:* X-rays are essential and should include tangential views (AP and axillary or scapular Y view). These are used to confirm the position of the humeral head in relation to the glenoid fossa but also to look for associated lesions such as glenoid rim injuries, Hill Sachs impaction fractures and greater tuberosity fractures. To further examine the integrity of the capsulo-labral tissues and rotator cuff, MRA is the gold standard investigation. CT can be used to better define any bony injuries as well as quantify any glenoid bone loss.
- *Management:* Definitive management of these injuries will depend on the level of function, any bony and soft tissue injuries, age, sport and frequency of instability. Athletes, especially those involved in overhead or collision sports, should be counselled with regard to the high recurrence risk with non-operative management. In most cases, early surgical referral should be considered to discuss intervention to reduce further dislocations. The nature of the surgical procedure is determined by many factors but with particular regard to capsulo-labral tears, glenoid bone loss and potential engagement of Hill Sachs lesions (On/Off track lesions).

CLINICAL CONSIDERATIONS

Shoulder dislocations have a high recurrence rate that correlates with the age at dislocation. Patients under 20 years have a 90% chance of recurrence, whilst patients older than 40 years have a 10% recurrence rate.

Posterior shoulder dislocations are commonly missed and only represent <5% of shoulder dislocations. Mechanisms involving forceful internal rotation such as with a seizure or electric shock can be a cause. AP X-ray view may show a 'Light Bulb' sign as the greater tuberosity is internally rotated.

Glenohumeral Joint Osteoarthritis (OA)

Osteoarthritis of the shoulder most commonly presents in those over 50 but can be seen in younger patients who have a history of traumatic instability. It is less common than hip or knee arthritis but can be managed by a similar, stepwise approach.

- *Presentation:* Individuals present with progressive pain that is deep in the joint, although many have difficulty localising this. The pain is worse with movement and can cause sleep disturbance and reduced function. A history of prior dislocation or previous shoulder instability may predispose to osteoarthritis in a younger patient.
- *Examination:* Patients often present with reduced active and passive movement in the shoulder, especially in external rotation.
- *Investigations:* X-ray is the first line investigation obtaining both an AP and axillary view. These may show evidence of joint space narrowing, subchondral sclerosis, cysts and osteophytes. CT scans can better define the bony anatomy and glenoid inclination and are useful to surgeons in pre-operative planning. MRI and US scans are both useful adjuncts in cases where the integrity of the rotator cuff needs to be determined.
- *Management:* First line management of osteoarthritis affecting the glenohumeral joint should be non-surgical. This includes analgesia and physiotherapy, which can help improve function and optimise the rotator cuff. Intra-articular injections may provide some temporary relief and may help improve range of motion if function is primarily limited by pain. These are not indicated in cases of radiographically established arthritis and repeated injections increase the risk of future infections if arthroplasty is considered. Hyaluronic acid may be a safer alternative and can have a role for young patients with early OA. Surgery should be considered in those who have severe arthritis or in whom

conservative measures have failed. Surgical options for glenohumeral arthritis include arthroscopic debridement, total shoulder arthroplasty (intact rotator cuff) or reverse shoulder arthroplasty (torn, non-functional rotator cuff).

Long Head of Biceps (LHB) Tendinopathy

The long head of biceps sits in the bicipital groove in the anterior aspect of the shoulder. Primary biceps tendinopathy can be seen in athletes participating in overhead sports such as volleyball and gymnastics. It is often associated with other shoulder pathologies such as degenerate rotator cuff disease or subacromial pain syndrome. Symptoms can also result from an inflammatory tenosynovitis of the LHB sheath.

- *Presentation:* Patients present with pain localised to their anterior shoulder, which may radiate down the course of the biceps tendon and can be similar to SAPS. It is often insidious in its onset and not associated with any trauma. Occupational history is often important as it can be seen in athletes participating in overhead sports, gym goers and occupations such as manual labourers.
- *Investigations:* X-rays will often be normal unless there is associated bony pathology. Ultrasound is useful as it can demonstrate LHB tendon thickening, tenosynovitis and excessive fluid in the biceps sheath. Furthermore, dynamic ultrasound assessment can look for LHB tendon instability. MRI can identify thickening of tendon and tenosynovitis but offers the advantage of being able to evaluate other soft tissue structures in the shoulder such as SLAP lesions and labral pathology.
- *Management:* Physiotherapy should be considered first line in conjunction with NSAIDs, if required. An image-guided steroid injection can be considered and is useful as both a diagnostic and therapeutic intervention. In those patients where conservative measures fail, then surgery should be considered. This may involve biceps tenodesis (fixing the tendon to the proximal humerus) or tenotomy (cutting/dividing the tendon). For active patients under the age of 40 then a tenodesis is preferred, whereas over the age of 40, a tenotomy yields reproducible outcomes. A tenotomy, however, can be associated with a cosmetic deformity (the Popeye sign).

ELBOW

Medial Elbow Pain

GOLFER'S ELBOW

Golfer's elbow is also known as medial epicondylitis. It occurs as a result of chronic overloading of the flexor-pronator tendons leading to a degenerative tendinopathy. It is seen in sports requiring repeated wrist flexion and forearm pronation such as golf and racquet sports. Golfer's elbow is also common in manual occupations.

- *Presentation:* Patients complain of pain in the medial aspect of the elbow at, or just distal to, the medial epicondyle. Pain may also radiate down the forearm to the wrist. There is tenderness on palpation of the medial epicondyle or common flexor tendon. Patients may also complain of weakness in the hand and wrist when gripping or carrying.
- *Investigations:* Golfer's elbow is a clinical diagnosis and therefore no routine radiological investigation is needed. X-ray may be used to rule out traumatic avulsions and ultrasound can be used to demonstrate common flexor tendon abnormalities such as degeneration, small tears and changes in vascularity. MRI is requested if there is concern around ligamentous injuries or if the diagnosis of medial elbow pain is unclear.
- *Management:* Management of this condition is conservative in the first instance. Physiotherapy (structured loading) and sporting technique evaluation, in combination with activity modification, has been shown to be effective in most cases. Other modalities such as Extracorporeal Shock Wave Therapy (ESWT) and acupuncture have been used with varying degrees of success. Steroid injections can be used as a diagnostic and short-term intervention, but patients should be counselled with regard to the effects of steroids on tendon tissue. Platelet Rich Plasma (PRP) injections are increasingly employed as an alternative to steroid injections to encourage tendon healing. Surgery is reserved for those who fail conservative management or those whose symptoms are severely affecting their quality of life.

Medial Collateral Ligament Sprain

The Medial Collateral Ligament (MCL) or Ulnar Collateral Ligament (UCL) of the elbow provides stability and restrains valgus forces across the elbow. It is made up of three components: the anterior oblique, posterior oblique and transverse ligaments.

- *Presentation:* MCL injuries arise from an acute trauma (e.g. elbow dislocations) or from chronic overuse. Repetitive valgus stress leading to MCL failure is seen in overhead throwing athletes such as baseball pitchers and volleyball players. Athletes will complain of medial elbow pain and poor throwing performance with a loss of velocity and power.
- *Examination:* There may be tenderness over the MCL origin and the valgus stress test may reveal increased laxity with soft end points of the medial joint.
- *Investigations:* X-rays will demonstrate if there are any bony injuries in acute trauma. Valgus stress X-rays can reveal excessive opening of the medial elbow when compared to the normal side. MRI is the gold standard for assessing the integrity of the medial soft tissues (sensitivity and specificity are increased with arthrography).
- *Management:* Physiotherapy, activity modification and rest are recommended in cases of degeneration, overload and partial tears. For complete ruptures then a surgical referral is advised for further assessment and consideration of ligament repair or reconstruction.

Cubital Tunnel Syndrome

The cubital tunnel (also known as ulnar tunnel) is a fibro-osseous space in the posteromedial aspect of the elbow. Cubital tunnel syndrome describes clinical symptoms and signs as a result of compression of the ulnar nerve within this tunnel. It is the second most common neuropathy affecting the upper limb after carpal tunnel syndrome. It is seen in individuals who perform repetitive overhead throwing motions or prolonged elbow flexion. Patients with excessive valgus carrying angles at the elbow are known to be more prone to ulnar neuropathy.

- *Presentation:* Patients occasionally report pain in the medial aspect of the elbow. In cases where

the nerve is unstable, patients may describe a clicking with elbow flexion. The most common complaint is paraesthesia in the fourth and fifth fingers. In later stages, patients may develop weakness and eventually atrophy of the intrinsic muscles of the hand, most notably the first dorsal interosseous.
- *Investigations:* Nerve conduction studies (NCS) are essential in confirming the diagnosis and establishing whether any permanent axonal loss has occurred. X-rays are useful where arthritis is suspected to be causing nerve compression.
- *Management:* In those that have mild symptoms, conservative management with night splinting is advised. Surgical intervention is reserved for those who fail conservative treatment or have progressive sensorimotor deficits.

LATERAL ELBOW PAIN

Tennis Elbow

Tennis elbow is the most common cause of lateral elbow pain. It is a degenerative tendinopathy affecting the proximal aspect of the extensor muscles of the forearm (most commonly extensor carpi radialis brevis). This arises as a result of an incomplete repair response to repetitive tendon microtrauma. It is commonly found in patients and athletes who perform repetitive upper limb movements involving wrist extension. This includes racquet sports (especially backhand groundstrokes) and manual jobs.

- *Presentation:* Patients will complain of a gradual onset of lateral elbow pain, which can radiate down the forearm into the wrist. It is often made worse on gripping activities with the wrist in extension.
- *Examination:* This will often reveal tenderness over the lateral epicondyle and, distal to this, in the area overlying the proximal tendon of extensor carpi radialis brevis. There is generally a full range of motion at the elbow but pain is reported on resisted wrist or middle finger extension (see elbow tests).
- *Investigations:* Diagnosis is usually made with history and examination and investigations are rarely required. X-ray may be used to rule out

other pathologies such as arthritis. Ultrasound or MRI can be used to demonstrate the degree of tendinopathy and any partial tears.

- *Management:* Conservative management should be first line in all cases. NSAIDs in conjunction with physiotherapy (structured loading) are used to improve pain and function. Athletes should have their techniques and equipment scrutinised. Extracorporeal Shockwave therapy (ESWT) and epicondylar clasps may provide symptom improvement in some patients. Corticosteroid injections can offer pain relief in the short term but may adversely affect long term outcomes. PRP injections are increasingly employed for this condition to try and improve tendon healing in the degenerate areas. Surgery should only be considered for severe cases and includes debridement and release/repair of the origin of the extensor carpi radialis brevis tendon.

OTHER

Distal Biceps Tendinopathy and Ruptures

Distal biceps pain occurs at, or near the insertion, of the biceps tendon onto the radius. It is a degenerate pathology that occurs in males more than females and between the ages of 25–55. It is seen in sports involving lifting and supination resistance movements. Traumatic ruptures of the distal biceps can occur and this is usually as a result of sudden eccentric loading.

- *Presentation:* Patients present with a gradual onset of pain localised to the biceps tendon in the antecubital fossa. The pain is made worse by resisted flexion or supination manoeuvres. Performing the Hook test of O'Driscoll reproduces the pain in the antecubital fossa. Acute ruptures present with sudden pain in the region of the distal biceps after sudden lifting or unexpected eccentric loading of the biceps, e.g. in a rugby tackle.
- *Examination:* There is often a tear or a 'pop' and a change in shape such that the biceps muscle belly migrates proximally. Bruising is commonly seen in the forearm a short time later.

- *Investigations:* Distal biceps tendinopathy and ruptures are largely a clinical diagnosis and X-ray rarely offers any additional information. MRI is the gold standard and will demonstrate signs of tendinopathy and thickening as well as bicipital bursitis. In acute ruptures, it is essential to arrange prompt imaging so as not to delay treatment.
- *Management:* The pain of distal biceps tendinopathy can be successfully managed with activity modification and analgesia. This should be supplemented with a structured physiotherapy loading programme. If pain persists then injections can be used to assist in rehabilitation. Both steroid injections and PRP are used, and the pros and cons of each should be discussed. Acute ruptures are time sensitive and, as such, require prompt identification and referral to a surgeon. Ideally, the patient will be offered surgical repair within 3 weeks of the initial injury.

Posterior Impingement

Posterior elbow pain (or impingement) occurs as a result of repetitive extension of the elbow. This movement causes the olecranon to forcefully contact the olecranon fossa on the back of the humerus, leading to inflammation and pain. It is most commonly seen in racquet sports, fencing and boxing.

- *Presentation:* Patients present with posterior elbow pain, which is exacerbated by full extension. This can occur during overhead tennis shots such as serving. As the condition progresses, a loss of terminal extension may be seen and a decrease in throwing or serving velocity.
- *Investigations:* X-rays can be normal but may reveal spurs of bone on the tip of the olecranon. MRI scans can show signs of inflammation in the olecranon fossa.
- *Management:* In most cases, posterior impingement can be successfully managed with analgesia, activity modification and physiotherapy. This can be supplemented by corticosteroid injections to enable good, pain free rehabilitation. When this fails and structural changes exist, surgery can be used to remove any spurs of bone.

MULTIPLE CHOICE QUESTION (MCQ) QUESTIONS

1. A 24-year-old rugby player injures his right shoulder during a tackle. He immediately feels pain and discomfort around the anterior shoulder and it appears asymmetrical to the other side. He is examined by the physiotherapist and any attempt at passive movement is painful for the player. The physiotherapist diagnoses a dislocated shoulder and they discuss management. The player is also complaining of tingling around the outer aspect of his shoulder. What nerve is most likely to be causing his symptoms?

   A. Radial nerve
   B. Axillary nerve
   C. Median nerve
   D. Ulnar nerve
   E. Musculocutaneous nerve

2. A 30-year-old boxer visits her GP complaining of pain in her posterior elbow. This is worse on straightening the elbow and at the end range of punching. On examination, there is a normal appearance to the elbow but there is a 10-degree deficit of full extension. What is the likely diagnosis?

   A. Golfer's elbow
   B. Posterior impingement of the elbow
   C. Tennis elbow
   D. Distal biceps rupture
   E. Cubital tunnel syndrome

3. A 15-year-old gymnast complains to her coach of lateral elbow pain. They ask her to see a physiotherapist. She complains of pain on the outside of her elbow when she goes into a handstand position, as well as a sensation of clicking. She is sent for an X-ray but this is normal. What would be the next best investigation?

   A. CT scan
   B. Ultrasound
   C. MRI
   D. MR Arthrogram
   E. Diagnostic injection

4. A 24-year-old baseball pitcher complains of 4 weeks of medial right elbow pain. The pain is worsened by pitching and overhead throwing. On examination, he is tender at the medial epicondyle, and valgus stress to the elbow causes pain. There is no locking or catching evident on movement. What is the most likely diagnosis?

   A. Medial epicondylitis
   B. Medial collateral ligament (MCL) sprain
   C. Cubital tunnel syndrome
   D. Flexor pronator injury
   E. Osteochondritis Dissecans of the elbow

5. A 63-year-old female attends clinic with 2 months of atraumatic left shoulder pain. She has a past medical history of well controlled Type 2 Diabetes Mellitus. On examination, there are no features of instability. There is no acromioclavicular joint tenderness. She appears to have globally restricted shoulder movements. There is a capsular restriction to passive external rotation. What is the most appropriate initial investigation?

   A. X-ray
   B. Ultrasound
   C. MRI
   D. MRI Arthrogram
   E. No investigations are required

MULTIPLE CHOICE QUESTION (MCQ) ANSWERS

1. **Answer B**
    In dislocation of any joint, it is important to consider the structures around the joint including the soft tissues, as these can be injured during the trauma of dislocation. The axillary nerve comes from the posterior cord of the brachial plexus and contains fibres from the C5 and C6 nerve roots. It wraps around the surgical neck of the humerus making it more prone to injuries such as humeral neck fractures and shoulder dislocations. Patients complain of tingling or numbness in the outer aspect of the shoulder over the deltoid (known as the 'regimental badge' in relation to soldiers' display of badges on uniform). Symptoms of axillary nerve damage should prompt quick relocation to reduce the damage to the axillary nerve. Not doing so may lead to weakness in shoulder abduction and atrophy of the deltoid muscles.

2. **Answer B**
    Posterior impingement is the most likely cause for this athlete's pain. Initial management should include conservative measures. Failure to progress should lead to imaging in the form of an MRI scan and a guided elbow injection. Occasionally, surgical debridement is needed.

3. **Answer C**
    This girl competes in gymnastics which often involves a lot of repeated overhand movements. Whilst tennis elbow could be considered in this age group, it is very unlikely and osteochondritis dissecans is more likely to be the diagnosis. X-ray may only show changes if the disease is unstable and there is a loose body present.

Therefore, in those in whom there is a high index of suspicion, MRI should be considered in the presence of a normal X-ray with persisting elbow pain. It is an important diagnosis not to be missed, particularly in a competitive athlete who may require surgical intervention.

4. **Answer B**
    Unlike the previous question, this athlete is not an adolescent, and there is an absence of mechanical symptoms, making answer E unlikely. Repetitive valgus stress leading to MCL failure is seen in overhead throwing athletes, such as in this case. Tenderness at the MCL origin with pain on valgus stress testing are also suggestive of MCL injury.

5. **Answer A**
    Although the most likely clinical diagnosis is frozen shoulder, as recommended by BESS guidelines (2021), an X-ray would differentiate this from other glenohumeral joint pathology such as osteoarthritis. NICE guidance states that a shoulder X-ray should be considered if there is reduced range of movement (NICE, 2022).

REFERENCES AND FURTHER READING

BESS, 2021. *Shoulder Pain—Primary, Community and Intermediate Care Guidelines.* Available from: https://bess.ac.uk/national-guidelines/

Cleland, J.C., Koppenhaver, S and J, Su. J. 2016. *Netter's Orthopaedic Clinical Examination: An Evidence-Based Approach.* 3rd ed. Philadelphia: Elsevier.

NICE, 2022. Osteoarthritis in over 16s: diagnosis and management. *National Institute for Health and Care Excellence.* Available from: https://www.nice.org.uk

Hand and Wrist **4**

Natalie Cheyne and Ian Gatt

INTRODUCTION

Hand and wrist injuries are relatively common in sport medicine and account for approximately 25% of all sporting injuries. As expected, incidence of hand and wrist injuries will vary vastly between the sports performed, with golf, climbing, gymnastics, boxing and tennis expected to have a higher incidence than lower limb dominant sports.

KEY ANATOMY

Bones and Joints

The carpal bones are separated into a proximal row—scaphoid, lunate, triquetrum, pisiform and trapezium—and a distal row—trapezoid, capitate and hamate (Figure 4.2). The metacarpal bones are numbered from radial to ulnar and consist of a head, neck and shaft. The phalanges comprise of proximal, middle, and distal phalanx (except for the thumb where there is no middle phalanx).

The wrist joint is formed of two articulations: the mid-carpal joint formed between the distal and proximal row of carpal bones, and the radiocarpal joint formed between the distal radius and the proximal row of carpal bones (except the pisiform). The ulnar does not form part of the wrist joint, although it provides stability and shock absorption through the triangular fibrocartilage complex (TFCC). It also articulates with the radius both proximally and distally, making up the proximal and distal radio-ulnar joints (these are important for pronation and supination).

Ligaments

There are four main ligaments found in the wrist, each on a separate side of the joint:

- *Palmar radiocarpal:* located on the palmar aspect of the hand. It extends from the radius to both carpal rows. The palmar radiocarpal ligament stabilises the wrist joint and limits over-extension of the wrist.
- *Dorsal radiocarpal:* located on the dorsal aspect of the hand. It extends from the radius to both carpal rows. It contributes to stability, but its main involvement is to limit excessive flexion of the wrist. Both the palmar and dorsal radiocarpal ligaments, together with the TFCC, create stability to allow the hand to follow the radius during pronation and supination.
- *Ulnar collateral:* extends from the ulnar styloid to the triquetrum and pisiform. It prevents excessive radial deviation of the hand.
- *Radial collateral:* extends from the radial styloid to the scaphoid and trapezium. It prevents excessive ulnar deviation of the hand.

Flexor Muscles

The flexor muscles are located on the volar aspect of the arm. They serve to flex the wrist and digits.

Wrist Flexors

- Flexor carpi radialis (FCR)
- Flexor carpi ulnaris (FCU)
- Palmaris longus (PL)

DOI: 10.1201/9781003179979-4

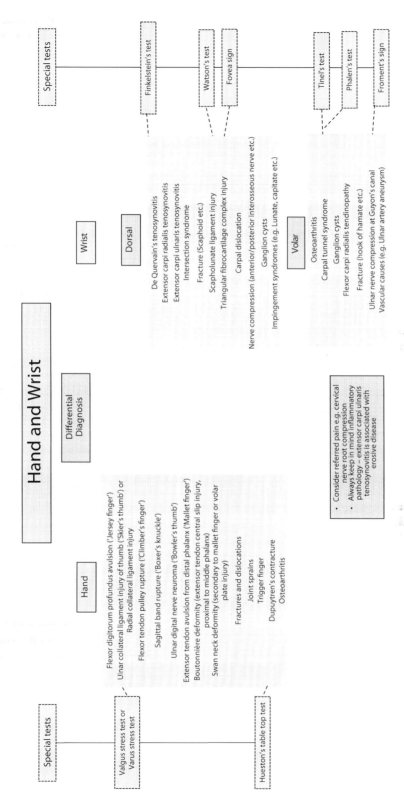

Figure 4.1 Differential diagnosis chart.

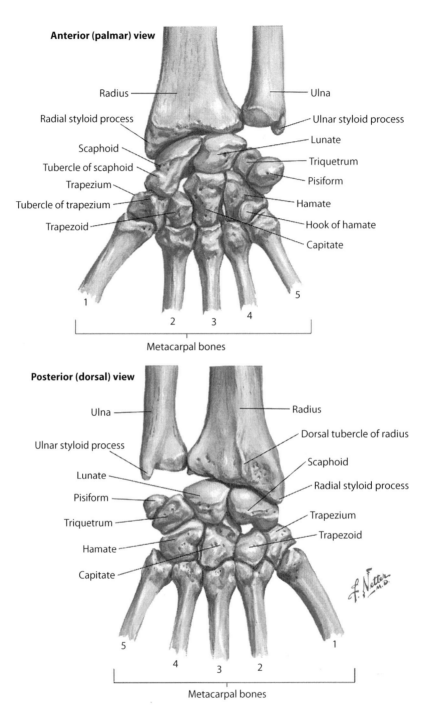

Figure 4.2 Carpal bones.

Source: Cleland et al. (2016). *Netter's Orthopaedic Clinical Examination: An Evidence-Based Approach.* 3rd ed. Philadelphia: Elsevier. With permission.

Digital Flexors

- Flexor digitorum superficialis (FDS)
- Flexor digitorum profundus (FDP)
- Flexor pollicis longus (FPL)

Wrist and Digital Extensors

The muscles on the dorsum of the forearm and hand serve to extend the wrist or digits. They are separated into compartments from one to six.

Compartments From Radial to Ulnar

1. Abductor pollicis longus (APL) and extensor pollicis brevis (EPB)
2. Extensor carpi radialis longus (ECRL) and extensor carpi radialis brevis (ECRB)
3. Extensor pollicis longus (EPL)
4. Extensor digitorum (ED) and extensor indicis (EI)
5. Extensor digiti minimi (EDM)
6. Extensor carpi ulnaris (ECU)

Muscles of the Hand

THENAR MUSCLES

Three muscles located at the base of the thumb make up the thenar eminence on the palmar aspect (Figure 4.3). They are innervated by the median nerve, although the flexor pollicis brevis deep head is innervated by the deep branch of the ulnar nerve. They can be remembered by the mnemonic 'OAF.'

- Opponens pollicis (OP)
- Abductor pollicis brevis (APB)
- Flexor pollicis brevis (FPB)

ADDUCTOR POLLICIS

This muscle also assists in control of thumb movement and lies deeper and more distal to FPB. However, it is not considered a part of the thenar group of muscles and is supplied by the ulnar nerve. Injuries to the median nerve affecting the thenar eminence would still allow opposition of the thumb through this muscle.

HYPOTHENAR MUSCLES

The hypothenar muscles make up the hypothenar eminence on the ulnar palmar aspect of the hand and control the little finger. They are innervated by the ulnar nerve.

- Opponens digiti minimi (OPD)
- Abductor digiti minimi (ADM)
- Flexor digiti minimi brevis (FDM)

Lumbricals

There are four lumbrical muscles in the hand, each corresponding to a finger. They link the flexor and extensor tendons and are innervated by both the ulnar and median nerve, depending on their location. The two at the ulnar aspect are supplied by the ulnar nerve and the two at the radial aspect are supplied by the median nerve. The lumbricals act to flex the finger at the MCPJ and extend at the interphalangeal joints, important for lumbrical grips.

Interossei

The interossei muscles are divided into dorsal and palmar groups and serve to abduct (dorsal) or adduct (palmar) the fingers at the MCPJ. This can be remembered via the mnemonic 'Pad and Dab.' Both groups of interossei are innervated by the ulnar nerve.

Vasculature

The hand is supplied by the radial and ulnar arteries. They combine to form the deep and superficial palmar arches. The main contributor to the deep arch is the radial artery, which primarily supplies the thumb and radial aspect of the index finger. The ulnar artery is the main contributor to the superficial palmar arch which supplies the rest of the digits.

Nervous Supply

ULNAR NERVE

This supplies sensation to the little and ulnar aspects of the ring fingers via its palmar and dorsal cutaneous branches. The nerve passes through Guyon's canal

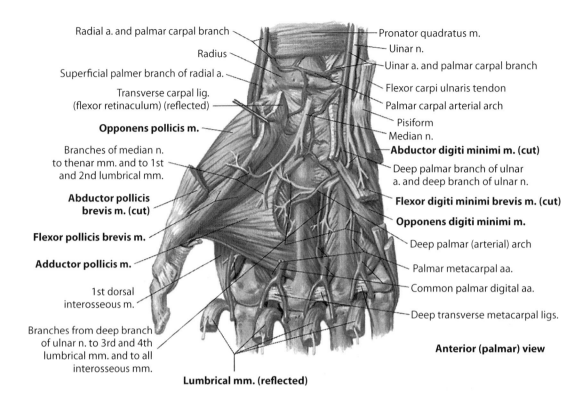

Radial a. and palmar carpal branch

Radius

Superficial palmer branch of radial a.

Transverse carpal lig. (flexor retinaculum) (reflected)

Opponens pollicis m.

Branches of median n. to thenar mm. and to 1st and 2nd lumbrical mm.

Abductor pollicis brevis m. (cut)

Flexor pollicis brevis m.

Adductor pollicis m.

1st dorsal interosseous m.

Branches from deep branch of ulnar n. to 3rd and 4th lumbrical mm. and to all interosseous mm.

Lumbrical mm. (reflected)

Pronator quadratus m.

Uinar n.

Uinar a. and palmar carpal branch

Flexor carpi ulnaris tendon

Palmar carpal arterial arch

Pisiform

Median n.

Abductor digiti minimi m. (cut)

Deep palmar branch of ulnar a. and deep branch of ulnar n.

Flexor digiti minimi brevis m. (cut)

Opponens digiti minimi m.

Deep palmar (arterial) arch

Palmar metacarpal aa.

Common palmar digital aa.

Deep transverse metacarpal ligs.

Anterior (palmar) view

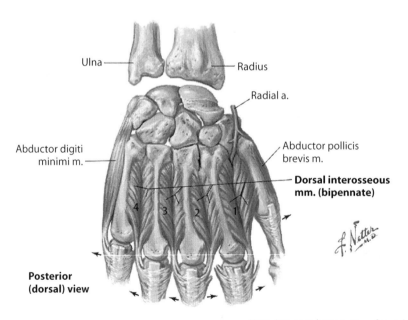

Ulna

Radius

Radial a.

Abductor digiti minimi m.

Abductor pollicis brevis m.

Dorsal interosseous mm. (bipennate)

4 3 2 1

Posterior (dorsal) view

Note: Arrows indicate action of muscles

Figure 4.3 Hands with intrinsic muscles.

Source: Cleland et al. (2016). *Netter's Orthopaedic Clinical Examination: An Evidence-Based Approach.* 3rd ed. Philadelphia: Elsevier. With permission.

(formed by the pisiform, hamate, transverse, and volar carpal ligaments) at the wrist and is compressed here. This is seen commonly in cycling.

The Ulnar Nerve Supplies:

- Hypothenar muscles
- Ulnar two lumbricals
- Palmar and dorsal interossei
- APL
- Ulnar portion of the FDP
- FCU

MEDIAN NERVE

The median nerve enters the wrist alongside the tendons of FPL, FDS and FDP at the carpal tunnel. This is formed between the hamate and pisiform at the ulnar aspect and the scaphoid and triquetrum at the radial aspect. The palmar cutaneous branch of the median nerve arises over the top of the carpal tunnel, innervating the skin over the thenar eminence. This is not affected in carpal tunnel syndrome, which is a useful differentiator between a true carpal tunnel syndrome vs. a neuropathy occurring more proximal to the wrist. In the former, sensation over the thenar eminence will not be affected.

The Median Nerve Supplies:

- Radial two lumbricals
- OP
- APB
- Forearm flexors (FCR, PL, FPL, FDS and median portion of the FDP)

RADIAL NERVE

In the hand, the only function of the radial nerve is to supply sensation to the first webspace on the dorsum, indicating that motor innervation is supplied to extrinsic muscles controlling the hand.

A branch of the radial nerve called the posterior interosseous nerve (PIN) has a motor function to supply the extensors of the wrist and digits.

The PIN supplies:

- ED
- EI
- EDM
- APL

- EPB
- EPL

HISTORY AND EXAMINATION OF THE HAND AND WRIST

History taking in an individual who presents with a hand injury should include the following:

- Hand dominance
- Occupation and sporting activities
- Mechanism of injury
- Chronicity (acute/chronic)
- Pain features (severity, irritability and 24-hour pattern)
- Associated symptoms e.g. swelling, deformity
- Mechanical symptoms e.g. locking, clicking, catching, stiffness
- Neurological symptoms e.g. numbness, altered sensation
- Previous injury status
- General health and systemic enquiry
- Known conditions e.g. rheumatoid arthritis and family history

Inspection

- Ensure the patient is adequately exposed with jewellery, watches and clothing removed, allowing for exposure from the elbow down.
- Skin: integrity, colour, erythema, scars, lesions
- Nails: colour, deformity, absence
- Muscular atrophy (mainly guttering of interossei or hypothenar/thenar regions)
- Joint position at elbows, wrist, and digits
- Deformity (flexion, extension, deformity)
- Ulnar or radial drift of digits
- Localised swelling (including Heberden's (DIPJ) and Bouchard's nodes (PIPJ)
- Effusion
- Ulnar or radial angulation at the distal radioulnar joint (DRUJ)

Movement

- Movement at the wrist occurs in three sets of patterns: flexion and extension, radial and ulnar deviation, pronation and supination. Movements of the hand and wrist should be performed both actively, passively and with resistance (Figure 4.4 and Table 4.1).

- Wrist flexion
- Wrist extension
- Ulnar deviation (wrist)
- Radial deviation (wrist)
- Pronation (forearm)
- Supination (forearm)
- Abduction (thumb)
- Opposition (thumb)
- Finger flexion (DIPJ/MCPJ/PIPJ)
- Finger extension (DIPJ/MCPJ/PIPJ)

Functional Tests

Functional assessments help to identify how an injury or pathology is impacting on day-to-day activities and can be tailored for the age of the individual.

- Unbuttoning a shirt
- Combing hair
- Writing with a pen
- Picking up a cup
- Waving goodbye
- Grip strength

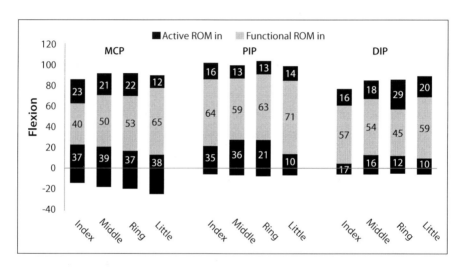

Figure 4.4 Active and functional range of movement in finger joints.

Source: Taken from Bain et al. (2015)

Table 4.1 Approximate Range of Motion

Joint	Flexion	Extension	Ulnar dev.	Radial dev.
Finger: Metacarpophalangeal Joint (MCPJ)	85°	0°	-	-
Finger: Proximal Interphalangeal Joint (PIPJ)	110°	0°	-	-
Finger: Distal Interphalangeal Joint (DIPJ)	80°	10°	-	-
Wrist	80°	75°	40	20
Thumb: Metacarpophalangeal Joint (MCPJ)	50°	0°	-	-
Thumb: Interphalangeal Joint	90°	10°	-	-

Palpation

- Radial and ulnar styloid
- Ulnar snuffbox for triquetral or triquetrolunate injury
- Radiocarpal joint
- Lister's tubercle (used as a pulley by EPL)
- Anatomical snuffbox and scaphoid tubercle (both useful in the assessment of scaphoid fracture)
- Carpals, metacarpals, and phalanges should be palpated anteriorly, posteriorly, medially, and laterally
- Extensor tendon compartments
- Flexor tendon sheaths
- Thenar and hypothenar eminences
- Palmar area
- Fingertips and nails
- Lumps or masses

Special Tests

SCAPHOID TESTS

- Palpation of the anatomical snuffbox dorsally for tenderness.
- Palpation of the scaphoid tubercle volarly for tenderness.
- Axially loading the thumb into the scaphoid and assessing for pain.
- These three tests have an 87–100% sensitivity and 74% specificity when all positive within 24 hours of injury.
- Scaphoid-lunate stress test (Watson's test)—to assess for scapholunate instability.

EXTENSOR TENDONS

- *Finkelstein's test:* to assess for De Quervain's tenosynovitis.

FLEXOR TENDONS

- *Flexor tendons:* if there is weakness to flex the PIPJ with the MCPJ stabilised in extension this could indicate an FDS or FDP injury. If there is a resultant inability to flex the DIPJ with the PIPJ stabilised in extension it is likely to be an FDP injury, whereas if the distal DIPJ is able to flex with good

strength then it is more likely there is an FDS injury.
- *Hueston's test:* to assess Dupuytren's contracture. If the patient's fingers are unable to be placed flat on the table, surgery (e.g. fasciectomy) is usually indicated with this level of restriction.

THUMB

- Valgus (or varus) stress test of the thumb—to assess for ulnar collateral ligament laxity and injury (or radial collateral ligament laxity and injury). A laxity of over 15° may indicate a complete rupture of the ligament.

NERVES

- *Phalen's test:* in order to reproduce symptoms of carpal tunnel syndrome.
- *Tinel's test:* at Guyon's canal for the ulnar nerve and at the volar centre of the wrist for carpal tunnel syndrome.
- *Froment's sign:* to assess for weakness of the adductors and possible ulnar neuropathy.
- Sensation check in the ulnar, median and radial nerve distributions.

OTHER

- Triangular fibrocartilage stress test (Scoop test)—to assess for TFCC tears.

IMAGING

In hand and wrist injuries, the initial imaging modality is usually a plain radiograph. Posteroanterior (PA), lateral and oblique views of the wrist, hand and digit will be sufficient to diagnose most bony injuries. In cases where disruption to the proximal carpal row is considered, an X-ray may be taken in a clenched fist, anteroposterior view. This will allow assessment of the scapholunate joint and highlight any widening between the two. For scaphoid injuries, further X-rays are taken specifically of the scaphoid bone. Although initial X-rays have a low sensitivity for scaphoid fractures, this also allows for direct comparison between initial and repeat X-rays in 14 days following the injury.

Magnetic resonance imaging (MRI) scans are the gold standard technique for occult scaphoid fractures. MRI scans are also used to assess for avascular necrosis, infections, soft tissue masses and ligamentous/cartilage injuries. In cases with joint involvement, MRI arthrograms or 3T MRI scans may be useful.

Computed tomography (CT) scans may be used to diagnose radiographically occult carpal fractures or to determine the extent of an injury. CT scans also demonstrate the presence of healing within a fracture, so may be indicated in the assessment of scaphoid fractures, when delayed union is of concern. In sports, delayed scaphoid unions should be considered for surgery to avoid complications.

Ultrasound imaging allows for dynamic assessment of the soft tissue structures in the hand and wrist. This quick diagnostic tool allows clinicians to visualise structures directly and confirm suspected diagnoses. Ultrasound imaging can be used to evaluate the healing of structures as rehabilitation progresses. It is useful in assessing tendon integrity and detecting joint effusions.

HAND AND WRIST PATHOLOGY

Fractures

DISTAL RADIUS/ULNA

Fractures at the wrist are more likely to occur in the elderly population and are typically caused by a fall onto an outstretched hand, leading to dorsal displacement (Colles fracture). If they happen when the wrist is flexed, there will often be volar displacement (Smith's fracture). Fractures of the distal radius and ulna are also categorised into extra- and intra-articular, which may influence their management.

In children, fractures at the joint may involve the growth plate (epiphyseal plate) leading to growth disruption at that site. If involving the metaphysis or diaphysis, due to the plasticity of the immature skeleton, there will often be bowing or an incomplete fracture through only one cortex (Greenstick).

- *Presentation:* Immediate pain and swelling at the site. Sometimes, deformity and crepitus are present at the fracture site.

- Examination should include a detailed neurovascular assessment, with emphasis on the median nerve. When there is median nerve involvement, there may be sensory disturbance (paraesthesia or numbness) at the radial and palmar aspects of the hand (thumb, index, middle and half of the ring finger), as seen in carpal tunnel syndrome. In this case, urgent reduction of the fracture is warranted under appropriate sedation.
- *Investigations:* Plain X-ray.
- Management can be categorised into non-surgical and surgical. Surgery is usually indicated in those fractures that are intra-articular, significantly displaced or involving an adolescent. Immobilisation involves a cast or wrist splint for comfort with appropriate control of load bearing activities for 3–6 weeks. Physiotherapy should commence at the earliest opportunity to facilitate restoration of function and plan a structured return to sporting activities.

SCAPHOID

The scaphoid bone is located in the proximal row of the carpal bones, proximal to the thumb.

- *Presentation:* Typical mechanism of injury is a fall onto an outstretched hand. Concurrent fractures of the scaphoid and distal radius are rare, occurring in approximately 2% of cases.
- *Examination:* There is tenderness in the anatomical snuffbox, pain on axial loading of the thumb and on ulnar deviation of the wrist. It is important not to miss a scaphoid fracture, as this commonly results in non-union and early osteoarthritis. The blood supply to the scaphoid is retrograde, meaning that when a fracture occurs in the centre (waist) of the scaphoid, the supply to the proximal pole is compromised, leading to avascular necrosis and delayed or non-union.
- *Investigations:* X-ray, with scaphoid views, is the initial investigation of choice. With clinical suspicion of a scaphoid fracture, the individual should be placed into a below elbow plaster of Paris cast, even with a negative X-ray. Repeat imaging should be sought in 10–14 days. MRI scans are the gold standard imaging modality for acute scaphoid fractures, but CT and nuclear medicine (bone scintigraphy) imaging are alternative modalities.

- *Management:* Treatment is largely non-surgical with a period of immobilisation in a cast to allow for healing, typically up to 6 weeks with a repeat X-ray recommended. Non-union occurs in approximately 10–15% of scaphoid fractures. These individuals will go on to have surgical fixation with possible bone grafting to promote healing. Displaced fractures are likely to require surgery immediately due to high non-union risk. Physiotherapy should commence as soon as immobilisation is removed.

HAMATE

- *Presentation:* The hamate is a carpal bone located at the ulnar aspect of the distal carpal row, consisting of a body and a hook. Hamate fractures usually occur as a result of direct impact and can be seen in racquet sports, golf and gymnastics due to high forces directly to this region. Grip and contact areas play a role in the mechanism of this injury.
- Examination is likely to reveal pain on the ulnar aspect of the wrist, over the hamate, with occasional involvement of the ulnar nerve. Symptoms would then include sensory disturbance to the ulnar aspect (little and half of ring fingers).
- *Investigations:* An X-ray should be performed but further imaging (e.g. CT) may be required.
- *Management:* Cast or splint immobilisation for 6 weeks and physiotherapy. In cases where the hook is fractured, an excision of this piece of bone may be considered if chronic pain develops.

METACARPAL

- *Presentation:* The metacarpal bones comprise of a head, shaft and base. These fractures may be intra- or extra-articular. A 'Boxer's fracture' is the name given to a fifth metacarpal body fracture, typically seen in punching injuries.
- Examination findings should evaluate for extensor lag (inability to fully extend as the extensor tendon is caught in the fracture), deformity and scissoring of the fingers, which would indicate a rotational deformity. These findings may indicate the need for surgical reduction and fixation.
- *Investigations:* X-ray

- *Management:* Non-displaced Boxer's fractures are usually managed in a splint for 2–4 weeks. Displaced intra-articular fractures may require splint or plaster of Paris cast immobilisation prior to (or instead of) surgical fixation to prevent deterioration in the fracture alignment.

  Typically, they are managed conservatively, with a return to sporting activities across most sports in approximately 3 weeks. Where surgery is required, rehabilitation is usually longer than this (e.g. 4 weeks).

PHALANGEAL

- *Presentation and examination:* As with metacarpal fractures, it is important to assess for deformity and malrotation by asking the individual to clench their fist. Phalangeal fractures may also be accompanied by tendon injuries. Therefore, it is important to assess both extension and flexion—specifically, the two functions of flexor digitorum superficialis and flexor digitorum profundus (flexion of the PIPJ and DIPJ respectively). Volar plate injuries are avulsions of the ligaments connecting the interphalangeal joints. They often accompany phalangeal fractures and dislocations.
- *Investigations:* X-ray
- *Management:* Phalangeal fractures can be 'neighbour' strapped to the next finger, which allows the finger to remain straight and splinted. Hand therapy can commence following a period of immobility; it is important to monitor progression as full function returns.

  Although conservative management is preferred, cases are typically managed operatively, with a return to play across most sports of approximately 4 weeks (Geoghegan et al., 2021).

KEINBÖCH'S DISEASE

Keinböch's disease is the term given to idiopathic avascular necrosis of the lunate bone.

- *Presentation and examination:* Cases are often associated with repetitive wrist trauma and present with dorsal wrist pain, loss of function, range of movement and grip. It is therefore important to consider sports where high force and repetition of the wrist are involved, like racquet and water sports. Differential diagnoses include lunate bone contusion, acute fracture or subluxation.

- *Investigations:* X-ray (although early changes may be missed). MRI is best for identifying early disease. CT is most useful once lunate collapse has occurred and can show the extent of necrosis.
- Management includes rest and off-loading the wrist with the use of braces or casts. Orthopaedic referral is recommended once imaging changes have been identified. Operative intervention depends on the level of necrosis present and may include bone grafting or joint levelling procedures if ulnar variance is present. Treatment for chronic pain includes wrist arthrodesis (fusion), which may lead to symptom chronicity.

ULNAR SIDED WRIST PAIN

Ulnar sided wrist pain may represent a number of conditions that can be difficult to diagnose. Therefore, a systematic approach is essential. It is important to assess for ulnar variance (the ulna is the main load bearing bone of the forearm). Any change in the length of the ulna will significantly alter the load bearing upon it and its biomechanics. For example, ulnar shortening (negative ulnar variance) can reduce the load to less than 5%. This is associated with conditions such as Keinböch's disease and ulnar impingement. Ulnar lengthening (positive ulnar variance) increases the load to over 40%. This is associated with ulnar impaction syndrome. X-rays may be useful to assess for ulnar variation.

Triangular Fibrocartilage Tear

- *Presentation:* The triangular fibro-cartilage complex (TFCC) is composed of fibro-cartilage and ligaments among the ulna, triquetrum and lunate bones. This arrangement of soft tissue contributes to the stability of the ulnar side of the wrist. The TFCC can be injured from either overuse or trauma. Individuals with positive ulnar variance are more likely to develop TFCC degeneration.
- *Examination:* Pain on the ulnar aspect of the wrist is common, with clicking and tenderness on palpation. Specifically, pain on palpation of the ulnar surface, between the ulna and pisiform, is called the 'fovea sign.' Wrist extension and ulnar deviation may exacerbate pain, with individuals often finding turning motions problematic, e.g. turning a key. Pronation may be more symptomatic due to compression on the fibrocartilaginous discus compared with supination, but with large tears, both motions can be equally impaired.
- *Investigations:* Diagnostic imaging is with an MRI scan.
- *Management:* Treatment includes splinting and offloading whilst considering appropriate rehabilitation targeting dynamic stability at the wrist. A corticosteroid injection may be required for moderate symptoms, where the conservative approach is not progressing as expected.
  Surgical intervention might be required, with debridement often indicated for central tears. Peripheral tears likely require repair, with acute athletic injuries more amenable. In individuals with positive ulnar variance, surgical osteotomy of the ulna (ulnar shortening) can be advised to prevent symptoms from returning.

Extensor Carpi Ulnaris (ECU) Tendonitis

- *Presentation:* The extensor carpi ulnaris tendon is situated in the sixth extensor compartment of the wrist and, like all tendons, is prone to overuse injury caused by repetitive movements and impaction. The ECU contributes to the stability of the wrist as its tendinous subsheath joins with the TFCC. Individuals may also describe a 'snapping' sensation at the ulnar aspect of the wrist. This is caused by subluxation of the ECU due to a tear of its subsheath.
- *Examination:* Pain associated with the ECU mainly occurs during pronation and supination. To assess for potential subsheath tears, ask the patient to flex their elbow, actively ulnar deviate and actively supinate and pronate. Look for tendon subluxation with any associated symptoms.
- *Investigations:* Dynamic assessment can be undertaken using ultrasound imaging. MRI evaluation will confirm the diagnosis and differentiate between TFCC pathology and ECU tendinopathy.

- *Management:* Pain and load management with analgesia and splinting are considered in moderate-to-severe cases. Injection therapy can be useful for symptoms.
- In prolonged cases, especially those with instability, surgical repair may be required.

Distal Radioulnar Joint Instability

- *Presentation:* The distal radioulnar joint (DRUJ) is the articulation between the distal radius and ulna at the wrist. It contributes to the stability of the wrist during pronation and supination. In pathological instability, it often presents with ulnar sided wrist pain due to its links with the TFCC. DRUJ instability, though a relatively common pathology, is often misdiagnosed or missed. DRUJ instability often occurs following distal radius fractures and can cause chronic pain.
- *Examination:* Clicking and snapping during pronation and supination, positive 'fovea' sign and weakened grip strength. Inability to load through the wrist, especially in extension.
- Investigations can consist of stress X-ray views (demonstrating joint widening) and MRI scans, depending on the aetiology of the DRUJ instability. This will also allow diagnosis of associated pathology e.g., TFCC tears.
- Management includes strapping or taping the wrist to approximate the radius and ulna, allowing the distal portion of the interosseous membrane to heal. This is typically performed for a 3–6 week period. Rehabilitation, with appropriate physical therapy, is important. If there is a high degree of instability and this has a significant impact on activities, surgical stabilisation may be warranted. In the absence of instability, injection therapy may be useful for pain management.

DIGITAL SOFT TISSUE INJURIES

Mallet Finger

- *Presentation:* This injury is seen in ball sports— when the tip of an extended finger is struck with a ball on its dorsal aspect, creating a flexion movement at the DIPJ—such as in catching. This action results in a rupture of the extensor tendon at its attachment to the distal phalanx.
- *Examination:* Inability to actively extend the fingertip and it sags in flexion.
- *Investigations:* X-ray can identify concurrent bony injury.
- *Management:* A fingertip mallet splint holds the DIPJ in extension for up to 6 weeks. When removed for bathing and washing, the individual must be careful not to allow the DIPJ to flex and the splint must be worn at all other times. Splinting may be considered in subacute injuries, such as those up to 3 months old—however, beyond 6 weeks, the prognosis is less favourable, especially in athletes. Therefore, after 6 weeks, in the absence of DIPJ instability, no treatment is usually performed.

Jersey Finger

- *Presentation:* This injury classically occurs when an individual's finger is caught in an opponent's clothing; while the athlete's finger is flexed, it is forced into extension.
- *Examination:* In contrast to a mallet finger, the individual will be unable to actively flex the DIPJ due to an avulsion of the flexor digitorum profundus tendon where it inserts onto the distal phalanx.
- *Investigations:* X-ray can identify concurrent bony injury.
- Management is commonly surgical, to re-attach the avulsed fragment, followed by splint immobilisation. DIPJ strength is important for many sporting activities.

Boutonnière Deformity

- *Presentation:* This is a disruption to the extensor digitorum tendon (the central slip) at the PIPJ, leading to an inability to actively extend at this joint, with compensation and resulting hyperextension of the DIPJ.
- *Examination:* Characterised by PIPJ flexion and DIPJ extension. There is an inability to actively extend the PIPJ. It can be passively extended with slight force unless the joint has been compromised.

- *Investigations:* X-ray can identify concurrent bony injury.
- *Management:* In acute injuries, the finger should be splinted in extension for 6 weeks to prevent a fixed-flexion deformity developing. Once established, correction is unachievable.

Boxer's Knuckle

- *Presentation:* This arises from a direct contact mechanism, either due to trauma or overuse, causing a tear to either one of the sagittal bands at the MCPJ (these anchor the extensor digitorum centrally over the knuckle). Joint capsule, as well as tendon injury, can also occur. The second and third MCPJ are the most commonly affected, as it is these knuckles which impact when a punch is thrown correctly.
- Examination findings include a flexion lag or—observed with capsular tears—hypermobility at the joint, with palpable tenderness and effusion on either side of the knuckle. Pain and tenderness can also be central in cases where a tendon injury or irritation occurs.
- *Management:* Traumatic injuries benefit from splinting for a period of 3-6 weeks with gradual return to loading activities. Overuse mechanisms benefit from addressing equipment used and loading volume. In chronic cases, injections can improve symptoms, especially when swelling is present. Surgery is typically reserved for those not responding to a conservative approach.

Skier's Thumb

- *Presentation:* The ulnar collateral ligament can be injured in many sports due to a valgus (abduction) force occurring at the first MCPJ. This can occur in both open (goalkeeper catching a ball) and closed (a fall onto an outstretched hand) kinetic chains.
- Examination will reveal reluctance to adduct. Testing for pinch grip (pulp of DIPJ of thumb moving toward pulps of DIPJ of index and middle finger) can be a useful objective measure. There will be tenderness to the ulnar aspect of the first MCPJ and increased laxity of the thumb when performing a UCL stress test.

- *Investigations:* X-ray may identify bony avulsion. Ultrasound and MRI can identify tendon tear and Stener lesions (interposition of the adductor pollicis aponeurosis between the MCPJ and the torn ligament, prohibiting healing).
- *Management:* Those with mild-to-moderate injuries can return back to full activity within days to weeks. This is dependent on symptoms, strength and the ability to protect the thumb (using taping or splinting). Surgical repair may be required in more significant injuries, such as when a Stener lesion is present. In chronic injuries, reconstruction is required.

WRIST SOFT TISSUE PATHOLOGY

De Quervain's Tenosynovitis

- *Presentation:* De Quervain's tenosynovitis is inflammation of the APL and EPB, at the first extensor compartment of the wrist, as they pass through the tight compartment at the radial styloid. The inflammation can occur due to overuse and is common in racquet sports and rowing.
- Examination may reveal pain and crepitus at the base of the thumb and a positive Finkelstein's test.
- *Investigations:* This is a clinical diagnosis, but ultrasound can show tendon sheath thickening, increased doppler activity and loss of normal tendon echotexture.
- Management includes analgesia, avoidance of aggravating activities and splinting of the wrist and thumb to allow for off-loading and rest. In some cases, the symptoms may become chronic and warrant corticosteroid injection, although the response is variable. Surgical decompression is a last resort.

Intersection Syndrome

- *Presentation:* Though similar to De Quervain's, intersection syndrome occurs more proximally on the forearm and can occur where the first and second extensor compartments cross over.
- Examination may produce tenderness and the individual may complain of 'squeaking' in the forearm on aggravating movements.

- Investigations are not usually required but ultrasound or MRI is diagnostic.
- Management includes analgesia, avoidance of aggravating activities and corticosteroid injections if symptoms are persistent. Surgical decompression is a last resort, although in some sports (like rowing or canoeing) this could be considered a primary approach as most do not respond well to conservative treatment.

Ganglion

- *Presentation:* Ganglions are cysts that either arise from a joint capsule or tendon sheath. Ganglions can occur on the volar or dorsal aspect, but most arise from the scapholunate ligament and joint.
- Examination usually reveals a firm swelling. There may be pain and weakness with certain movements, depending on the location, and some concerns will be purely cosmetic.
- *Investigations:* Though a clinical diagnosis, X-ray can detect underlying osteoarthritis, which may be a cause. Ultrasound is diagnostic.
- *Management:* Many ganglions resolve spontaneously so 'watching and waiting' is reasonable. Aspiration is possible, sometimes followed by a steroid injection, but there is a risk of recurrence. Surgical excision can take out the entirety of the ganglion but, again, recurrence is still possible.

NEUROLOGICAL IMPAIRMENT

Ulnar Nerve Compression

- *Presentation:* Along the course of the peripheral nerves, there are areas which can be compressed by surrounding structures. For example, at Guyon's canal in the wrist, the ulnar nerve can be compressed as it traverses through the space between the hamate and the pisiform bones.

Cyclists are prone to developing ulnar nerve compression due to the position of their wrists on the handlebars.
- *Examination:* As the ulnar nerve has both sensory and motor function in the hand, the result can be a sensory disturbance to the ulnar one and a half digits and/or weakness of finger abduction.
- *Investigations:* Nerve conduction studies can be used to diagnose ulnar nerve compression.
- Management includes splinting and padding or changing hand position, along with analgesia. In severe cases, surgical decompression of the nerve can be considered.

Carpal Tunnel Syndrome

- *Presentation:* The median nerve enters the wrist at the carpal tunnel (formed between the hamate and pisiform at the ulnar aspect and the scaphoid and triquetrum at the radial aspect), accompanied by the tendons of FPL, FDS and FDP. It is at this site that the nerve can become compressed. Carpal tunnel syndrome is more prevalent in individuals who have diabetes or hypothyroidism and in those who are pregnant.
- Examination may reveal altered sensation and wasting of the thenar eminence. Phalen's and Tinel's may be positive.
- *Investigations:* Diagnosis is usually clinical but can be confirmed with nerve conduction studies.
- Management options include splinting, avoidance of aggravating activities, analgesia, physiotherapy, corticosteroid injections and surgical carpal tunnel decompression.

CLINICAL CONSIDERATIONS

With neurological symptoms affecting the hand and wrist, it is important to consider other differential diagnoses such as cervical spine pathology or medical conditions predisposing to neuropathy such as alcoholism, hypothyroidism, diabetes and renal disease.

MULTIPLE CHOICE QUESTION (MCQ) QUESTIONS

1. A 28-year-old basketballer attends your clinic with wrist pain following a fall mid-match. She is tender at the anatomical snuff-box. Plain X-rays are unremarkable. Which of the following is considered the gold standard to confirm the diagnosis?

    A. Magnetic resonance imaging (MRI)
    B. Repeat X-ray in 7–10 days
    C. Ultrasound
    D. Magnetic resonance arthrography (MRA)
    E. Computed Tomography (CT)

2. A 40-year-old female with 3 months of dorsal and distal forearm pain attends for review. A recent ultrasound scan comments on 'hypoechoic features and loss of typical fibrillar pattern of the first and second extensor compartments, with some hypervascularity and thickening of the surrounding tendon sheaths.' What is the most likely diagnosis?

    A. De Quervain's tenosynovitis
    B. Vaughan-Jackson Syndrome
    C. Intersection Syndrome
    D. Extensor Carpi Ulnaris tendinosis
    E. Extensor Pollicis Longus tenosynovitis

3. A 20-year-old indoor sprint cyclist presents 2 weeks after a fall from his bike, with dorsal wrist pain. He has an X-ray, which reveals an increased capitolunate angle, an increased scapholunate angle and no fractures. Which of the following statements is true regarding this injury?

    A. Magnetic resonance imaging (MRI) is the gold standard for diagnosis

    B. A painful 'clunk' during Watson's test helps support the diagnosis
    C. VISI (volar intercalated segment instability) is commonly associated with this condition
    D. The scapholunate ligament is likely to be intact
    E. Dynamic Ultrasound is the gold standard for diagnosis

4. A 38-year-old female presents to you with a painful 1 cm swelling on the palmar aspect of her index finger, near the DIPJ. It is firm and smooth to palpate and the patient thinks it has increased in size over the past 2 months. You examine it with ultrasound, which reveals a well-defined hypoechoic lesion with internal vascularity. What is the most appropriate action?

    A. Advise her to watch and wait
    B. With full consent and with aseptic technique, aspirate using needle and syringe, ensuring to counsel her about the risk of recurrence
    C. Arrange X-ray
    D. Arrange MRI
    E. Refer to a hand surgeon for further assessment

5. You are leading a revision session for your colleagues on the extensor wrist compartments. Which two extensor tendons of the wrist typically lie either side of Lister's tubercle?

    A. ECRB and EPL
    B. ECRL and EPB
    C. EPB and APL
    D. EPL and EI
    E. EDM and ECU

MULTIPLE CHOICE QUESTION (MCQ) ANSWERS

1. Answer A

MRI is considered the gold standard investigation in suspected scaphoid fractures. Although follow-up plain radiograph (B) is used in some settings, it has relatively poor sensitivity.

2. Answer C

The ultrasound report describes features in keeping with tendinopathy and tenosynovitis of the first and second extensor compartments, which typically takes place in Intersection syndrome.

3. Answer B

Watson's (or the Scaphoid-Lunate shift) test can help diagnose scapholunate instability, despite a relatively low sensitivity. Scapholunate instability can lead to Dorsal intercalated segment instability (VISI usually occurs due to disruption of the radiocarpal ligaments at the ulnar wrist), so B is incorrect. Arthroscopy is the gold standard for diagnosis.

4. Answer D

Although many of the features described could suggest a ganglion cyst (where answers A and B would be reasonable), there would not be vascularity present on ultrasound. This makes a giant cell tumour, fibromatosis or glomus tumour more likely. Although E may be an appropriate answer, an MRI scan (D) would help determine the urgency of referral depending on the likely diagnosis.

5. Answer A

ECRB of the second extensor compartment and EPL, the third extensor compartment, lie either side of Lister's tubercle in most individuals.

FURTHER READING AND REFERENCES

Bain, G.I., Polites, N., Higgs, B.G., Heptinstall, R.J., McGrath, A.M. (2015). The functional range of motion of the finger joints. *J Hand Surg Eur*, 40(4), 406–411.

Cleland, J.C., Koppenhaver, S and J, Su. J. 2016. *Netter's Orthopaedic Clinical Examination: An Evidence-Based Approach*. 3rd ed. Philadelphia: Elsevier.

Geoghegan, L., Scarborough, A., Rodrigues, J.N., Hayton, M.J., Horwitz, M.D. (2021). Return to sport after metacarpal and phalangeal fractures: A systematic review and evidence appraisal. *Orthop J Sports Med*, 9(2), p. 2325967120980013.

Foot and Ankle 5

Raymond Leung, Suzy Speirs, Andrew Howse and Peter Rosenfeld

INTRODUCTION

Foot and ankle injuries account for about 27% of musculoskeletal injuries amongst athletes. The assessment of these injuries are best divided based on anatomical region.

EXAMINATION OF THE FOOT AND ANKLE

Inspection

- Standing and supine
- Inspect footwear
- Look for swelling, discolouration, asymmetry and lower limb muscle loss
- Look for potential issues in each section—the ankle, hindfoot, midfoot and forefoot. e.g. hindfoot valgus or varus, high arch or midfoot collapse, forefoot supination or pronation, hallux valgus or varus, lesser toe malalignment (e.g. toe clawing), nail deformities or onychocryptosis, and skin lesions (e.g. calluses or plantar warts)

Movements

- Ankle plantarflexion and dorsiflexion; hindfoot inversion and eversion, midfoot adduction and abduction; forefoot supination and pronation; toe flexion and extension
- The above needs to be assessed actively, passively and against resistance

Functional Tests

- Squats
- Lunges
- Knee to wall
- Hopping
- Heel raises
- Balance
- Gait
- Sport specific movements

Palpation

The key structures should be palpated systematically (Figures 5.2–5.4).
- Anterior ankle structures

  o Talocrural joint
  o Antero-inferior tibiofibular ligament (AITFL)
  o Talus

- Lateral ankle structures

  o Proximal to distal fibula and lateral malleolus
  o Lateral ligaments (anterior talofibular, calcaneofibular and posterior talofibular)
  o Peroneal tendons
  o Peroneal tubercle
  o Base of fifth metatarsal
  o Lateral talar process
  o Anterior calcaneal process
  o Subtalar joint
  o Sinus tarsi
  o Bifurcate ligament

DOI: 10.1201/9781003179979-5

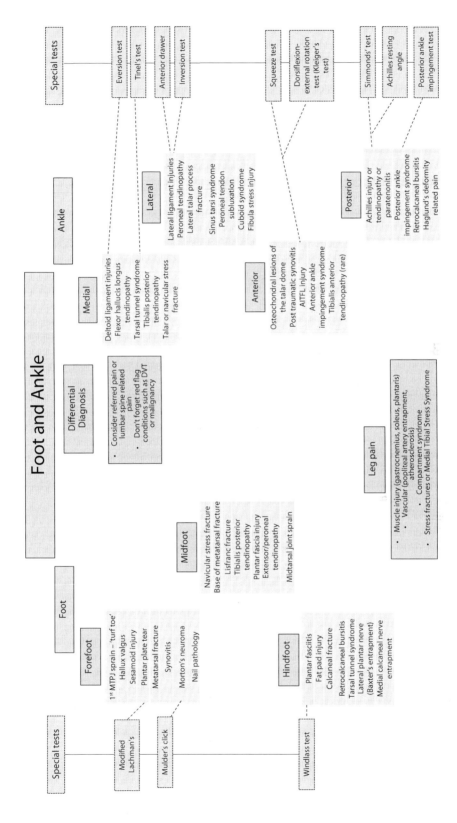

Figure 5.1 Differential diagnosis chart.

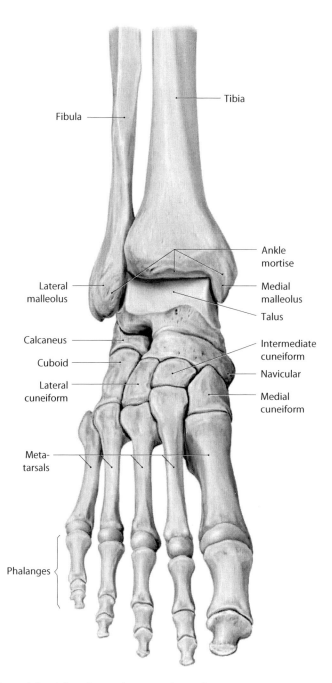

Figure 5.2 Anterior view of the right talocrural joint in plantarflexion.

Source: Schuenke, E. and Schumacher, U. (2010). *Thieme—Atlas of Anatomy: General Anatomy and Musculoskeletal System*. New York. Thieme. p. 402.

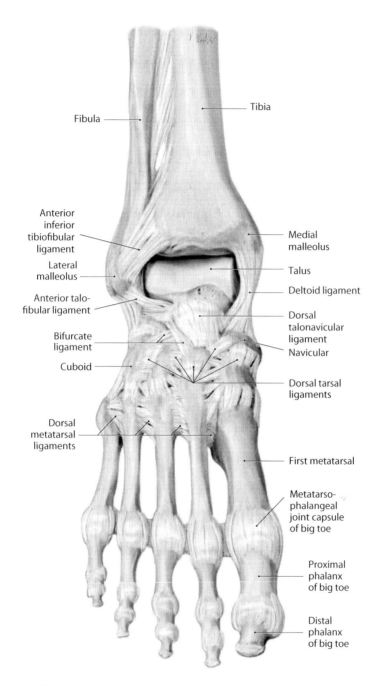

Figure 5.3 Ligaments of the right foot and ankle.

Source: Schuenke, E. and Schumacher, U. (2010). *Thieme—Atlas of Anatomy: General Anatomy and Musculoskeletal System*. New York. Thieme. p. 409.

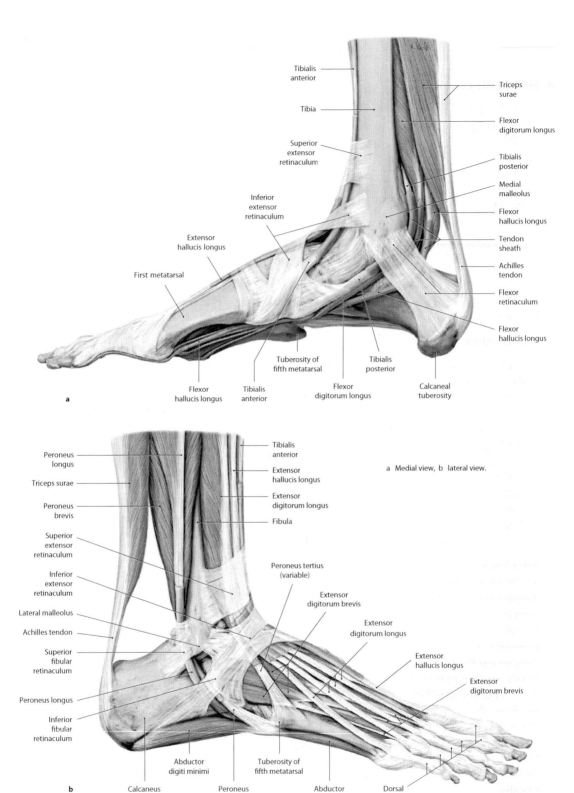

Figure 5.4 The tendons and muscles of the right foot and ankle (a medial view, b lateral view).

Source: Schuenke, E. and Schumacher, U. (2010). *Thieme—Atlas of Anatomy: General Anatomy and Musculoskeletal System*. New York. Thieme. p. 455.

- Medial ankle structures

  - Medial malleolus
  - Deltoid ligament
  - Tibialis posterior
  - Flexor digitorum longus
  - Flexor hallucis longus
  - Sustentaculum tali
  - Navicular tubercle
  - Neurovascular bundle

- Posterior ankle structures

  - Achilles tendon
  - Calcaneum
  - Haglund's
  - Retrocalcaneal bursa

- Foot structures

  - Navicular
  - Cuboid
  - Cuneiforms
  - Metatarsals
  - Sesamoids
  - Phalanges
  - Joint spaces (talonavicular, calcaneocuboid, navicular-cuneiform, tarsometatarsal, metatarsophalangeal, and interphalangeal)
  - Medial calcaneal tuberosity
  - Navicular tuberosity

Special Tests

- Anterior drawer test for anterior talofibular ligament laxity
- Inversion test (Talar tilt test) for calcaneofibular ligament laxity
- Eversion test for deltoid laxity
- Tinel's test for posterior tibial nerve entrapment
- Squeeze test and dorsiflexion-external rotation test for syndesmosis injury
- Simmonds' test and Achilles tendon resting angle for ruptured Achilles tendon
- Posterior ankle impingement test (forced plantar-flexion of ankle in prone)
- Windlass test (passive dorsiflexion of the first metatarsophalangeal joint, in standing, for plantar fasciopathy)
- Modified Lachman's anterior-posterior drawer of metatarsophalangeal joint for plantar plate tear
- Mulder's click test for Morton's neuroma

POSTERIOR ANKLE

Achilles Tendinopathy

The Achilles tendon (AT) starts near the mid-calf and provides distal attachment of the gastrocnemius (lateral and medial heads) and soleus muscles. The AT inserts onto the posterior surface of the calcaneum. Tendinopathy is most commonly located in the mid-portion of the free AT, but in older athletes or those with inflammatory pathology, it may occur at the calcaneal insertion. The risk factors for tendinopathy include increased training load, recent footwear alteration, calf muscle weakness, excess foot pronation, more supinated foot types (with less rearfoot motion), metabolic conditions (e.g. diabetes) and family history.

- *Presentation:* gradual or subacute onset pain in the AT exacerbated during or after strenuous activity such as running. It may be relieved by heat or warm-up activities. Morning stiffness and start up pains are common. There is tendon swelling in the mid-portion or insertion.
- *Examination:* active ankle dorsiflexion pain and tenderness over the affected AT area. AT swelling or an insertional spur is often palpable.
- *Investigations:* mid-portion AT on ultrasound scan (USS) typically shows fusiform thickening, hypoechogenic or heterogenous changes and sometimes neovascularity. Insertional AT on USS may show disruption of distal fibres and cortical irregularity at the posterior aspect of the calcaneum. Insertional spurs are often present.
- *Management:* Optimise biomechanics, review footwear and adjust training load initially. Then a progressive AT loading programme should be implemented starting with isometric exercises, then isotonic exercises such as slow concentric and eccentric heel raises. Addressing other biomechanical deficits, such as posterior chain weakness, is required for long term recovery. Extracorporeal shockwave therapy may be used as an adjunct to rehabilitation. Surgery for resistant cases (e.g. tendoscopy, plantaris release or AT debridement).

Achilles Tendon Rupture

AT rupture affects about 1 in 8000 competitive athletes and is more common in male athletes in their

40's. It usually occurs after an explosive ankle dorsiflexion movement (e.g. push-off during running).

- *Presentation:* sudden acute pain in the AT area (like being kicked) with a possible audible pop. There is usually bruising and swelling.
- *Examination:* impaired active plantarflexion, inability to tiptoe walk, and a palpable gap in the AT. The AT resting angle is vertical (lack of normal tension/plantarflexion) and Simmonds' test is positive, whereby squeezing the calf in prone does not elicit plantarflexion movements.
- *Investigations:* USS or MRI can confirm the diagnosis. A dynamic USS allows evaluation of the gap between tendon ends (in neutral and plantarflexion), establishing whether surgery may be required.
- *Management:* Non-surgical treatment involves immobilisation in plantarflexion with an equinus cast or a rigid boot with equinus wedges. Full weight-bearing is permitted, with the equinus reduced each week to neutral over 8–10 weeks. Surgery is indicated if the USS reveals a gap in plantarflexion or for professional athletes. This involves repairing the ruptured ends of the AT with sutures, performed using either open or minimally invasive techniques that have lower risks. Surgery has a lower risk of AT re-rupture and improved power.

Posterior Ankle Impingement Syndrome

This syndrome refers to pain from impingement of soft tissue, or repetitive stress to bone, at the posterior ankle, between the tibia and posterior aspect of the talus. Bony causes relate to os trigonum (unfused lateral tubercle of the posterior process of the talus), with or without cartilaginous synchondrosis,or a Stieda process (enlarged lateral tubercle of the posterior process of the talus). Soft tissue causes are from excessive synovitis, scarring, low lying flexor hallucis longus (FHL) muscle belly or presence of anomalous muscles. Impingement occurs with activities resulting in extremes of plantarflexion, common in ballet dancers, gymnasts, swimmers and kicking sports such as football.

- *Presentation:* pain in the posterior ankle (sometimes felt over the AT) exacerbated by plantarflexion movements such as kicking or standing on

tiptoes. It may present acutely with forceful plantarflexion which fractures the posterior process of the talus.
- *Examination:* pain with passive ankle plantarflexion particularly with overpressure (posterior impingement test).
- *Investigations:* MRI scan is preferable to X-ray as it can evaluate the presence of bone or soft tissue oedema including synovitis.
- *Management:* relative rest, activity modification and a short course of oral anti-inflammatories can be helpful. Orthoses can relieve soft tissue impingement. USS or fluoroscopic guided corticosteroid injections can be curative or provide temporary symptomatic relief. If these measures fail, then arthroscopic surgery to excise the bony impingement is often effective.

ANTERIOR ANKLE

Osteochondral Lesions of the Talar Dome

Osteochondral lesions of the medial talar dome often develop gradually with no history of trauma. However, lesions of the lateral talar dome are typically seen following ankle injuries, particularly inversion injuries. The risk factors include a cavus hindfoot alignment and lateral ankle ligamentous instability. Many osteochondral lesions are asymptomatic and do not require treatment.

- *Presentation:* ongoing pain and swelling around the anterior aspect of the ankle particularly after an initial sprain. There may be catching or locking sensations.
- *Examination:* ankle effusion, anterior joint line tenderness and a reduced ankle range of motion with or without ligament laxity.
- *Investigations:* MRI can classify these lesions to determine treatment and CT may be helpful for pre-operative planning.
- *Management:* non-displaced stable lesions require a period of non-weight bearing and immobilisation in a cast or boot between 3 weeks to 4 months followed by progressive weight bearing. Surgical options include arthroscopic debridement or microfracture (bone marrow stimulation). Rarely, large or acute fragments can be fixed. In large or recurrent lesions, osteochondral grafting is successful.

Post Traumatic Synovitis

Post-traumatic synovitis is the most common presentation of ankle pain following any ankle injury such as a sprain. It may persist due to early return to sport or inadequate rehabilitation, and can occur in those with chronic ankle instability.

- *Presentation:* ongoing pain and swelling following an original ankle injury.
- *Examination:* anterior joint tenderness especially in the medial or lateral gutter with associated swelling. Anterior drawer and inversion stress tests may demonstrate laxity or pain.
- *Investigations:* USS may show signs of synovitis. MRI is not as reliable but will show other lesions, and both can detect associated ankle ligamentous injuries.
- *Management:* a period of relative offload from impact activities, oral anti-inflammatories and an ultrasound-guided corticosteroid injection may be required alongside ankle rehabilitation. Arthroscopy with partial synovectomy is sometimes needed for resistant cases.

Anterior Inferior Tibiofibular Ligament (AITFL) Injury

The AITFL runs obliquely from the anterior tubercle of the distal tibia to the anterior fibular at the lateral malleolus. It is one of three major ligaments that provide stability to the distal tibiofibular syndesmosis joint. The other two ligaments are the posterior inferior tibiofibular ligament and the interosseous ligament. AITFL injuries (high ankle sprains) often do not occur in isolation and may be associated with other ankle ligament injuries e.g. deep deltoid ligament, medial malleolar or proximal fibula fractures (Maisonneuve injury).

- *Presentation:* Anterolateral ankle pain after a moderate to severe ankle injury involving sudden external rotation and forced dorsiflexion on a planted foot.
- *Examination:* Tenderness and swelling over the anterolateral ankle and syndesmosis, extending proximally a few centimetres above the ankle joint (High ankle sprain). Passive dorsiflexion and external rotation (Kleiger's test) is positive and

syndesmosis squeeze test (proximal tibiofibular compression produces distal pain) may be positive in more severe injuries. Reduced range of ankle dorsiflexion is common.

- *Investigations:* X-rays with AP and Mortise views may show syndesmosis widening and any associated fractures. USS can assess the AITFL integrity, but MRI is the overall investigation of choice.
- *Management:* AITFL sprains without ankle diastasis should be managed in a controlled ankle motion walking boot for 2–3 weeks with non-weight bearing or weight-bearing as tolerated. Syndesmosis taping can help. Physiotherapy rehabilitation should include progression of loading, mobility exercises and proprioception. In unstable cases, surgery is essential, with compression and fixation of the syndesmosis using a synthetic ligament (tightrope) or screw fixation, non-weight-bearing for 4–6 weeks.

Anterior Ankle Impingement Syndrome

The syndrome refers to soft tissue or bony impingement between the anterior tibiotalar joint during dorsiflexion. It is caused by bone spurs (exostoses) in the anterior rim of the tibia or the anterior neck of the talus. Soft tissue impingement is due to thickening of anterior soft tissues, hypertrophy of the ATFL or synovitis. It can be seen in sports such as football, dance and ballet.

- *Presentation:* gradual onset anterior ankle pain exacerbated by dorsiflexion movements. Stiffness and swelling may be associated.
- *Examination:* tenderness to palpate the anterior joint line, pain with forward lunges or squats, and pain with passive and forced dorsiflexion.
- *Investigations:* X-rays can detect bony spurs and MRI can reveal soft tissue collections or loose bodies.
- *Management:* activity modification, heel lifts, taping to reduce ankle dorsiflexion and short-course oral anti-inflammatories. An ultrasound guided corticosteroid injection can provide symptomatic relief. Arthroscopic surgery may be needed to remove soft tissues or bone spurs.

LATERAL ANKLE

Lateral Ligament Injuries

Acute ankle sprains account for 16% to 40% of all sports-related injuries and the majority affect the lateral ligaments. The anterior talofibular ligament (ATFL) is most commonly injured, followed by the calcaneofibular ligament (CFL). The posterior talofibular ligament (PTFL) is less commonly injured. The usual mechanism of injury is forced inversion of the ankle.

- *Presentation:* acute lateral ankle pain following an inversion injury. There is usually swelling and sometimes an audible snap.
- *Examination:* tenderness in the anterolateral aspect of the ankle and over the fibula insertion with a positive anterior drawer test if there is ATFL disruption.
- *Investigations:* consider X-rays if a fracture is suspected using Ottawa ankle rules. USS can grade the lateral ligament injury but can be limited in the early stages due to swelling. MRI will identify ligament injuries as well as other injuries, but it does not diagnose instability.
- *Management:* protection (e.g. use of ankle stirrup), optimisation of loading, ice, compression (e.g. elasticated support) and elevation initially. Crutches may be needed temporarily if too painful to weight bear. Active range of motion exercises should be started early. Strengthening and proprioceptive retraining should be incorporated once pain allows. Functional then sport-specific exercises should occur in the late phases of rehabilitation. Surgery is rarely needed acutely but has high success rates in chronic instability.

CLINICAL CONSIDERATIONS

Ankle inversion injuries can cause more than lateral ligamentous sprains. Sprains not responding to initial management should raise suspicion for osteochondral injury, fracture (e.g. anterior calcaneal process), peroneal tendon injury, posteromedial impingement lesions or sinus tarsi syndrome.

Peroneal Tendinopathy

The peroneus longus and brevis tendons share a common synovial sheath and travel posterior to the lateral malleolus in the retromalleolar groove. Tendinopathy may occur in those with previous ankle inversion injuries and sports that require frequent change of direction. The risk factors include increased training load, change in footwear, weak peroneal muscles, or a pes cavus foot type.

- *Presentation:* gradual onset lateral ankle pain during or after exercise, and maybe worse the morning after exercise. Pes cavus may be evident.
- *Examination:* there may be swelling over the lateral ankle and hindfoot. There may be tenderness over the lateral calcaneum or posterolateral ankle. Functional assessment may reveal weakness, with varus tilt on single heel raise and pain during resisted eversion. It may be tender at the peroneal tubercle, the base of the fifth metatarsal or the cuboid tunnel.
- *Investigations:* USS shows tendinopathic changes such as loss of linear fibrillar pattern, and the common tendon sheath may be thickened with synovial hypertrophy. MRI is useful but can be confused by magic angle effects (artefact) below the malleolus.
- *Management:* optimise biomechanics, review footwear and adjust training load initially. Stretching and strengthening of the peroneal muscles and implementing proprioceptive ankle exercises are essential. Surgery (e.g. tendon debridement, tendoscopy or re-alignment of cavus) for resistant cases.

Lateral Talar Process Fracture

Typically occurs with forced dorsiflexion and inversion of the ankle which causes the lateral aspect of the talus to be jammed against the fibula. It is also known as a Snowboarder's fracture and is often misdiagnosed as a lateral ankle sprain.

- *Presentation:* acute lateral ankle pain with swelling and inability to fully weight bear.

- *Examination:* generalised or localised pain in the lateral talar process area (antero-inferior to the tip of the lateral malleolus).
- *Investigations:* X-ray with lateral views can be diagnostic, but MRI is more sensitive. A CT can assess the extent of the fracture.
- *Management:* an orthopaedic opinion is required. Minimally displaced fractures <2 mm can usually be managed conservatively with a non-weight bearing cast for 6 weeks. Surgical options include open reduction internal fixation or fragment excision.

Sinus Tarsi Syndrome

The sinus tarsi is an anatomical landmark, over the anterolateral aspect of the ankle, formed by the articulation of the talus and calcaneus. It is a tunnel through the rearfoot, formed by the sulcus calcanei as the floor and the sulcus tali as the roof. It separates the anterior and posterior parts of the subtalar joint; containing nerves, fat, blood vessels and ligaments. Sinus tarsi syndrome (more recently described as sinus tarsitis) refers to painful irritation of the tissues within the tarsal canal due to impingement or injury. It is either the result of other injuries or related to foot function and alignment. Pain in this area can be due to a number of issues: ligamentous injury associated with a lateral ankle sprain; soft tissue compression from forced eversion and overpronation in a flatter foot type; related to tarsal coalition or inflammatory arthropathies, such as rheumatoid arthritis.

- *Presentation:* anterolateral ankle pain exacerbated by exercise particularly on uneven surfaces with an instability sensation.
- *Examination:* tenderness in the sinus tarsi opening at the lateral ankle with or without swelling. There is usually pain with combined plantarflexion and inversion, or with eversion.
- *Investigations:* MRI scan is most helpful as it can detect injury to the ligaments in the sinus tarsi, inflammation and scar tissue formation.
- *Management:* initial management will be similar to an ankle sprain if this has occurred. Rehabilitation includes mobilisation of the ankle and subtalar joint, muscle strengthening and proprioceptive training. Ultrasound-guided corticosteroid and local anaesthetic injection may help with persistent pain. Surgery involves removal of scar tissue in the sinus tarsi if all other measures fail.

MEDIAL ANKLE

Tibialis Posterior Tendinopathy

The tibialis posterior muscle runs through the deep posterior compartment of the leg and its tendon travels behind the medial malleolus before inserting onto the navicular tuberosity then the plantar aspect of the medial and lateral cuneiforms. It supports the medial arch of the foot, inverts the heel and plantarflexes the ankle. Tendinopathy is most commonly due to chronic flat foot (pes planus) deformity. It also occurs with muscle overuse (e.g. ballet dancers), trauma, tightness in other lower limb muscles (e.g. calf and hamstring) and foot overpronation.

- *Presentation:* gradual onset medial ankle pain exacerbated during or after activity such as running or prolonged walking. There may be a snapping sensation and swelling.
- *Examination:* typically, flat foot deformity with tenderness behind and under the medial malleolus. There is pain and weakness with resisted inversion and reduced hindfoot inversion with heel raises.
- *Investigations:* USS shows tendinopathic changes such as thickening, loss of linear fibrillar pattern and sometimes neovascularity. The tendon sheath may be thickened with fluid and synovial hypertrophy. MRI can also be diagnostic and show tendon splits.
- *Management:* optimise biomechanics, review footwear, orthoses or ankle foot orthoses (AFO) to reduce hindfoot valgus, support the midfoot and improve ambulation. Adjustments to training load are important in the initial stages of management. Tibialis posterior strengthening in a graded manner is essential. Surgical treatment for resistant cases includes debridement or reconstruction with tendon transfers.

Flexor Hallucis Longus Tendinopathy

The FHL muscle originates from the posterior fibula, runs through the deep posterior compartment of the leg and its tendon travels across the posterior ankle joint between the medial and lateral talar tubercles, then inserts onto the base of the distal phalanx of the great toe. It assists with plantarflexion of the ankle and inversion of the foot, but also flexion of the great toe. Tendinopathy can occur with overuse of the muscle (e.g. ballet dancers), trauma, poor fitting footwear (e.g. oversized shoes) and overpronation of the foot.

- *Presentation:* gradual onset posteromedial ankle pain exacerbated during or after activities involving the great toe such as forefoot balance, toe-off when running, and jumping and landing on the forefoot. Triggering of the great toe may be a feature.
- *Examination:* pain at posteromedial ankle with resisted flexion of the hallux interphalangeal joint and associated weakness. Crepitus may be felt at the posteromedial aspect of the ankle with plantarflexion and hallux flexion.
- *Investigations:* USS can show tendinopathic changes such as thickening, loss of linear fibrillar pattern and sometimes neovascularity. The tendon sheath may be thickened with fluid and synovial hypertrophy. MRI is useful as posterior impingement can be associated with this condition.
- *Management:* optimise biomechanics, review footwear and adjust training load initially. Strengthening of both the FHL and calf muscles are helpful. Ultrasound-guided corticosteroid or hyaluronic acid injections if no improvement. Surgery (e.g. arthroscopic release) for resistant cases.

Tarsal Tunnel Syndrome

The tarsal tunnel is a fibro-osseous canal between the medial malleolus, talus, calcaneus and the flexor retinaculum. It contains the tibialis posterior tendon, flexor digitorum longus tendon, posterior tibial neurovascular bundle and the FHL tendon. The syndrome refers to a compressive neuropathy of the posterior tibial nerve. The causes may include trauma, osteophytes from ankle arthroses, soft tissue masses (e.g. lipoma, ganglions), varicose veins, foot overpronation, and rarely systemic conditions (e.g. diabetes, hypothyroidism).

- *Presentation:* paraesthesia on the sole of the foot, often including the toes and heel. Involvement of medial or lateral plantar nerve in isolation gives symptoms affecting one half of the sole. The symptoms worsen with exercise, prolonged standing or walking and can be aggravated by ankle dorsiflexion.
- *Examination:* a positive Tinel's sign when percussing over the nerve behind the medial malleolus, causing radiation to the foot or heel. Sensation may be decreased or absent over the plantar surface of the foot (medial and/or lateral aspects).
- *Investigations:* Often normal. MRI can show a compressive lesion or atrophy of the small muscles of the foot. USS may show changes around the nerve. Nerve conduction studies may be positive in up to two thirds of cases.
- *Management:* orthoses can reduce nerve compression in those with foot pronation. Neural glides can be tried. Ultrasound-guided corticosteroid and local anaesthetic injections can provide symptomatic relief. Surgical decompression may be required.

Deltoid Ligament Injuries

The deltoid ligament is a strong medial ankle ligament with superficial and deep layers. The superficial layer consists of the anterior tibionavicular ligament, tibiospring ligament, tibiocalcaneal ligament and superficial posterior tibiotalar ligament. The deep layer consists of the anterior tibiotalar ligament and deep posterior tibiotalar ligament. Deltoid ligament injury is usually due to an eversion mechanism, but rarely occurs in isolation.

- *Presentation:* acute medial ankle pain with a significant eversion injury. There may be an audible snap and associated swelling.

- *Examination:* medial ankle pain with tenderness over the whole border of medial malleolus. Pain is exacerbated by passive eversion and may show laxity.
- *Investigations:* X-ray is required as deltoid ligament injuries are associated with ankle fractures (e.g. talus). USS is limited to view the entire deltoid ligament. MRI scan is recommended.
- *Management:* protection (e.g. use of ankle stirrup), optimisation of loading, ice, compression (e.g. elasticated support) and elevation initially. Crutches temporarily if too painful to weight-bear. If there are associated ankle fractures or ankle instability, then the patient should be non-weight bearing and an orthopaedic opinion should be sought. Ankle mobility exercises, strengthening (particularly of the medial structures) and proprioceptive retraining should be incorporated if stable and once pain allows. Functional, then sport-specific exercises should occur in the late phases of rehabilitation.

HINDFOOT

Plantar Fasciopathy

The plantar fascia is a thick connective tissue which supports the foot arch and absorbs shock. Plantar fasciopathy develops as a result of collagen degeneration and the condition is very common, affecting one in ten people in their lifetime. Risk factors include pes cavus, pes planus, poor footwear, increased weight, increased age, increased load (e.g. runners, military personnel), calf muscle tightness and inflammatory arthropathy.

- *Presentation:* gradual onset plantar heel pain that is typically worse in the mornings and at the end of the day, with start-up pains after any period of rest. It is exacerbated by lots of standing, walking or running.
- *Examination:* focal tenderness over medial calcaneal tubercle in the heel pad. Passive dorsiflexion of the first metatarsophalangeal joint (MTPJ) provokes pain (Windlass test positive).

- *Investigations:* USS shows thickening of the plantar fascia (usually >4 mm) at the medial calcaneal tuberosity with heterogenous changes.
- *Management:* review footwear and adjust training load if required. Orthotics or heel lifts may be helpful. Eccentric calf stretches, plantar fascia stretches, and ankle joint mobilisation can be effective. Shockwave therapy should be considered as an adjunct.

Calcaneal Stress Fracture

Stress fractures develop from repetitive submaximal forces applied to a bone over time. It can be associated with low bone mineral density or have a metabolic component (e.g. relative energy deficiency in sport). Calcaneal stress fractures may occur in military personnel, runners and in sports that involve lots of jumping and landing.

- *Presentation:* gradual onset heel pain exacerbated by weight-bearing activities that progressively worsen. There is usually a history of increased training load.
- *Examination:* palpation tenderness of the posterior calcaneus when squeezed or localised tenderness on either side. Unable to heel walk.
- *Investigations:* X-ray is usually normal but may show calcaneal sclerotic changes. MRI is diagnostic showing a focal area of intraosseous oedema and sometimes a fracture line. Blood tests (e.g. bone profile and vitamin D) can be helpful.
- *Management:* relative rest from physical activities is required for 4–6 weeks. Address other risk factors (such as low calcium or vitamin D) and consider metabolic or endocrinology review in relevant cases. If there is pain with walking, then a walker boot should be used and crutches to non-weight bear should be considered temporarily depending on symptom severity. Normal weight bearing with a well cushioned pair of shoes is recommended once pain settles. Physiotherapy rehabilitation such as calf stretches and joint mobilisation should be implemented, then graduated progression back to sport or exercise can commence once the stress fracture has healed.

MIDFOOT

Navicular Stress Fracture

Stress fractures develop from repetitive submaximal forces applied to a bone over time. Navicular stress fractures are at risk of non-union because it typically occurs at a relatively avascular area. Athletes that do lots of high impact activities such as running and jumping are at risk.

- *Presentation:* gradual onset pain around the navicular (or maybe poorly localised) exacerbated by weight-bearing activities that progressively worsen. There is usually a history of increased training load.
- *Examination:* tenderness on the dorsal surface of the navicular bone with or without swelling.
- *Investigations:* X-ray may appear normal. MRI is diagnostic showing a focal area of intraosseous oedema and sometimes a fracture line. CT has prognostic value. Blood tests (e.g. bone profile and vitamin D) can be helpful.
- *Management:* A walker boot and strict non weight-bearing with crutches is recommended for 6–8 weeks. If it is still symptomatic afterwards, then a further period of non-weight-bearing is required. Address other risk factors (such as low calcium or vitamin D) and consider metabolic or endocrinology review in relevant cases. Physiotherapy rehabilitation such as calf stretches and joint mobilisation should be implemented, then graduated progression back to sport or exercise can commence once the stress fracture has healed. Surgery is warranted if there is no improvement with conservative management.

Lisfranc Joint Injuries

The Lisfranc joint is the articulation between the cuneiform bones and the metatarsal bases (tarsometatarsal joints). The Lisfranc ligament extends obliquely from the medial cuneiform to the base of the second metatarsal bone to stabilise the first and second tarsometatarsal joints. Injury can occur from direct trauma (crush injury) or indirect trauma such as longitudinal compression, whilst the foot is plantarflexed.

- *Presentation:* acute onset pain in the midfoot exacerbated by forefoot weight-bearing following direct or indirect trauma.
- *Examination:* tenderness in the dorsal mid-foot with bruising and sometimes swelling. Ecchymosis may be seen plantarly under the arch of the foot. with delayed diagnosis. There is pain with rotation of the forefoot and passive eversion/abduction of the foot. The second TMT joint may be unstable dorsally.
- *Investigations:* weight-bearing X-ray of the foot shows a diastasis between the first and second metatarsal bases, discontinuity of a line drawn from the medial base of the 2nd metatarsal to the medial side of the middle cuneiform, and a 'fleck' sign maybe seen representing avulsion of the Lisfranc ligament. MRI can be diagnostic and a CT is useful for pre-operative planning.
- *Management:* an orthopaedic opinion is required. In stable non-displaced Lisfranc joint injuries, non-weight bearing in a boot or a cast for 6–8 weeks may be adequate. Displaced or unstable injuries require open reduction and internal fixation.

CLINICAL CONSIDERATIONS

These injuries are often missed on first presentation and can cause significant long term disability with progressive midfoot malalignment and degenerative change.

Midtarsal Joint Sprains

The midtarsal (Chopart) joint is made up of the calcaneocuboid and talonavicular joints that represents the functional articulation between the midfoot and hindfoot. A sprain of this joint can involve the dorsal calcaneocuboid ligament and or bifurcate ligament (Y shaped band that divides into calcaneonavicular and calcaneocuboid ligament). Dorsal calcaneocuboid ligament sprain is often due to an inversion injury whereas a bifurcate ligament sprain is due to a more severe inversion injury with forceful plantarflexion.

Bifurcate ligament injuries are associated with anterior calcaneal process fractures.

- *Presentation:* acute onset lateral midfoot pain.
- *Examination:* pain in the dorsal lateral aspect of the midfoot that is painful with inversion movements.
- *Investigations:* X-ray to identify any associated fractures. MRI can confirm a midtarsal joint sprain and detect a fracture.
- *Management:* relative rest, comfortable footwear, cold therapy and elevation for initial management. A walker boot and crutches may be needed for 1–2 weeks if there is severe pain. An orthopaedic opinion is warranted if there is an associated fracture of the anterior calcaneal process. Physiotherapy rehabilitation should target foot and ankle mobility, strengthening and proprioception.

FOREFOOT

Metatarsal Stress Fractures

These are common stress fractures that occur in athletes, particularly runners. The second and third metatarsal bones are often affected. Risk factors include increased training load, alterations in footwear, and altered foot or running mechanics. It can be associated with low bone mineral density or have a metabolic component (e.g. relative energy deficiency in sport).

- *Presentation:* gradual onset forefoot pain exacerbated by weight-bearing exercises and relieved with rest.
- *Examination:* localised tenderness at the affected metatarsal bone sometimes with swelling.
- *Investigations:* X-rays may appear normal in the early stages or show periosteal changes later on. MRI is the investigation of choice. Blood tests (e.g. bone profile and vitamin D) can be helpful.
- *Management:* rest from weight-bearing exercises for 4–6 weeks with review of footwear. A forefoot offloading shoe may be needed temporarily if it is painful to walk or the fracture is unstable. Address other risk factors (such as low calcium or vitamin

D) and consider metabolic or endocrinology review in relevant cases. Both stress fractures at the base of the second metatarsal bone and the base of the fifth metatarsal bone are at high risk of complications, so these require initial non weight-bearing for 4 weeks with crutches.

Base of Fifth Metatarsal Avulsion Fracture

The mechanism of injury is usually due to forceful inversion of a plantarflexed foot. The peroneus brevis muscle forcefully contracts resulting in a bony tuberosity avulsion, although some argue it is disruption to the lateral cord of the plantar aponeurosis that causes an avulsion.

- *Presentation:* acute onset lateral forefoot pain with difficulty weight-bearing.
- *Examination:* localised tenderness at the base of the fifth metatarsal bone with pain and weakness during resisted eversion.
- *Investigations:* X-ray is diagnostic, needing anterior-posterior, oblique or lateral views.
- *Management:* a walker boot or a forefoot offloading shoe may be needed temporarily if there is pain with walking. These can be removed once pain free with walking. Foot and ankle mobility and balance exercises should be implemented. Most heal in 4–6 weeks.

Jones Fracture

The fracture is a transverse fracture at the base of the fifth metatarsal bone between the metaphyseal and diaphyseal junction. There is a risk of non-union due to watershed areas of poor blood supply. The mechanism of injury is usually due to forceful forefoot adduction (or inversion) with the ankle plantarflexed.

- *Presentation:* acute onset lateral forefoot pain with difficulty weight-bearing.
- *Examination:* localised tenderness at the proximal fifth metatarsal bone with possible swelling and crepitus.
- *Investigations:* X-ray is diagnostic in anterior-posterior, oblique or lateral views.

- *Management:* an orthopaedic opinion is warranted. Conservative treatment requires non-weight bearing cast immobilisation for 6–8 weeks. Intramedullary screw fixation is the surgical treatment of choice.

First MTPJ Sprain (Turf Toe)

The mechanism of injury is extreme hyperextension of the big toe that results in trauma to the plantar capsuloligamentous complex and plantar plate (e.g. with the heel off the ground, pushing off to sprint). Risk factors include playing on artificial turf, soft flexible footwear, reduced MTPJ motion, and overpronation.

- *Presentation:* acute onset localised pain and swelling at the first MTPJ which is exacerbated by weight-bearing or big toe movements.
- *Examination:* tenderness to palpate the first MTPJ especially the sesamoid region and pain with dorsiflexion.
- *Investigations:* X-ray may show retraction of the sesamoids or a sesamoid fracture with diastasis. MRI to assess for any injury to the plantar capsuloligamentous complex, sesamoid bones, plantar plate and toe flexors. It can also help grade the injury.
- *Management:* initial treatment is relative rest, ice, elevation and analgesia. Grade 1 injuries with no tear of the plantar structures can be managed with taping and activity modification until pain free. Orthoses can be used to offload the first MTP joint. Grade 2 injuries with partial tear of the plantar structures may require a walker boot for 2 weeks. Grade 3 injuries with complete tear of the plantar structures require immobilisation in a boot or cast for 4–6 weeks. A surgical opinion is required for grade 2 and 3 injuries, or if there is vertical instability of the first MTPJ, avulsion fracture, sesamoid bone injury or loose body.

Sesamoid Injuries of the Great Toe

There are two sesamoid bones (medial and lateral) that lie within the flexor hallucis brevis tendons on the plantar aspect of the first MTPJ and form part of the plantar plate complex. They absorb weight-bearing pressure and contribute to MTPJ plantarflexion power. The flexor hallucis longus tendon runs in between the two sesamoid bones. Types of sesamoid injuries include sesamoiditis (chondromalacia), stress fracture, fracture (hyperextension and axial loading mechanism), subluxation, dislocation and osteochondritis (avascular necrosis).

- *Presentation:* acute or gradual onset sesamoid pain with weight-bearing particularly during toe-off. Swelling may be present and first MTPJ movements are painful or restricted.
- *Examination:* tenderness on palpation of the medial or lateral sesamoid. The medial sesamoid is more commonly affected. There is pain and weakness with resisted plantarflexion of the great toe.
- *Investigations:* X-rays including sesamoid views can detect an acute fracture or evidence of avascular necrosis. Bipartite sesamoids are present in 10–25% of people so must not be misinterpreted as a fracture. MRI can detect stress fractures and distinguish between sesamoid pathologies.
- *Management:* conservative measures include adjustments to training load, posterior chain flexibility improvement, stiffer or rocker soled shoes and podiatry input for orthoses to reduce pressure under the sesamoid complex. Sesamoiditis may benefit from non-steroidal anti-inflammatory medications. Sesamoid stress fractures require non weight-bearing and immobilisation in a boot for 4–6 weeks. If non-operative interventions fail, then surgery should be considered.

Plantar Plate Tears

Plantar plates in the foot are fibrocartilaginous structures situated across MTPJ and interphalangeal joints that absorbs compressive loads and restrict hyperextension movements. It can present acutely (e.g. turf toe) or chronically with attenuation and degeneration due to repeated hyperextension or long-term joint overload. The risk factors include high impact activities, foot overpronation, hallux valgus and alterations in the metatarsal parabola i.e. long second metatarsal.

- *Presentation:* acute or gradual onset pain in the plantar aspect of the MTPJ with or without swelling exacerbated by dorsiflexion.
- *Examination:* tenderness at the base of the affected MTPJ and proximal phalanx. There is usually pain with active dorsiflexion and weakness on resisted plantarflexion. There may be joint laxity with dorsal translation of the proximal phalanx, or abnormal toe alignment.
- *Investigations:* X-ray can show subluxation or dislocation of the proximal phalanx. USS can identify plantar plate tears and allow for dynamic evaluation. MRI visualises plantar plate tears, is useful for assessing ligamentous injury and can reveal associated bone marrow oedema and chondral defects.
- *Management:* relative rest, ice, elevation, plantarflexion strapping and analgesia initially followed by forefoot strengthening exercises. A stiff or rocker soled shoe and orthoses with appropriate joint offload e.g. a metatarsal dome may be required. A walker boot for 2 weeks if it is too painful to weight-bear. Surgical repair of the plantar plate is indicated if there is no improvement with conservative measures or there is severe toe deformity and dislocation.

LEG PAIN

Muscle Injury

Calf injuries are common and the classical mechanism involves a sudden acceleration. The majority affect the medial head of gastrocnemius and specifically, the myotendinous junction. There are numerous risk factors including poor biomechanics, reduced ankle dorsiflexion and a lack of conditioning.

- *Presentation:* sudden onset calf pain, sometimes with a 'tearing' or 'pop' sensation.
- *Examination:* tenderness to palpation, sometimes with a defect and visible bruising. Pain and weakness with ankle dorsiflexion. Limited ability to heel raise. The AT should also be assessed.

- *Investigations:* Ultrasound is particularly useful in medial gastrocnemius injuries. MRI may be required.
- *Management:* initial management includes relative rest, optimisation of loading with early weight bearing as tolerated or crutches temporarily if too painful, ice, compression and elevation. A progressive physiotherapy rehabilitation programme is needed to restore movement and strength in the muscle. Ultrasound-guided haematoma aspiration may be appropriate in some cases. A surgical opinion is rarely required but may be warranted for complete ruptures or those that fail to improve.

Vascular Causes

Claudicant-type calf pain may indicate a vascular cause such as popliteal artery entrapment, where anatomical variations lead to compression on the popliteal artery (usually from the medial head of gastrocnemius), or atherosclerotic disease in older athletes. Deep vein thrombosis (DVT) should always be considered in an acutely swollen limb.

- *Presentation:* exertional calf pain or cramp with or without discoloration (pallor), paraesthesia and coolness.
- *Examination:* Calf hypertrophy may be a feature. Post-exertion popliteal artery bruit may be heard and peripheral pulses may be absent.
- *Investigations:* Doppler ultrasound and ankle-brachial pressure indices. Magnetic resonance angiography (MRA) is sometimes required to identify anatomical variations.
- *Management:* vascular opinion required as management may include angiographic dilatation or stenting.

Chronic Exertional Compartment Syndrome (CECS)

Often seen in endurance athletes, it is thought that repetitive muscle use leads to inflammation and thickened fascia, which restricts tissue expansion during exercise. The anterior compartment is most

Table 5.1 Leg Compartments

Compartment	Contents
Anterior	Tibialis anterior, extensor digitorum longus, extensor hallucis longus, peroneus tertius, deep peroneal nerve, anterior vessels
Lateral	Peroneus longus and brevis, superficial peroneal nerve
Superficial Posterior	Gastrocnemius, soleus, plantaris, sural nerve
Deep Posterior	Tibialis posterior, popliteus, flexor hallucis longus, flexor digitorum longus, tibial nerve, posterior vessels

commonly affected, followed by the lateral and deep posterior compartment. Superficial posterior compartment involvement is rare (Table 5.1).

- *Presentation:* increasing leg pain or 'tightness' with exercise that resolves quickly with rest. Anterior compartment pain usually occurs lateral to the anterior shin.
- *Examination:* usually normal at rest, but affected compartments may feel tender and exhibit sensory changes with exertion. Sometimes small areas of muscle herniation are a feature.
- *Investigations:* Pre and post exertional MRI may show signal changes. Intracompartmental pressure testing is considered diagnostic if post-exertional readings >25 mmHg or baseline readings that increase >10 mmHg during exercise.
- *Management:* reduction in training load and modification of biomechanical risk factors via gait retraining. Orthoses can increase compartment pressures. Soft tissue massage may be helpful. Surgery (e.g. fasciotomy) if no improvement.

Medial Tibial Stress Syndrome (MTSS)

MTSS is an overuse injury causing exercise induced pain over the medial tibia. The risk factors for this condition include female status, hard running surfaces and an increase in any of the following factors: training load, BMI, navicular drop, external hip rotation and range of ankle plantarflexion. A muscle imbalance may also be related (e.g. strong plantar flexors, ankle equinus). It is suggested that repetitive impact forces that

eccentrically fatigue the soleus causing tibial bending and therefore overload, may be a cause.

- *Presentation:* unilateral diffuse pain along the medial tibia after exercise with relief during warm-up.
- *Examination:* typically, diffuse tenderness on palpation of the lower one third of the medial or posteromedial edge of the tibia.
- *Investigations:* X-rays are usually normal. MRI is the most sensitive investigation demonstrating bone marrow oedema or periosteal reaction.
- *Management:* relative offload or activity modification, ice, analgesia and address risk factors. Rehabilitation to address muscle imbalance and ankle strength. Footwear modification, biomechanical assessment, gait retraining and orthoses.

Stress Fractures

These injuries commonly occur in high impact exercises that involve running or jumping. Risk factors include increased training load, hard surfaces, pes cavus, excessive pronation, relative energy deficiency in sport (RED-S) and reduced bone mineral density. Most tibial stress injuries affect the posteromedial tibia; however, anterior tibial cortex stress fractures tend to have more issues with delayed union and complete fracture.

- *Presentation:* gradual onset pain that worsens with exercise.

- *Examination:* localised area of tenderness over the tibia.
- *Investigations:* X-rays are often normal in the early weeks of symptom onset. MRI is the investigation of choice as oedema and cortical breach can be characterised. Bone scans and CT scans are sometimes indicated. Blood tests (e.g. bone profile and vitamin D) should be considered.
- *Management:* relative rest and offload from impact activities is required for about 6 weeks until pain free. A pneumatic boot is sometimes needed. Address other risk factors (such as low calcium or vitamin D) and consider metabolic or endocrinology review in relevant cases. Training is gradually reintroduced in the late phases of rehabilitation. Surgical opinion is needed if at risk of non-union or delayed union especially for anterior tibial cortex stress fractures.

MULTIPLE CHOICE QUESTION (MCQ) QUESTIONS

1. A 19-year-old football player reports a four-month history of gradual onset dull pain in the back of the left ankle that occurs when he kicks the ball with power. The pain can also occur if he pushes off too quickly or when he jogs down the stairs. There has not been any recent trauma or changes to his footwear. You assess the player and there is pain in the left posterior ankle with heel raises and pogo jumps. There is tenderness on palpation deep to the mid-portion of the left Achilles tendon. Active plantarflexion of the left ankle is reduced compared to the right side and passive plantarflexion at end range is painful on the left side. What is the most useful investigation of choice?

   A. Ultrasound scan of the left ankle
   B. MRI of the left ankle
   C. X-ray of the left ankle
   D. CT of the left ankle
   E. Bone scan of the left ankle

2. A 42-year-old recreational runner has developed a gradual dull ache in the back of the right heel after increasing her training load over 3 months in preparation for a marathon in 4 weeks' time. She develops symptoms after running about 10 km, but would normally be able to run through the pain. The day after a run her right Achilles tendon typically feels painful and stiff. You assess her and find localised tenderness on palpation of the right Achilles tendon in its mid-portion. An ultrasound scan demonstrates a hypoechoic thickened right mid-portion Achilles tendon with increased vascularity. What would be your initial management plan?

   A. Offer extracorporeal shockwave therapy
   B. Rest from running for 2 weeks
   C. Prescribe eccentric exercises for the Achilles tendon
   D. Offer a corticosteroid injection
   E. None of the above

3. A 23-year-old jumped over a wall about 1 metre in height during parkour and twisted his left ankle when he landed. He describes an inversion type injury. He was seen in A+E and had a left ankle X-ray that excluded a fracture. He was given a pair of crutches for 1 week and some ankle mobility exercises. You are now seeing him 6 weeks post-injury where he still has pain in the anterolateral aspect of the left ankle, bruising has resolved but there is some swelling still present. Whilst he can mobilise independently, he describes giving way sensations. You assess his left ankle and find laxity on passive inversion stress, a positive anterior drawer test, and pain with passive dorsiflexion and external rotation. There is tenderness to palpate the anterior joint line, lateral calcaneal area and anterolateral aspect of the left ankle. What is the most likely diagnosis?

   A. High grade sprain of the ATFL and CFL
   B. Osteochondral lesion of the talar dome
   C. High grade sprain of the ATFL, CFL and syndesmosis injury
   D. Sinus tarsi syndrome related to the original injury
   E. Plantaris rupture

4. A 26-year-old volleyball player develops progressively worsening localised right forefoot pain. She has increased her training volume and intensity in the last 8 weeks in addition to playing multiple competitive matches. Her past medical history includes a previous stress fracture of the sacrum. She is on a vegetarian diet and does not consume much dairy products. She has regular menstrual cycles but takes the combined oral contraceptive pill for dysmenorrhoea. Examination demonstrates focal tenderness in the distal aspect of the right second metatarsal bone. An MRI scan of her right foot confirms a right second metatarsal neck stress fracture. Which of these are unlikely to be a risk factor for her developing a stress fracture?

   A. Increased training volume
   B. Poor dietary intake of calcium
   C. Combined oral contraceptive pill use
   D. Previous history of a stress fracture
   E. Increased training intensity

5. You are managing a 42-year-old female runner with persisting ankle pain following a sprain 6 months ago. Sinus tarsi syndrome is the working differential diagnosis. What is the most likely anatomical location of this patient's pain?

   A. Anterolateral hindfoot
   B. Posterolateral forefoot
   C. Anteromedial hindfoot
   D. Posteromedial forefoot
   E. Posterolateral hindfoot

MULTIPLE CHOICE QUESTION (MCQ) ANSWERS

1. Answer B

The most likely clinical condition here is posterior ankle impingement syndrome (PAIS). An MRI scan is the investigation of choice for PAIS as it can detect os trigonum, enlarged posterior tubercle of the talus, soft tissue impingement and evaluate for any active bone oedema or synovitis. An ankle X-ray can often miss os trigonum and it would not be able to detect soft tissue causes of PAIS. Whilst an ultrasound is helpful to exclude other causes of posterior ankle pain such as Achilles tendinopathy, the diagnosis is unlikely in this age group. Ultrasound can also visualise an os trigonum but not in sufficient detail. A CT scan (or bone scan) risks high dose radiation. CT is perhaps only helpful if an X-ray demonstrates a possible fracture that needs further exploration or for surgical planning.

2. Answer E

The initial management for this runner should be to modify her training load, review her running mechanics and modify other intrinsic or extrinsic factors that might be contributing to the development of her Achilles tendinopathy. Shockwave therapy can be used as an adjunct to her management plan later on if there is no improvement with training modifications and rehabilitation. Rest from running for 2 weeks is unlikely to be helpful in this case unless there is a severe flare-up of symptoms. There is evidence that eccentric loading programmes are effective for Achilles tendinopathy but some people may respond better to other exercises such as heavy slow resistance training or a combination of concentric and eccentric exercises.

3. Answer C

Whilst a high-grade lateral ankle ligament sprain is often symptomatic after 6 weeks, the mechanism of injury from a height and a positive Kleiger's test would suggest an associated syndesmosis injury, so C is the correct answer. Acute osteochondral lesions of the talar dome and sinus tarsi syndrome are both associated with ankle inversion injuries but these diagnoses are least likely in the context of the given scenario.

4. Answer C

Stress fractures develop from repetitive submaximal forces on bone over time so increased training load is a definite risk factor. Calcium is important for bone health and low daily dietary calcium intake is correlated with increased rates of stress fractures, although further research is required to explore this link. Previous history of stress fractures is a risk factor for future stress fractures. Combined oral contraceptive pill appears to be associated with lower risk of stress fractures in some studies and there is overall insufficient evidence to suggest it is a risk factor, so therefore the answer is C.

5. Answer A

Sinus tarsi pain is typically anterolateral hindfoot pain, often exacerbated by exercise.

REFERENCES AND FURTHER READING

Thieme—Atlas of Anatomy: General Anatomy and Musculoskeletal System. (2010). Authors: Michael Schuenke, Erik Schulte and Udo Schumacher.

Knee and Hip 6

Sean Carmody, James Noake and Jonathan Power

KNEE

Knee injuries make up about one third of musculo-skeletal injuries amongst athletes. The assessment of knee injuries are best divided based on anatomical region.

Examination of the Knee

INSPECTION

- Standing and supine
- Look for swelling, discoloration, deformity, asymmetry, wounds, previous scars, and lower limb muscle loss (e.g. loss of quadriceps muscle bulk)
- Assess for genu varum or valgus, gross deformity or malalignment
- Examine gait, looking for signs of an antalgic gait or flexed knee gait
- Observe for any obvious effusion

MOVEMENTS

- Knee flexion and extension actively, passively and then with resistance
- Always consider assessing the joints above and below (the hip can often be a source of knee pain, especially in children)

FUNCTIONAL TESTS

- Double-leg squat
- Single-leg squat control
- Lunges
- Hop tests—hop for height, distance, side shuffle (if tolerant of hop on the spot)

- Duck-walk
- Analysis of running gait

PALPATION

Key structures need to be palpated systematically (Figures 6.2–6.3).

- Joint lines
- Tibial tuberosity
- Patella (e.g. translation, facet pain to palpation)
- Patella tendon (ligament)
- Quadriceps tendon
- Fat pad—compression test
- Distal pes anserine complex/insertion
- Popliteal fossa
- Iliotibial band (ITB) at lateral femoral condyle and Gerdy's Tubercle
- Check for effusion—sweep test
- Superior tibiofibular joint—glide
- Distal, lateral and medial hamstring tendons

SPECIAL TESTS

Collateral Ligaments

- Valgus stress test for Medial collateral ligament (MCL) injury—in 0 and 30 degrees of flexion
- Varus stress for Lateral collateral ligament (LCL) injury

Cruciate Ligaments

- Posterior drawer/posterior sag for Posterior cruciate ligament (PCL) injury—check first before ACL tests to avoid a false positive
- Lachman's test, anterior drawer, Lever sign, pivot shift for Anterior cruciate ligament (ACL) injury

DOI: 10.1201/9781003179979-6

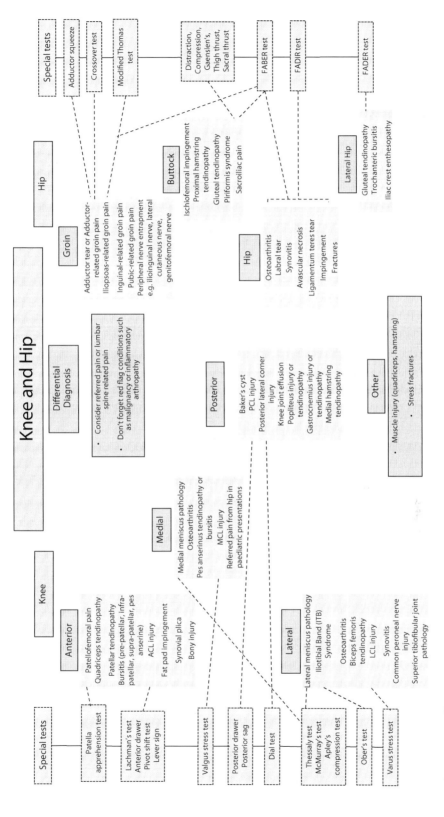

Figure 6.1 Differential diagnosis chart.

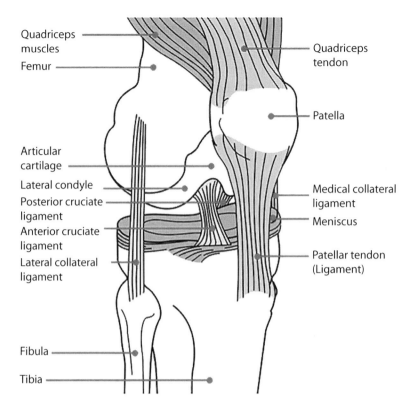

Figure 6.2 Anatomy of the knee.

Source: Mysid, 'Knee diagram,' https://commons.wikimedia.org/wiki/File:Knee_diagram.svg. Public domain.

Other

- McMurray's test for meniscal injury
- Apley's compression test for meniscal injury
- Thessaly test for meniscal injury
- Dial test—Posterolateral corner injury
- Patellar apprehension test for MPFL or medial retinacular injury

Anterior Knee

ACL INJURY

ACL injuries are relatively common, high-burden knee injuries leading to anterior and lateral rotatory instability of the knee. The mechanism can be contact or non-contact and the patient typically describes their knee giving way or buckling (forced valgus mechanism).

- *Presentation:* feeling a 'pop' in the knee accompanied by pain deep in the knee, swelling (haemarthrosis), a feeling of instability and difficulty weight-bearing.
- Examination may reveal an effusion, reduced range of motion (ROM) and a positive Lachman's/anterior drawer/pivot shift test. There are often concomitant injuries (e.g. meniscal, MCL).
- *Investigations:* X-rays are often normal, although the presence of a Segond fracture is pathognomonic for an ACL tear. MRI is the gold-standard investigation for ACL injury, and is also useful to exclude coexisting pathology. MRI usually demonstrates discontinuity of ACL fibres and more than half of ACL tears will have accompanying bone bruising visible on MRI in a typical pivot shift pattern.

Right knee in flexion: anterior view

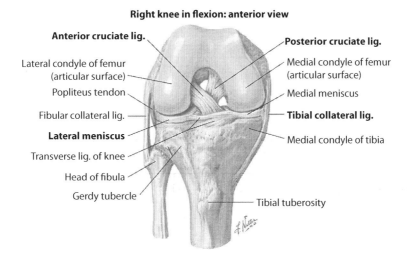

Anterior cruciate lig.

Lateral condyle of femur
(articular surface)

Popliteus tendon

Fibular collateral lig.

Lateral meniscus

Transverse lig. of knee

Head of fibula

Gerdy tubercle

Posterior cruciate lig.

Medial condyle of femur
(articular surface)

Medial meniscus

Tibial collateral lig.

Medial condyle of tibia

Tibial tuberosity

Inferior view

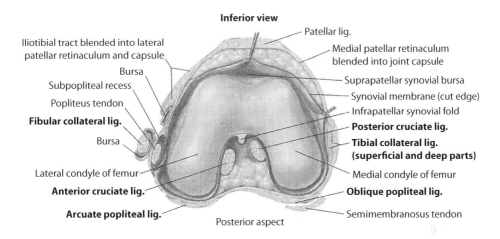

Iliotibial tract blended into lateral
patellar retinaculum and capsule

Bursa

Subpopliteal recess

Popliteus tendon

Fibular collateral lig.

Bursa

Lateral condyle of femur

Anterior cruciate lig.

Arcuate popliteal lig.

Patellar lig.

Medial patellar retinaculum
blended into joint capsule

Suprapatellar synovial bursa

Synovial membrane (cut edge)

Infrapatellar synovial fold

Posterior cruciate lig.

**Tibial collateral lig.
(superficial and deep parts)**

Medial condyle of femur

Oblique popliteal lig.

Semimembranosus tendon

Posterior aspect

Superior view

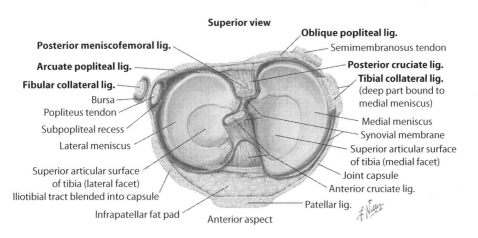

Posterior meniscofemoral lig.

Arcuate popliteal lig.

Fibular collateral lig.

Bursa

Popliteus tendon

Subpopliteal recess

Lateral meniscus

Superior articular surface
of tibia (lateral facet)

Iliotibial tract blended into capsule

Infrapatellar fat pad

Oblique popliteal lig.

Semimembranosus tendon

Posterior cruciate lig.

Tibial collateral lig.
(deep part bound to
medial meniscus)

Medial meniscus

Synovial membrane

Superior articular surface
of tibia (medial facet)

Joint capsule

Anterior cruciate lig.

Patellar lig.

Anterior aspect

Figure 6.3 Further anatomy of the knee.

Source: Cleland et al. (2016). *Netter's Orthopaedic Clinical Examination: An Evidence-Based Approach.* 3rd ed. Philadelphia: Elsevier. With permission.

- *Management:* Treatment decisions will depend on patient age, presence of concomitant injury and activity levels. Management options can generally be divided into operative versus non-operative. For athletes looking to return to high level cutting/pivoting sports, surgery is usually the treatment of choice with graft options including bone-patellar tendon-bone and hamstring. The principles of rehabilitation are similar for operative and non-operative management, with the main focus being on reducing swelling, increasing range of motion, developing strength and neuromuscular control, and graded return to sport-specific activity. Rehabilitation generally takes six to twelve months, depending on patient goals and resources.

CLINICAL CONSIDERATIONS

Traumatic knee injury with immediate effusion should raise the suspicion for a severe intra-articular injury; most commonly, this is ACL disruption.

PATELLAR TENDINOPATHY

Patellar tendinopathy is a relatively common sporting injury characterised by anterior knee pain.

- *Presentation:* the characteristic features of patellar tendinopathy are pain localised to the inferior pole of the patella, load-related pain that increases with the demand on the knee extensors, notably in activities that store and release energy in the patellar tendon (e.g. plyometrics).
- *Investigations:* diagnosis of patellar tendinopathy remains clinical, as asymptomatic tendon pathology may exist in people who have pain from other anterior knee sources. Imaging can be helpful to include or exclude potential alternate diagnoses of anterior knee pain when the clinical picture is unclear. Characteristic ultrasound findings include a thickened, hypoechoic area, calcification, and neovascularisation on doppler. Ultrasound should not be used to monitor patient progress, as many patients improve clinically but have persistent sonographic findings. A normal US means that anterior knee pain is very unlikely to be tendinous in origin.
- *Management:* Management should focus on progressively developing tendon load tolerance (e.g.

developing strength, power and energy storage or release). Developing the musculoskeletal unit and the kinetic chain, as well as addressing key biomechanical and other risk factors (e.g. training load) is also important (Malliaras et al., 2015).

PATELLA DISLOCATION

Patella dislocation is typically a traumatic knee injury characterised by a lateral shift of the patella, leaving the trochlea groove of the femoral condyle. This mostly occurs as a disruption of the medial patellofemoral ligament (MPFL). Risk factors may include previous injury, hypermobility, ligament laxity, patella alta and patellofemoral dysplasia.

- *Presentation:* a patella dislocation may be as a result of contact or may be non-contact. The patient will report pain and a feeling of instability in the knee. There is usually immediate swelling.
- Examination may reveal an obvious deformity and patella hypermobility or apprehension.
- *Investigations:* X-rays can rule out any associated fractures, and can also indicate any underlying risk factors such as patella alta. MRI is useful to exclude any associated injuries, in particular osteochondral injury, and usually reveals a tear of the MPFL.
- *Management:* Acute management involves relocation of the patella. Consideration of surgical management depends on the number of previous dislocations +/− underlying risk factors. Principles of rehabilitation include reducing swelling, improving range of motion, developing strength and neuromuscular control, and restoring sport-specific function.

PATELLAR FRACTURE

Patellar fractures are relatively rare, making up about 1% of all skeletal injuries. The usual mechanism is direct trauma or rapid contracture of the quadriceps with a flexed knee that can lead to loss of the extensor mechanism. Patellar stress fractures can also occur in at-risk groups e.g. Relative Energy Deficit in Sport (RED-S) athletes, which can then progress to full fractures.

- *Presentation:* following a history of trauma, the patient presents with knee pain, swelling and may also have laceration/abrasion in the presence of an open fracture.

- *Examination:* ROM will be reduced, with patients classically unable to perform a straight leg raise.
- *Investigations:* X-ray should be performed initially to assess for displacement of fracture and any other factors which may influence treatment (e.g. patella alta). CT scan is the most useful test to appreciate the extent of injury.
- *Management:* for non-operative management, the knee is braced in extension (full weight-bearing). This management is usually reserved for nondisplaced or minimally displaced fractures, or for those in whom surgery would not be appropriate (e.g. significant medical comorbidities). Surgical management is needed for more complex injuries, and the approach will be determined based on the extent of injury, and surgical and patient preference.

PATELLOFEMORAL JOINT PAIN

Patellofemoral joint pain is a term that encompasses anterior knee pain in the absence of other pathology. A number of structures around the patellofemoral joint are vulnerable to overload and are pain sensitive. Risk factors include poor lumbopelvic control, increased femoral anteversion, increased hip adduction, abnormal patella position, quadriceps dysfunction, age or previous injury (e.g. patellofemoral joint chondropathy).

- *Presentation:* insidious anterior knee pain is the most common symptom, with pain exacerbated by activities which load the patellofemoral joint including running, squatting, and ascending stairs. Prolonged sitting can also aggravate symptoms. Pain is typically localised to the peri-patellar or retro-patellar area.
- *Examination:* may reveal restricted medial glide or posterior tilt of the patella. Patellofemoral joint compression may be painful.
- *Investigations:* Imaging is usually unremarkable but may reveal anatomical risk factors. X-ray and CT are limited modalities for assessing chondral changes. MRI is the modality of choice for assessing patellar cartilage, which may reveal patellofemoral joint osteoarthritis.
- *Management:* Treatment is generally conservative, with analgesia, activity modification, patella

taping, orthotics, biomechanical assessment and appropriate strengthening exercises (e.g. for quadriceps dysfunction). Patient education regarding the source of their pain, treatment options and disease course is also key.

Medial Knee

MCL INJURY

MCL injuries are one of the most common knee injuries, and the typical mechanism is a valgus force on the knee. It is sometimes associated with other injuries such as patellofemoral dislocation, meniscal and ACL injuries. Chronic MCL deficiency is associated with calcification at the femoral origin site (Pellegrini-Stieda lesion).

- *Presentation:* usually with medial joint line pain, a feeling of instability and occasionally difficulty weight bearing.
- *Examination:* Valgus stress test is positive plus tenderness to the MCL. There may also be an effusion present.
- *Investigations:* MRI can identify the location and extent of injury. MRI can also assess for the presence of concomitant injuries. The most obvious sign of medial collateral ligament injury on MRI is ligament discontinuity in the form of a partial or complete tear. Other signs include a wavy form of the ligament. Ultrasound can allow dynamic stress testing to be performed to demonstrate ligamentous disruption.
- *Management:* principles of rehabilitation include reducing swelling, increasing range, developing strength, and progression from linear to change of direction movements and, ultimately, return to sport-specific activity. Some injuries might require a formal period of ROM bracing. High-grade MCL injuries involving the distal ligament insertion may require surgical intervention.

Posterior Knee

PCL INJURY

PCL injuries are traumatic knee injuries that may lead to knee instability. They are less common than ACL injuries. The usual mechanism is a direct blow to the proximal tibia with a flexed knee which is why they are sometimes termed a 'dashboard injury.' They are often accompanied with other injuries (e.g. ACL injury).

- *Presentation:* the patient usually presents with posterior knee pain and a feeling of instability (although this may be subtle for isolated PCL injuries).
- *Examination:* There may be an associated effusion. A positive posterior sag sign or positive posterior drawer test is usually indicative of a PCL injury.
- *Investigations:* MRI is the investigation of choice for suspected PCL injuries. MRI can also exclude other pathology. There may be complete or partial ligamentous disruption seen on MRI.
- *Management:* Depending on the extent of injury, management may be operative or non-operative. Non-operative management may involve a period of bracing which should be initiated soon after injury to be successful. The principles of rehabilitation include reducing swelling, increasing range of motion, developing quadriceps strength and return to sport-specific activity.

BAKER'S CYST

A Baker's cyst (also known as a popliteal cyst) is a fluid-filled swelling that is developed at the back of the knee in the popliteal fossa. They are usually due to distension of the semimembranosus-gastrocnemius bursa, with fluid content within. In adults, a Baker's cyst is often found in combination with other intra-articular pathologies and inflammatory conditions (e.g. osteoarthritis). Serious conditions (e.g. DVT) should be excluded in the individual presenting with posterior knee pain or swelling.

- *Presentation:* vague posterior knee pain or tightness, which may be associated with a palpable mass in the popliteal space. The most frequent complication is spontaneous rupture which may mimic the symptoms of thrombophlebitis or DVT.
- *Investigations:* Ultrasound of a Baker's cyst can identify the three parts of the cyst (neck, body, base). MRI is the gold standard as it can differentiate Baker's cysts from other conditions such as meniscal cysts or myxoid tumours.

- *Management:* Depending on the nature of the cyst (and its causative factors) management may involve NSAIDs, activity modification, US-guided aspiration, and surgical removal for large or troublesome cysts.

Lateral Knee

LCL INJURY

The primary purpose of the LCL is to prevent excess varus and posterior-lateral rotation of the knee. LCL injuries of the knee typically occur due to a sudden varus force to the knee, and isolated LCL injuries are rare—with ACL, PCL or posterior-lateral corner (PLC) injuries often coexisting.

- *Presentation:* the patient describes a history of a high-energy impact to the anteromedial aspect of the knee resulting in lateral joint line pain, swelling and a feeling of instability.
- *Examination:* may also reveal tenderness over the LCL insertion with a positive varus stress test.
- *Investigations:* MRI is the imaging modality of choice to grade severity and location of LCL injury. Depending on the severity, MRI may identify fluid surrounding the LCL, partial discontinuity or complete disruption of the LCL fibres. MRI will also assess for other injuries.
- *Management:* Treatment options include non-operative and operative approaches and will mainly depend on the presence of associated injuries and the grade of injury. The principles of rehabilitation include reducing swelling, a period of immobilisation if appropriate, increasing ROM, developing quadriceps strength and return to sport-specific activity.

ILIOTIBIAL BAND SYNDROME

Iliotibial band syndrome is an atraumatic overuse injury commonly seen in runners and cyclists.

- *Presentation:* usually presents with pain on palpation of the lateral aspect of the knee, superior to the joint line at the lateral femoral epicondyle.
- *Investigations:* It is usually a clinical diagnosis. Ultrasound is a useful point of care tool. MRI is reserved for when the diagnosis is unclear and

to exclude other causes of lateral knee pain such as a meniscal tear or lateral collateral ligament injury.

- *Management:* load modification and correcting training errors is key. Although foam rolling of the ITB is commonly suggested, there is little evidence that this hastens recovery or lengthens the ITB. Assessment and correction of biomechanical factors and strengthening of the proximal kinetic chain are the mainstay of treatment. Other management options include NSAIDs and corticosteroid injections, podiatry interventions and running re-education.

Other

KNEE OSTEOARTHRITIS

Knee osteoarthritis is a joint disorder, which occurs when damage triggers repair processes leading to structural changes within a joint. Joint damage may occur through repeated excessive loading and stress of the joint over time, or by injury (e.g. ACL, meniscal injury etc).

- *Presentation:* Knee osteoarthritis is a clinical diagnosis, and it should be suspected in those presenting with activity-related joint pain and functional impairment.
- *Examination:* there may be restricted and painful range of joint movement, joint deformity, effusion or crepitus.
- *Investigations:* Imaging is not generally required to confirm a diagnosis of knee osteoarthritis, however, weight bearing X-ray (including Rosenberg view) may reveal loss of joint space, osteophytes, subchondral sclerosis and cysts.
- *Management:* should include education, advice on self-care strategies (such as weight loss), local muscle strengthening exercises and aerobic fitness training, appropriate footwear, local heat or cold packs, or transcutaneous electrical nerve stimulation (TENS) (NICE CKS, 2022). Patients should receive advice on analgesia. Intra-articular injections, usually steroid or hyaluronic acid, may provide pain relief for several months. Involvement of the wider interdisciplinary team should be considered at appropriate stages; orthopaedics (e.g. for consideration of joint replacement), physiotherapy (e.g. for advice re. exercise) or pain services.

MENISCAL INJURIES

Meniscal injuries are common sports-related injuries in young athletes and can also present as a degenerative condition in older patients.

- *Presentation:* patient may report pain localised to the medial or lateral aspect of the knee. They may also experience mechanical symptoms (e.g. locking).
- *Examination:* Joint line tenderness is the most sensitive physical examination finding, but may be accompanied by an effusion or a positive special test (e.g. McMurray's, Thessaly's or Apley's).
- *Investigations:* X-ray is generally normal for meniscal injuries. MRI is the most useful diagnostic test, and can assess the presence of other pathology. High signal extending to the surface of the meniscus or the presence of a parameniscal cyst usually indicates meniscal injury.
- *Management:* Conservative management may include NSAIDs, activity modification and appropriate rehabilitation. Consideration of surgery is patient dependent, especially in the presence of mechanical symptoms, and options may include partial meniscectomy, meniscal repair, total meniscectomy or meniscal transplantation (Borque et al., 2022).

HIP

Hip pain is a common cause of time-loss in athletes. The likelihood of a sportsperson sustaining a hip injury is increased in sports which require repetitive hip flexion, adduction, and rotation. There is considerable evidence that the presence of hip pathology increases the risk of hip, groin and pelvic pain in young adults.

Key Anatomy

An overview is provided in Figures 6.4–6.6

Examination of the Hip

INSPECTION

- Standing and supine.
- Inspect for any discoloration, wounds, swelling or obvious deformity.

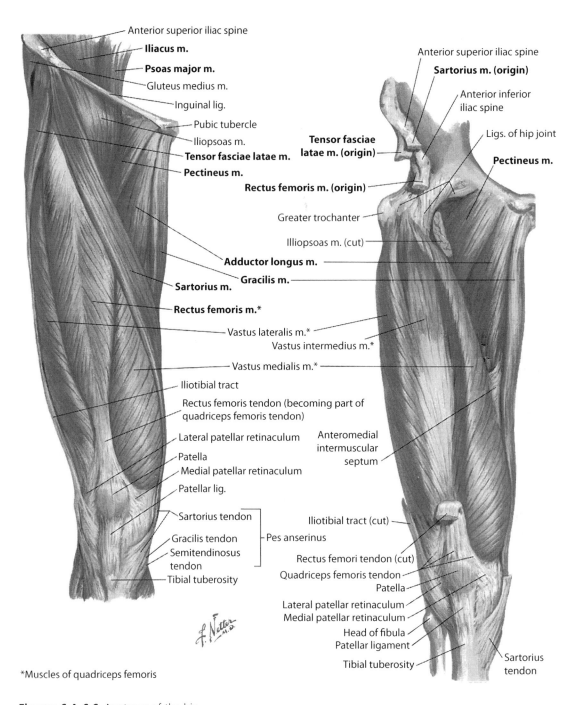

Anterior superior iliac spine
Iliacus m.
Psoas major m.
Gluteus medius m.
Inguinal lig.
Pubic tubercle
Iliopsoas m.
Tensor fasciae latae m.
Pectineus m.
Rectus femoris m. (origin)
Greater trochanter
Illiopsoas m. (cut)
Adductor longus m.
Gracilis m.
Sartorius m.
Rectus femoris m.*
Vastus lateralis m.*
Vastus intermedius m.*
Vastus medialis m.*
Iliotibial tract
Rectus femoris tendon (becoming part of quadriceps femoris tendon)
Lateral patellar retinaculum
Patella
Medial patellar retinaculum
Patellar lig.
Sartorius tendon
Gracilis tendon
Semitendinosus tendon
Tibial tuberosity
Pes anserinus

Anterior superior iliac spine
Sartorius m. (origin)
Anterior inferior iliac spine
Ligs. of hip joint
Pectineus m.
Tensor fasciae latae m. (origin)
Anteromedial intermuscular septum
Iliotibial tract (cut)
Rectus femori tendon (cut)
Quadriceps femoris tendon
Patella
Lateral patellar retinaculum
Medial patellar retinaculum
Head of fibula
Patellar ligament
Tibial tuberosity
Sartorius tendon

*Muscles of quadriceps femoris

Figures 6.4–6.6 Anatomy of the hip.

Source: Cleland et al. (2016). Netter's *Orthopaedic Clinical Examination: An Evidence-Based Approach.* 3rd ed. Philadelphia: Elsevier. With permission.

Superficial dissection

Deeper dissection

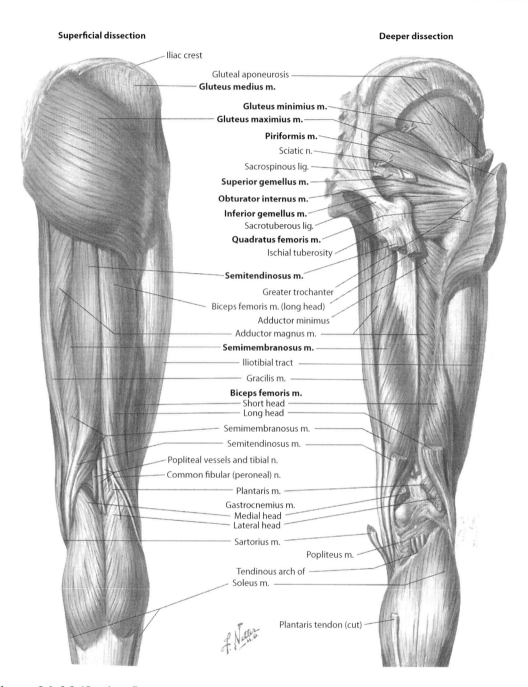

Iliac crest

Gluteal aponeurosis

Gluteus medius m.

Gluteus minimius m.

Gluteus maximius m.

Piriformis m.

Sciatic n.

Sacrospinous lig.

Superior gemellus m.

Obturator internus m.

Inferior gemellus m.

Sacrotuberous lig.

Quadratus femoris m.

Ischial tuberosity

Semitendinosus m.

Greater trochanter

Biceps femoris m. (long head)

Adductor minimus

Adductor magnus m.

Semimembranosus m.

Iliotibial tract

Gracilis m.

Biceps femoris m.

Short head

Long head

Semimembranosus m.

Semitendinosus m.

Popliteal vessels and tibial n.

Common fibular (peroneal) n.

Plantaris m.

Gastrocnemius m.

Medial head

Lateral head

Sartorius m.

Popliteus m.

Tendinous arch of

Soleus m.

Plantaris tendon (cut)

Figures 6.4–6.6 (Continued)

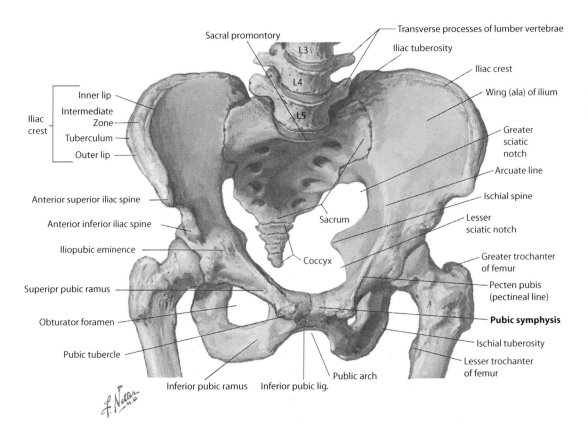

Figures 6.4–6.6 (Continued)

- Assess general lower limb alignment, femoral alignment, pelvic symmetry, muscle tone and symmetry in standing.
- Perform a detailed assessment of the patient's gait, evaluating for the presence of an antalgic gait or a Trendelenburg gait. Observe the stride length, foot rotation, pelvic rotation, stance phase.
- Examine leg length, and compare the contralateral side. Assess for any external rotation of the leg in supine.

MOVEMENTS

- Hip flexion, extension, abduction, adduction, internal and external rotation should be assessed passively, actively, and with resistance.

- Consider internal rotation: external rotation ratio.
- Examine the lumbar spine—referred pain may travel into the hip, groin and buttock.

FUNCTIONAL TESTS

- Squats (including single leg)
- Lunges
- Hopping
- Straight-leg raise
- Kicking/leg-swings
- Running pattern

PALPATION

- Greater trochanter

- Anterior superior iliac spine (ASIS) and anterior inferior iliac spine (AIIS)
- Ischial tuberosity
- Iliac crest
- Tensor fasciae latae/ITB
- Symphysis pubis and pubic tubercle
- Cough impulse at deep and superficial rings to assess for herniae
- Adductor muscles, tendons

SPECIAL TESTS

- Thomas test: to test hip flexors and for Iliopsoas-related pain
- Combined testing

  - FADIR test: hip flexion, adduction and internal rotation for hip pathology (e.g. labral pathology, femoroacetabular impingement)
  - FABER test: hip flexion, abduction and external rotation for hip pathology, sacroiliac pain or iliopsoas strain/bursitis
  - FADER-R test: for gluteal tendinopathy

- Ober's test: to assess tensor fasciae latae or iliotibial band tightness
- Trendelenburg's sign: contralateral drop of the pelvis whilst standing on one-leg can indicate hip pathology or a weakness in hip abductors on the side being tested
- Adductor squeeze tests: for adductor-related groin pain
- Cross over sign: for adductor-related groin pain

LATERAL HIP PAIN/GLUTEAL TENDINOPATHY

Gluteal tendinopathy, often referred to as trochanteric bursitis or greater trochanteric pain syndrome, has a prevalence of 10–25% and is experienced by one in four women aged over 50 years.

- *Presentation:* The disorder presents as pain and tenderness over the greater trochanter and often interferes with sleep and physical function.
- *Examination:* In addition to tenderness on palpation, positive examination findings may include a combination of single-leg stance test, FADER-R test (flexion/adduction/external rotation with static resisted internal rotation of the hip) and

ADD-R test (End-of-range hip adduction in side-lying with resisted isometric abduction).
- *Investigations:* This is usually a clinical diagnosis; however, imaging may be useful to confirm the diagnosis and exclude other pathology such as hip OA (X-ray, MRI) or referred lumbar spine pain (MRI).
- *Management:* a programme of load management education plus exercise has been shown to be the most effective approach for the management of gluteal tendinopathy. Corticosteroid injection has also been shown to have some benefit (Mellor et al., 2018). Despite limited evidence, Platelet Rich Plasma (PRP) injections can be used as an alternative to steroid injections to encourage tendon healing. Consideration should be given to optimising hormonal status in peri/post-menopausal women.

HIP OSTEOARTHRITIS

Hip osteoarthritis is a joint disorder, which occurs when damage triggers repair processes leading to structural changes within a joint. Joint damage may occur through repeated excessive loading and stress of the joint over time, by injury (e.g. FAI), or instability (e.g. dysplasia).

- *Presentation:* hip osteoarthritis is a clinical diagnosis, and it should be suspected in those presenting with activity-related joint pain and functional impairment. The patient may report deep pain in the groin on walking or climbing stairs, with possible referred pain to the lateral thigh and buttock, anterior thigh, knee, and ankle.
- *Examination:* there may be painful restriction of internal rotation with the hip flexed, an antalgic or Trendelenburg gait.
- *Investigations:* Imaging is not generally required to confirm a diagnosis of hip osteoarthritis; however, X-ray may reveal loss of joint space, osteophytes, subchondral sclerosis and cysts.
- *Management:* should include education and advice on self-care strategies such as: weight loss, local muscle strengthening exercises and aerobic fitness training, appropriate footwear, local heat or cold packs, or transcutaneous electrical nerve stimulation (TENS). Patients should receive advice on analgesia. Involvement of the wider

interdisciplinary team should be considered at appropriate stages: orthopaedics (e.g. for consideration of joint resurfacing and joint replacement), physiotherapy (e.g. for advice re exercise) or pain services.

FEMOROACETABULAR IMPINGEMENT SYNDROME

Femoroacetabular impingement (FAI) syndrome is a motion-related clinical disorder of the hip with a triad of symptoms, clinical signs and imaging findings. It represents a symptomatic, premature contact between the proximal femur and the acetabulum (Griffin et al., 2016).

- *Presentation:* patients may present with motion or position related hip or groin pain, buttock or thigh pain. They may report clicking, catching, locking, stiffness, restricted range of motion or giving way.
- *Examination:* hip ROM may be reduced, with a positive FADIR test.
- *Investigations:* AP X-rays of the pelvis and a lateral femoral neck view of the symptomatic hip may identify cam or pincer morphologies, as well as other potential causes of hip pain. Where a more detailed assessment of hip morphology, associated cartilage and labral lesions is desired, cross-sectional imaging (e.g. MRI) may be appropriate.
- *Management:* depending on patient goals and activity levels, management may include some of or a combination of rehabilitation, surgery or non-operative care. Non-operative care includes education, watchful waiting, lifestyle and activity modification. Rehabilitation strategies should be focussed on improving hip stability, neuromuscular control, strength, range of motion and movement patterns. Surgery (typically arthroscopic) can improve the hip morphology (e.g. cam osteotomy) and repair damaged tissue.

HIP LABRAL TEARS

An acetabular labral tear is a defect in the labral surface, intralabral surface or chondrolabral junction, most commonly seen in patients with developmental dysplasia of the hip or femoroacetabular impingement. It may be traumatic or atraumatic. Up to twenty-two percent of athletes with groin pain have a labral tear.

- *Presentation:* may be asymptomatic or present with mechanical hip pain and snapping, vague groin pain or a sensation of locking. If trauma preceded onset, patients may describe an audible pop or a sensation of subluxation at the time of trauma.
- *Examination:* symptoms may be replicated by provocative tests (e.g. FADIR, FABER, quadrant sweep) and an altered gait may be noted.
- *Investigations:* Radiological investigations are relatively unreliable, and diagnosis generally requires an MR arthrogram of the hip joint in question. Hip arthroscopy remains the gold standard for diagnosis of labral pathology.
- *Management:* Treatment is a nonoperative trial to include NSAIDs, activity modification and progressive rehab. Intra-articular injections (which also add diagnostic value) may also be trialled. Surgical management includes arthroscopic labral debridement versus repair and is indicated for patients with progressive symptoms who have not improved despite conservative care.

LIGAMENTUM TERES TEARS

The ligamentum teres is an intra-articular ligament which is covered by synovium within the hip. The mechanism of injury for ligamentum teres most commonly involves forced flexion and adduction, and pivoting on a fixed foot.

- *Presentation:* patients generally report deep groin or medial/anterior thigh pain, mechanical symptoms (e.g. catching), reduced ROM and night pain.
- *Examination:* there will generally be increased tone of the adductor muscle group.
- *Investigations:* Imaging is limited for identifying these injuries, and hip arthroscopy remains the gold-standard in diagnosis.
- *Management:* principles of rehabilitation include restoration of neuromuscular control, proprioception training, manual therapy (adductor muscles) and activity modification.

FEMORAL STRESS FRACTURE

The femur, due to its size and multiple muscle origins and insertions is at risk of stress injury due to training overload. Stress injuries develop from repetitive loading forces (bone strain) coupled with inadequate recovery and adaptation time. This leads to progressive microscopic disruption of the bony architecture and ultimately, a stress fracture. Underlying bone pathology e.g. osteoporosis, lowers the threshold for developing a stress injury (insufficiency fracture). Lateral (tension side) femoral neck stress fractures are considered high-risk for complications (particularly displacement), whereas femoral shaft stress fractures are low-risk.

- *Presentation:* a patient usually presents with groin or proximal thigh pain, which can be diffuse and radiate into the pelvis and lateral hip. There may be an antalgic gait, pain and loss of power on single-leg hopping, with limited ROM e.g. into FADIR.
- *Investigations:* Although there may be evidence of a stress fracture seen on several modalities, MRI has the highest sensitivity and specificity for these injuries. On MRI, a stress injury is characterised by periosteal inflammation and bone marrow oedema like signals in different stages. Linear or globular cortical signal changes are seen in case of a stress fracture.
- *Management:* Provided there is no complete cortical break or displacement, management is typically non-operative. This includes a period of relative off-load and activity modification, before progressively re-loading using pain and function as a guide. Treatment of underlying factors including training error, metabolic conditions, predisposing biomechanics, vitamin D deficiency and RED-S should be included in the management plan.

GROIN PAIN

Groin pain is complex and can be driven by multiple musculoskeletal, urogenital, gynaecological and gastrointestinal structures. Risk factors for injury include twisting sports such as hockey and football, as well as previous groin injury and higher level of competition.

Groin pain can be hip joint-related, referred from the lumbar spine or may be related to other structures:

- *Pubic-related groin pain:* the pubic symphysis is a secondary cartilaginous joint and a location for multiple muscular attachments, stabilising the pelvis. It is vulnerable to shear stress. Point tenderness of this structure, in addition to bone oedema seen on MRI may point to this diagnosis. Reducing load before gradually reintroducing it (using pain and function as a guide), is key to management.
- *Adductor-related groin pain:* adductor longus, brevis, magnus, gracilis and pectineus adduct the hip. All of these muscles may be injured, with injury to adductor longus the most common. Chronic pain in this area is the most common cause of groin pain in athletes. Pain with palpation of the adductor insertion and with resisted adduction aids diagnosis. There may be pain with twisting or kicking. Conservative management includes an exercise programme with initial isometric exercises, before introducing resistance training and proprioception work. Surgical release of the tendon may be considered.
- *Iliopsoas-related groin pain:* the iliopsoas muscle is closely related to the hip joint and can cause pain in isolation or alongside neighbouring pathology. Stretching the hip flexors and pain with resisted hip flexion, or on palpation, can indicate iliopsoas-related pain. Rehabilitation with hip flexor strengthening and improving pelvic stability can improve symptoms. Occasionally, ultrasound guided corticosteroid injections are helpful. Rarely, this pain can present alongside coxa saltans (snapping psoas tendon) where hip extension causes an audible snapping. Rehabilitation is effective. Rarely, surgical release of the tendon is indicated when exercise therapy fails.
- *Inguinal region:* this site is anatomically complex with merging of urogenital structures as well as transversus abdominis, internal and external oblique, rectus abdominis and the conjoint tendon. Pain on palpation of the inguinal canal and invagination of the external ring, resisted sit up and cross over test can aid diagnosis. The actual pathology is variable and bulging or weakness of the posterior wall or tearing of the external oblique aponeurosis have been implicated; however, a true direct or indirect inguinal hernia should be excluded as a source of pain. Management includes lumbopelvic and core

rehabilitation and addressing hip adductor-abductor muscle imbalances. Surgical repair (with numerous techniques described) has shown good outcomes in returning to sport compared with exercise, but the literature is limited.

CLINICAL CONSIDERATIONS

'Groin pain in athletes' is the currently accepted terminology and preferred to athletic pubalgia, sports hernia and others. It is also important to consider non-musculoskeletal causes such as prostatitis, UTI, gynaecological pain, appendicitis or cancers with groin pain (Weir et al., 2015).

Muscular Causes

HAMSTRING INJURY

Acute hamstring injuries are common, with biceps femoris most commonly affected, followed by semimembranosus and then semitendinosus. The most common mechanism is sprinting, but injuries can occur with extremes of knee extension and hip flexion, such as when sliding. Intramuscular tendon involvement is associated with a longer return to sport.

- *Presentation:* posterior thigh pain may start suddenly when sprinting, causing an athlete to stop abruptly, or it may present more insidiously with 'slow stretch' mechanism injuries e.g. in dancers (these tend to be more proximal). Tracking bruising and a focal defect or retraction may be visible and indicate more significant injury.
- *Examination:* reveals tenderness to palpation, either mid belly through the long head of biceps femoris or more proximally toward the ischial tuberosity, involving the proximal semimembranosus. There may be pain and tenderness in the inferior gluteal area with a proximal tendon avulsion. Resisted knee flexion and hip extension may be weaker and generate pain.
- *Investigations:* diagnosis is clinical, but Ultrasound or MRI can be used for further information,

particularly when tendon involvement is suspected.
- *Management:* should follow POLICE principles; protection, optimally loading, icing, compression and elevation (Bleakley et al., 2012). Simple isometrics should be introduced followed by a graded strengthening programme that should be criteria-driven, not time-dependent. Given the high risk of recurrence, ensuring full range of movement, pain-free isometric contraction, satisfactory power and functional tests, and psychological readiness are important prior to return to activity. Avulsion proximally or distally may warrant surgical repair.

QUADRICEPS INJURY

Sprinting, decelerating, kicking or jumping can frequently cause a quadriceps muscle injury. The rectus femoris muscle is most commonly injured, being more susceptible as the only biarthrodial quadricep muscle and exposed to high eccentric forces.

- *Presentation:* local pain and tenderness is present, potentially with a focal muscle defect or gap, with the distal rectus femoris the most common site. Pain is generally accompanied by loss of range and reduced muscle strength. A proximal strain, involving the tendon, carries a worse prognosis.
- *Examination:* there may be pain on palpation at or close to the AIIS origin. A burning pain or paraesthesia may indicate femoral nerve injury.
- *Investigations:* diagnosis is clinical, but ultrasound and MRI can be useful in identifying tendon involvement and haematoma location.
- *Management:* initial management should follow POLICE principles to control swelling and bleeding. Static isometrics and stretching should aim to restore range of movement, with concentric, eccentric and more functional exercises then introduced. Surgery is rarely needed, but repair of a significant tendon injury, e.g. the proximal common or central tendon may be required.

MULTIPLE CHOICE QUESTION (MCQ) QUESTIONS

1. A female footballer sustains an ACL injury. Which graft type or technique is most commonly associated with post-operative anterior knee pain?

   A. Bone-patellar tendon-bone autograft
   B. Central quadriceps tendon graft
   C. Cadaver (donor) graft
   D. Hamstring tendon graft
   E. Bridge-enhanced ACL repair

2. A 26-year-old professional footballer sustains a traumatic knee injury. Video footage reveals a contact mechanism of anterolateral impact causing knee valgus. Which structure is most vulnerable to injury in this mechanism?

   A. Posterior cruciate ligament
   B. Lateral collateral ligament
   C. Patellar tendon
   D. Medial meniscus
   E. Medial collateral ligament

3. A 22-year-old female amateur netballer lands awkwardly from a jump and feels her left knee give way. She reports she felt a 'pop.' Lachman's test is positive. Which of the following is true in relation to this injury?

   A. Surgical repair is necessary in this athlete
   B. Undergoing surgical repair will reduce the risk of developing osteoarthritis in later life
   C. The primary function of the injured structure is to prevent anterior translation of the tibia relative to the femur
   D. Females are less prone to this injury than males
   E. The pivot shift test is not a useful test to detect this injury

4. An 18-year-old cyclist falls off their bike, and the ground makes direct contact with their proximal tibia whilst their knee is flexed. On examination, there is an abrasion overlying their anterior knee and a moderate effusion. Clinical examination is limited due to swelling. Which structure do you suspect has been injured?

   A. Patella
   B. Tibial plateau fracture
   C. Posterior cruciate ligament
   D. Anterior cruciate ligament
   E. Medial meniscus

5. An elite inter-county Gaelic footballer describes a 6-month history of hip and groin pain. Which of the following would NOT typically be used to support a diagnosis of femoroacetabular impingement syndrome?

   A. AP radiograph showing evidence of a cam lesion
   B. Positive FADIR test
   C. A reduced adductor squeeze score
   D. Hip pain with reduced range of motion
   E. AP radiograph showing evidence of a pincer lesion

MULTIPLE CHOICE QUESTION (MCQ) ANSWERS

1. Answer A

   The correct answer is bone-patellar tendon-bone autograft. The most common complication of this type of graft is ongoing anterior knee pain. Complications, risk of re-rupture and surgeon experience will differ for each graft type. Patients should be counselled as to the merits of each option in the context of their athletic goals in order to help them make an informed decision.

2. Answer E

   This mechanism may put several knee structures at risk, including MCL, ACL and medial meniscus. However, the anterolateral impact and forced valgus mechanism is the typical mechanism for MCL injuries. LCL injuries are usually as a result of an anteromedial impact.

3. Answer C

   The injury described here is an ACL injury. Although surgery may be required for the patient (as their sport demands cutting/pivot movements), it is not always required. Osteoarthritis is an anticipated sequelae, irrespective of whether the injury is managed operatively or non-operatively. Females are more at risk of this injury for a number of potential reasons: hormonal, biomechanical, anatomical or socioeconomic (e.g. restricted access to gyms, quality training etc.). Pivot shift is a sensitive special test to diagnose ACL injury, although is often performed under anaesthetic as it can be distressing for the patient and is more technically difficult to perform than Lachman or anterior drawer tests. The primary purpose of the ACL is to prevent anterior translation of the tibia relative to the femur.

4. Answer C

   This mechanism describes the typical 'dashboard injury'—a direct force applied to the proximal tibia on a flexed knee. PCL injuries are common with this mechanism. There may be a positive posterior drawer or posterior sag sign.

5. Answer C

   The condition described here is femoroacetabular impingement (FAI) syndrome . According to the Warwick Agreement on FAI syndrome, it is a motion-related clinical disorder of the hip with a triad of symptoms (e.g. hip pain, stiffness), clinical signs (e.g. reduced ROM, positive FADIR test) and imaging findings (e.g. morphological changes). While reduced adductor squeeze scores may be present, they are not diagnostic of FAI syndrome.

FURTHER READING AND REFERENCES

Bleakley CM, Glasgow P, MacAuley DC PRICE needs updating, should we call the POLICE? *British Journal of Sports Medicine 2012*; 46, 220–221.

Borque KA, Jones M, Cohen M, Johnson D, Williams A. Evidence-based rationale for treatment of meniscal lesions in athletes. *Knee Surg Sports Traumatol Arthrosc. 2022 May*; 30(5), 1511–1519. doi: 10.1007/s00167-021-06694-6. Epub 2021 Aug 20. PMID: 34415368.

Cleland, J.C., Koppenhaver, S and J, Su. J. (2016). *Netter's Orthopaedic Clinical Examination: An Evidence-Based Approach.* 3rd ed. Philadelphia: Elsevier.

Griffin DR, Dickenson EJ, O'Donnell J, et al. The Warwick agreement on femoroacetabular impingement syndrome (FAI syndrome): an international consensus statement. *Br J Sports Med* 2016; 50, 1169–76.

Malliaras, P., Cook, J., Purdam, C. & Rio, E. (2015). Patellar tendinopathy: clinical diagnosis, load management, and advice for challenging case presentations. *J. Orthop. Sports Phys. Ther.* 45, 887–898.

Mellor, R. et al. Education plus exercise versus corticosteroid injection use versus a wait and see approach on global outcome and pain from gluteal tendinopathy: prospective, single blinded, randomised clinical trial. *BMJ* 361, k1662 (2018).

NICE CKS (2022). Osteoarthritis: https://cks.nice.org.uk/topics/osteoarthritis/diagnosis/diagnosis/

Weir A, Brukner P, Delahunt E, et al Doha agreement meeting on terminology and definitions in groin pain in athletes. *British Journal of Sports Medicine 2015*; 49, 768–774.

Spine **7**

Steven Whatmough, K Pumi Senaratne and Craig Zalecki

INTRODUCTION

Low back pain is common, affecting one in three of the British population. The lifetime prevalence of low back pain is 84% and of those affected, around 20% will seek the attention of their GP annually.

Low back pain is defined as pain in the lumbosacral area, between the bottom of the ribs and the top of the legs. It is divided into acute low back pain, lasting less than 6 weeks; subacute low back pain, lasting 6–12 weeks; and chronic low back pain, lasting over 12 weeks.

KEY ANATOMY

The spine consists of a column of 33 bones called vertebrae. Each vertebra is separated by an intervertebral disc (Figures 7.2–7.3). The column can be divided into five regions:

- Cervical vertebrae (seven vertebrae)
- Thoracic vertebrae (twelve vertebrae)
- Lumbar vertebrae (five vertebrae)
- Sacrum (five fused vertebrae)
- Coccyx (four fused vertebrae)

The spine has four main functions:

- Spinal cord protection
- Supporting and carrying the weight of the body above the pelvis
- Forming the central axis of the body
- Movement and posture

Vertebrae

Despite each region demonstrating unique differences, all vertebrae share a common structure:

- Spinous process (central posterior protrusion)
- Transverse process (two lateral protrusions—in the thoracic region, these articulate with the ribs)
- Pedicles (connect the transverse process with the vertebral body)
- Lamina (connect the spinous process with the transverse process)
- Articular process (forms the facet joints, or the joints between vertebral bodies)

Ligaments

The ligaments of the spine are responsible for strengthening the spinal column and preventing excessive movement. The anterior and posterior longitudinal ligaments run the length of the spine, anterior and posterior to the vertebral bodies. The ligamentum flavum extends between the lamina of adjacent vertebrae. The interspinous and supraspinous ligaments attach between the spinous processes along the length of the spinal column.

Intervertebral Discs

Found between the vertebral bodies of the spine, they function as a cushion and shock absorber between the two vertebrae. The disc is made up of two structures:

- Annulus fibrosus
- Nucleus pulposus

The annulus fibrosus consists of concentric layers of collagen fibres called lamellae. These fibres contain the nucleus pulposus, a gel-like structure sitting in the disc centre. The compressive nature of the nucleus pulposus assists in the spine's flexibility.

DOI: 10.1201/9781003179979-7

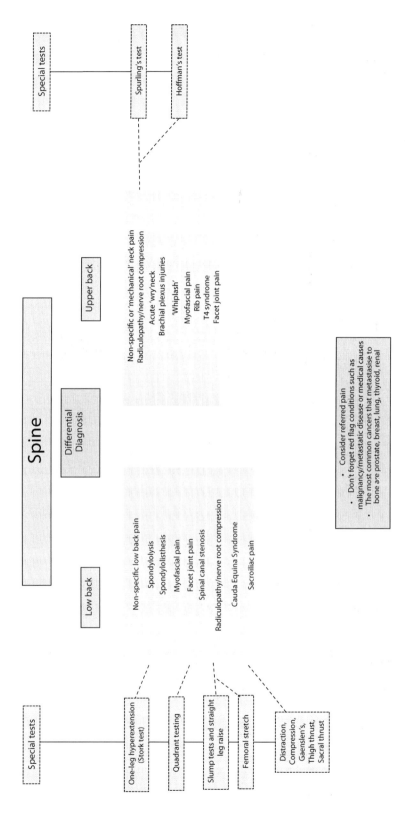

Figure 7.1 Differential diagnosis chart.

The Nervous System

The spinal cord travels through the vertebral foramen. Branches of nerves leave the spinal cord at each level, through the intervertebral foramen. These branches of nerves are called nerve roots. The cervical spine has eight nerve roots (C1–C8). There are seven cervical vertebrae, but eight cervical nerve roots. Each cervical nerve root leaves the cord above the corresponding vertebrae (i.e. the C4 nerve root exits above the C4 vertebrae), and the C8 nerve root exits below the C7 vertebrae. Therefore, the T1 nerve root exits below the T1 vertebrae. From T1 down, each nerve root leaves below their corresponding vertebrae.

Each nerve root can be mapped to a sensory and motor area and are referred to as dermatomes and myotomes, respectively (Figure 7.4). There can be variation between individuals in the areas of dermatomes

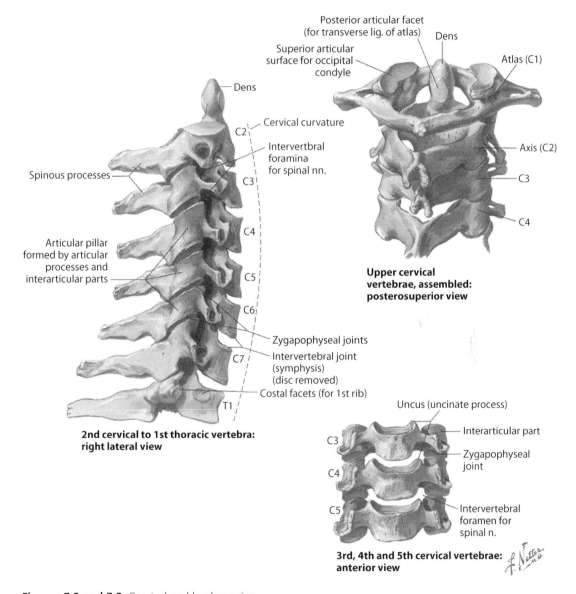

Figures 7.2 and 7.3 Cervical and lumbar spine.

Source: Cleland et al. (2016). Netter's *Orthopaedic Clinical Examination: An Evidence-Based Approach*. 3rd ed. Philadelphia: Elsevier. With permission.

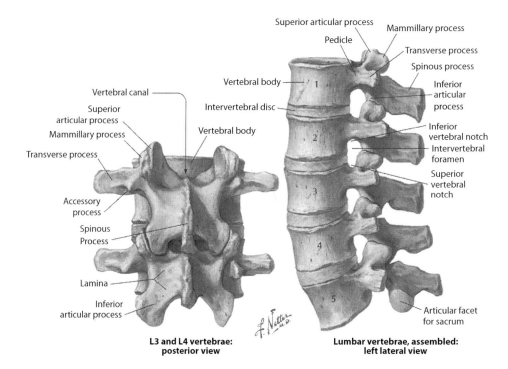

L3 and L4 vertebrae:
posterior view

Lumbar vertebrae, assembled:
left lateral view

Figures 7.2 and 7.3 (Continued)

and myotomes. Muscles have multiple nerve root innervations and certain movements can be the action of multiple muscles, making mapping difficult.

DERMATOMES

- *C1:* Typically, no sensory function
- *C2:* Lower jaw
- *C3:* Upper neck
- *C4:* Upper shoulders (area over the trapezius muscle)
- *C5:* Area over the clavicles
- *C6:* Lateral area of upper limbs toward the thumb
- *C7:* Posterior aspect of upper limbs, index and middle finger
- *C8:* Medial aspect of upper limb, ring and little finger
- *T1-T12:* Levels down the trunk with T4 commonly thought to supply the area of the nipples and T10 the area of the umbilicus
- *L1:* Hips and groin
- *L2:* Anterior and medial thigh
- *L3:* Anterior thigh down past the medial knee
- *L4:* Lateral thigh down through the central knee
- *L5:* Lateral knee down to the great toe

- *S1:* Little toe and posterior leg
- *S2:* Posterior leg and genitalia
- *S3–5:* Buttocks and genitalia

MYOTOMES

- *C5:* Elbow flexion
- *C6:* Wrist extension
- *C7:* Elbow extension
- *C8:* Finger flexion
- *T1:* Finger abduction
- *L2:* Hip flexion
- *L3:* Knee extension
- *L4:* Ankle dorsiflexion
- *L5:* Great toe extension
- *S1:* Ankle plantarflexion

Reflexes are also mediated by nerve roots, but there are variations:

- *C5:* Biceps
- *C6:* Brachioradialis
- *C7:* Triceps
- *L2–4:* Patellar
- *S1:* Achilles tendon

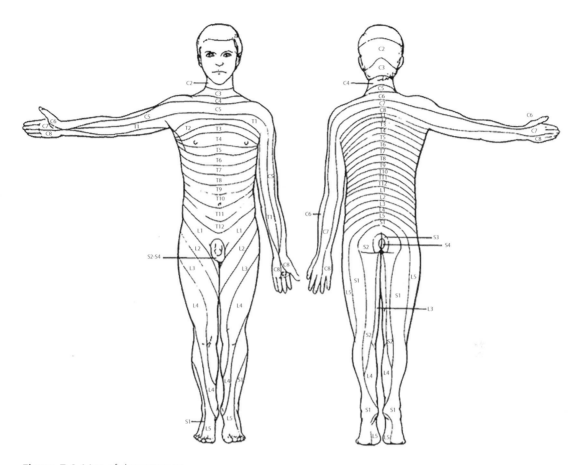

Figure 7.4 Map of dermatomes.

Source: Taken from Agache P. (2017) Dermatomes. In: Humbert P., Fanian F., Maibach H., Agache P. (eds) Agache's Measuring the Skin. Springer, Cham.

SPINAL CORD ANATOMY

The spinal cord has several tracts, divided into ascending and descending pathways. Ascending pathways transport sensory information from the peripheral nerves to the cerebral cortex. Descending pathways transport motor information from the brain to muscle tissue.

The main ascending pathways are the dorsal columns and the spinothalamic tracts (anterior and lateral). The dorsal columns carry fine touch, vibration and proprioception information. The pathway is formed by three groups of neurones (first, second and third order). The first order neurones enter the cord at each vertebral level and end in the medulla oblongata.

Second order neurones start at the medulla and end at the thalamus. Third order neurones take information from the thalamus to the sensory cortex of the brain. The neurones run at the posterior aspect of the spinal cord. The second order neurones decussate at the medulla oblongata.

The spinothalamic tract is divided into the anterior and lateral tracts, carrying crude touch/pressure information, and pain/temperature information, respectively. The first order neurones enter at each vertebral level. They will ascend one to two vertebral levels and synapse with second order neurones. The second order neurones decussate within the spinal cord and travel to the thalamus. Third order neurones connect the thalamus to the sensory cortex of the brain.

The main descending tract is the corticospinal tract. This carries information from the motor cortex to the muscles, and is divided into anterior and lateral tracts. The anterior tract is predominantly involved in providing motor information to extremity muscles, whereas the lateral tract is involved in sending motor information to the trunk or axial muscles. The lateral tract decussates at the medulla, whereas the anterior tract decussates within the cord.

HISTORY

Pain is often the primary presenting symptom of problems in this area and is therefore an appropriate starting point. A particular importance in spinal conditions is establishing whether back pain is radicular or not i.e. is the pain radiating down a dermatome. Then it should be established whether there is associated numbness or paraesthesia. Is the patient complaining of weakness? With this information a hypothesis may be formed of a particular nerve root compression. During examination, this hypothesis may be confirmed by testing the relevant dermatomes and myotomes.

Flexion-related back pain may point to a discogenic cause, whereas extension-related pain is associated more with spinal stenosis or a facet joint issue.

Past medical/surgical history will provide further clues to the underlying diagnosis. A patient with a history of spinal fusion is likely to develop disc disease above and below the level of fusion. Whereas, an elderly patient with a past history of osteoporosis presenting with sudden onset back pain would raise your suspicion of an osteoporotic fracture.

Family history is important when considering medical causes of low back pain. In particular, a young person with pain who has a family history of inflammatory arthritis would raise suspicion of an inflammatory cause to the pain.

Social history and occupational/sporting history will assist in the identification of populations of people that are at risk of certain conditions. For example, gymnasts or cricket fast bowlers are at risk of pars defects.

CLINICAL CONSIDERATIONS

Red flags are symptoms associated with serious pathology and are therefore essential questions to consider with all patients. The serious pathologies in the spine are:

- Malignancy (Metastatic Spinal Cord Compression (MSCC), Multiple Myeloma)
- Infection (Spinal Tuberculosis, Vertebral Osteomyelitis, Discitis)
- Spondyloarthropathy
- Osteoporotic Vertebral Compression Fracture
- Craniocervical Instability
- Cervical Myelopathy
- Cervical Vascular Lesions
- Cauda Equina Syndrome (CES)
- Abdominal Aortic Aneurysm (AAA)

Other important questions to consider include:

- Unexplained weight loss and night sweats (suggestive of a malignant process)
- Perineal numbness, urine and faecal incontinence, bilateral radicular symptoms (suggestive of cauda equina)
- Clumsiness of hands, change in gait, loss of balance (suggestive of cervical myelopathy)

Identifying patients' ideas, concerns and expectations (ICE) can be a useful way of managing more complex patients. A patient with chronic back pain who has exhausted all treatment options may initially present as challenging. It may well be that the patient is only looking for reassurance that their low back pain is not a cancer and discussion about the complexity of pain can be useful.

EXAMINATION

Cervical Spine

INSPECTION (STANDING)

- Gait, including the patient's static (standing) and dynamic (walking) posture.

INSPECTION (SITTING)

- Observe the patient's static posture: look for protrusion of the chin or protraction (rounding) of the shoulders.

SCREENING EXAMINATIONS

- Thoracic screen including rotation, flexion, extension, lateral flexion.
- Shoulder screen including abduction, forward flexion, internal rotation and external rotation.

MOVEMENTS

- Assess active cervical movements, making note of the range and quality.
- Flexion, extension, rotation, lateral flexion, protraction/retraction, combined movements/quadrant.

NEUROLOGICAL TESTS

- Motor (cervical myotomes)
- Sensory (cervical dermatomes).
- Reflexes (cervical reflexes)

PALPATION

- Palpate each spinous process running down the cervical and upper thoracic spine, assessing for tenderness and malalignment. Then palpate the paraspinal muscles for tenderness. This should also be done in prone, as this relaxes the muscles around the cervical spine, making palpation easier.

SPECIAL TESTS

- Thoracic outlet tests (Adson's stress test and Roos test)
- Upper limb neural tension tests (radial, median and ulnar)
- Spurling's test to assess for nerve root pain
- Hoffman's test to assess for cervical corticospinal tract dysfunction

Thoracic Spine

INSPECTION (STANDING)

- Observe in standing and whilst walking. Assess posture.
  - Hyperkyphosis may be linked to poor posture (e.g. protracted shoulders, protruding

head position) or spinal pathology such as Scheuermann's disease.
  - Assess for scoliosis.

SCREENING EXAMINATIONS

- Lumbar spine screen including flexion, extension, lateral flexion, quadrant.
- Shoulder screen including abduction, forward flexion, internal rotation, external rotation.
- Cervical spine screen including flexion, extension, rotation, lateral flexion and quadrant.

MOVEMENT

- Assess the thoracic spine active movements for range and quality. Over pressure can be used to assess end range. Flexion, extension, lateral flexion, rotation and rib expansion.

NEUROLOGICAL TESTS

- Upper or lower limb neurology tests, depending on distribution of symptoms: Motor, sensory, reflexes.

PALPATION

- In supine, palpate the sternocleidomastoid, chest wall structures and rib expansion.
- In prone palpate the thoracic spine and paraspinal muscles for superficial and deep tenderness.

SPECIAL TESTS

- If there is upper limb symptom distribution, perform upper limb neural provocation tests.
- If there is lower limb symptom distribution consider a slump test for neural sensitivity.
- Thoracic outlet tests (Adson's stress test and Roos test).

Lumbar/Sacral Spine

INSPECTION (STANDING)

- Observe in standing and whilst walking. Assess posture, noting the lumbar spine.

○ Hyperlordosis may be linked to poor posture (e.g. tight hip flexors, anterior pelvic tilt) or spinal pathology such as spondylolisthesis.

○ Assess for scoliosis.

SCREENING EXAMINATIONS

• Cervical spine screen including flexion, extension, rotation, lateral flexion and quadrant.

• Hip screen including flexion, quadrant testing, internal and external rotation at 90 degrees of hip flexion.

MOVEMENT

• Assess lumbar spine active movements for range and quality. Flexion, extension, lateral flexion.

NEUROLOGICAL TESTS

• Motor (lumbar/sacral myotomes)
• Sensory (lumbar/sacral dermatomes)
• Reflexes (lumbar/sacral reflexes)

PALPATION

• In prone palpate the lumbar spine and paraspinal muscles for superficial and deep tenderness. Palpate the sacroiliac joints, piriformis and gluteal muscles for trigger points.

SPECIAL TESTS

• Slump test and straight leg raise for nerve root sensitivity
• Obturator slump for obturator nerve sensitivity
• Femoral stretch to assess for upper lumbar nerve root sensitivity
• Sacroiliac joint pain provocation tests (thigh thrust, sacral thrust, compression, distraction, Gaeslen's)
• Quadrant testing (lumbar hyperextension and lateral flexion/rotation whilst controlling the patient's shoulder) to assess for lumbar facet pain
• One-leg standing hyperextension (or 'Stork test') to assess for facet pain and pars interarticularis injury, with passive rotation toward the weight bearing side

MECHANICAL

Torticollis/Wry Neck

Torticollis is thought to be due to minor local musculoskeletal irritation causing pain and spasm in the muscles of the neck. The cause is often unknown, but poor posture (e.g. sat at the computer, during sleep, etc.) is common. Symptoms usually resolve within 24–48 hours.

• *Presentation:* Typically, an acute onset of a unilateral painful, stiff neck with an absence of trauma. Patients with torticollis will not have neurological symptoms or other systemic compromise, but serious pathology should be excluded.

• *Examination:* Reduced cervical movement with palpable trigger points.

• *Investigations:* Not required unless an alternative diagnosis is suspected.

• *Management:* Simple analgesia to allow range of movement exercises to take place is advised. Soft collars are not recommended. Long term management would aim to identify risk factors, particularly in posture, and prescribe appropriate exercise programs.

Facet Joint Disease

Facet joints are formed by the superior and inferior articular processes of the two adjacent vertebrae. The joint contains synovial fluid, which is held in place by an inner membrane. They allow spinal flexion and extension whilst limiting rotation and preventing the vertebrae from slipping over each other. The sensory nerve of these joints is the medial branch of the dorsal spinal ramus. Chronic low back pain can result from facet joint disease.

• *Presentation:* Facet joint disease is a clinical diagnosis. Facet-mediated pain is typically non-radicular and is often worse in the mornings, upon awakening, or during periods of inactivity.

• *Examination:* The pain may also increase with spine extension, facet joint palpation, and spinal rotation.

• *Investigations:* Imaging of patients with facet joint disease is often not helpful. X-ray, CT, and MRI may show degeneration, joint space narrowing, facet joint hypertrophy, joint space calcification and osteophytes. These findings, however, may be present in both symptomatic and asymptomatic patients. Data shows that 89% of patients in the 60 to 69 years of age population studied have facet joint osteoarthritis, although not all were symptomatic (Kalichman and Hunter, 2007).

- *Management:* Conservative management is used as first-line therapy to treat facet-mediated pain. Weight loss and physical therapy are the mainstay of treatment. When conservative measures fail there are interventional options. The following criteria for medial branch blocks are suggested by NICE (NICE, 2020):

  ○ Non-surgical treatment has not worked **and**
  ○ The main source of pain is thought to come from structures supplied by the medial branch nerve **and**
  ○ They have moderate or severe levels of localised back pain (rated as five or more on a visual analogue scale, or equivalent) at the time of referral

A diagnostic medial branch block involves injecting local anaesthetic around the medial branches, often under fluoroscopic guidance. Each facet joint has sensory innervation from the nerve root above and below (i.e. the L4/5 facet joint receives sensory innervation from the L4 and L5 nerve root). If a patient has a positive response to a diagnostic block, radiofrequency ablation can be done to ablate the medial branch nerves. Radiofrequency ablation uses heat to temporarily destroy the medial branch of the sensory nerve, thus reducing pain. Nerve regeneration can result in a gradual return of symptoms, usually around 6–12 months later. Denervation can be repeated.

Stress Fracture of Pars Interarticularis/ Spondylolysis and Spondylolisthesis

Spondylolysis is a defect in the pars interarticularis, an area between the spinal lamina and pedicle. If this defect is bilateral, slippage (spondylolisthesis) can occur. The pars interarticularis is the weakest part of the vertebral body and therefore prone to stress fractures. Individuals that repetitively extend the spine (e.g. gymnasts) are therefore at risk.

Spondylolisthesis is where one vertebral body slips forward onto another. It can be caused by bilateral pars defects, as well as degeneration in the lumbar spine (usually in patients over the age of 50). Spondylolisthesis is graded depending on the amount of slippage that has occurred.

- Grade 1: <25% of the vertebral body has slipped forward
- Grade 2: 25–50% slippage
- Grade 3: 50–75% slippage
- Grade 4: 75–100% slippage
- Grade 5 (Spondyloptosis): >100% slippage (i.e. the superior vertebral body has completely fallen off the inferior vertebral body)
- *Presentation:* It is important to differentiate between active bone stress and chronic, asymptomatic defects. Symptoms can include localised back pain worse after activity and extension of the back, or with pain radiating into the buttock and down the hamstring. Cases may present after changes to training volume or technique. Spondylolisthesis may be asymptomatic and is often found incidentally on imaging in later-life. However, the slippage can cause nerve root impingement resulting in radicular back pain.
- Examination will identify pain on lumbar extension and rotation. Neural tension tests (straight leg raise and slump tests) may be positive if nerve root compression is present. Depending on the degree of impingement, the patient may have positive findings on neurological assessment. A reproduction of a patient's symptoms on stork testing can suggest either a spondylolysis or spondylolisthesis.
- *Investigations:* Anteroposterior and lateral plain films, as well as lateral flexion-extension plain films, are standard for the initial diagnosis of spondylolisthesis. It is important to consider that the slippage can be dynamic, such as worsening with lumbar flexion. This suggests instability. A defect in the pars interarticularis may be seen on X-ray and is often referred to as the 'Scottie dog sign.' CT imaging provides the highest sensitivity for identifying pars defects. MRI scanning has advanced in recent years and various sequencing can take place to visualise pars defects, having the advantage of reduced radiation. This is important considering that most patients presenting

with this condition will be young. MRI is helpful in identifying other pathology that may be contributing to the patients' symptoms (e.g. disc prolapse).

MRIs can classify spondylolysis into the Hollenberg classification:

- ○ Grade 0: normal pars interarticularis; MRI: no signal abnormality, pars interarticularis intact
- ○ Grade I: stress reaction; MRI: marrow oedema; intact cortical margins
- ○ Grade II: incomplete stress fracture; MRI: marrow oedema; incomplete cortical fracture or fissure
- ○ Grade III: acute complete stress fracture; MRI: marrow oedema; complete cortical fracture extending through pars interarticularis
- ○ Grade IV: chronic stress fracture; MRI: no marrow oedema. Fractures completely extend through pars interarticularis

Risk factors of stress fractures should be investigated, with DEXA considered to assess bone density, as well as blood tests including Vitamin D and bone profile. Relative Energy Deficiency in Sport (RED-S) may present with a stress fracture.

- *Management:* spondylolysis management will depend on whether the fracture is acute, chronic, or complete and the patient's symptoms and level of activity. If acute and symptomatic, spondylolysis is initially managed with rest. Bracing is occasionally used to prevent hyperextension. After the initial healing phase, range of movement exercise and strengthening is introduced (particularly of the trunk and gluteal muscle groups). Load is gradually introduced before sport-specific movements. Depending on the sport, technique and training load should be optimised to prevent recurrence.

Spondylolisthesis management depends on symptoms, nerve compression and level of slippage. Non-operative treatment is the treatment of choice in most cases of spondylolisthesis, with or without neurological symptoms. Rehabilitation should aim to improve lumbar flexion, including pelvic control exercises. Stationary cycling promotes spinal flexion, deconstruction of the thecal sac, and allows for more exercise before the development of neurogenic claudication is present.

Epidural injections have been used historically for spondylolisthesis. These injections may be beneficial in the short term but are unlikely to provide long-lasting benefits. Surgical stabilisation (or fusion) is the surgery of choice should conservative management fail, but most cases will not require surgery.

Non-Specific Low Back Pain (LBP)

Non-specific low back pain is a symptom rather than a diagnosis. The term is controversial and usually refers to back pain without a recognisable, known pathology (e.g. infection, tumour, fracture, disc prolapse, etc.). Any of the many structures in the back can cause pain and making a specific diagnosis can be challenging.

Non-specific low back pain is usually categorised into three subtypes: acute, sub-acute and chronic low back pain. This subdivision is based on the duration. Acute low back pain is an episode of low back pain for less than 6 weeks, sub-acute low back pain between 6 and 12 weeks and chronic low back pain for 12 weeks or more.

Low back pain is a self-limiting condition:

- 90% of people with LBP will recover in 3–4 months with no treatment.
- 70% of people with LBP will recover in 1 month with no treatment.
- 50% of people with LBP will recover in 2 weeks with no treatment.
- 5% of the remaining 10% will not respond to conservative care (such as physiotherapy).
- The final 5% are the more challenging cases that do not naturally improve.
- Despite LBP often being self-limiting, it has a high recurrence rate of about 60%.
- *Presentation:* Given the high rates of recurrence, the history of low back pain can be prolonged. Patients will often present with many years of back pain. There is often no trauma or specific time of onset. It is, therefore, important to work out exacerbating and alleviating factors. Ask about patient mobility and activity (e.g. what sports or hobbies do they have). Improving activity in sedentary patients can significantly improve symptoms. Asking about their social history is also important. Working at a non-ergonomic desk all day can be a cause of low back pain.

Suboptimal postures when lifting and carrying a child can also cause low back pain. A thorough history can often identify activities that drive the back pain. It is essential to go through the red flags of low back pain and ensure that a serious diagnosis is not missed. Enquiring about yellow flags and psychological factors is also useful.

- Examination in non-specific low back pain should be similar to other spinal conditions. It is important to pay attention to posture, muscle patterning and gait. Screening the hip is also important as hip pathology can cause low back pain. A neurological assessment to ensure no serious pathology is missed should be performed.
- *Investigations:* radiological investigations should not be routinely requested in patients with non-specific low back pain. There have been many papers showing that abnormal findings on MRI do not correlate well with symptoms. Savage et al. (1997) reported that 32% of their asymptomatic subjects had 'abnormal' lumbar spines (evidence of disc degeneration, disc bulging or protrusion, facet hypertrophy, or nerve root compression).
- Management should take a holistic, biopsychosocial approach with multidisciplinary input. Weight loss (if overweight) and exercise advice is the mainstay. Patients should be empowered to take control of their own rehabilitation. The Keele STarT back tool is a useful way to risk stratify patients (Table 7.1). Those at low risk of chronicity should be encouraged to self-manage, whereas those at high risk of chronicity should be referred onto specialists.

Questions 1–8 are given a score if you agree with the statement. Question 9 is divided into: Not at all, Slightly, Moderately, Very much and Extremely. A score of 1 is given for answers of 'Very much' or 'Extremely.' Questions 5-9 are added to give a sub score. A total score of less than 3 means there is a low risk of chronicity. A total score of 4 or more is divided into medium and high risk depending on the sub-score. A sub score less than or equal to 3 is a medium risk. A sub score more than 3 gives a high risk of chronicity.

Sacroiliac Pain

The sacroiliac joints aim to provide a stable, yet flexible support for the transmission of force through the lower back and pelvis. They are diarthrodial synovial joints with a fibrous capsule. Sacroiliac joint dysfunction is often a non-specific diagnosis that may be used when other diagnoses have been excluded.

- *Presentation:* Often a unilateral or bilateral deep buttock pain that can worsen after activity.
- *Examination:* Pain provocation tests may be positive including passive hip extension, Gaenslen's test, (Hip) flexion, abduction and external rotation (FABER), distraction test, compression test and the thigh thrust test.
- *Investigations:* Imaging will often be unremarkable but is useful in excluding other diagnoses. MRI is sensitive in detecting sacroiliitis in inflammatory pathology.
- *Management:* Biomechanical and psychosocial factors should be addressed, but strengthening and functional rehabilitation is key. Improving functional movements and lumbo-pelvic control with strengthening exercises is useful.

Table 7.1 Keele STarT Back Screening Tool (Hay et al., 2008)

1. My back pain has spread down my leg(s) at some time in the last 2 weeks.
2. I have had pain in the shoulder or neck at some time in the last 2 weeks.
3. I have only walked short distances because of my back pain.
4. In the last 2 weeks, I have dressed more slowly than usual because of back pain.
5. It's not really safe for a person with a condition like mine to be physically active.
6. Worrying thoughts have been going through my mind a lot of the time.
7. I feel that my back pain is terrible and it's never going to get any better.
8. In general, I have not enjoyed all the things I used to enjoy.
9. Overall, how bothersome has your back pain been in the last 2 weeks?

Abnormal movement patterns and poor sport technique should be addressed. In those with high impact activity, improving lower limb strength may negate ground reaction forces. Guided corticosteroid injections may provide pain relief.

Coccydynia

The coccyx is the terminal section of the spine and is an insertion site for multiple ligaments, muscles and tendons. Pain can often present in this location and is more common in females or in those with hypermobility.

- *Presentation:* Focal coccyx pain that may worsen with sitting, standing from a seated position, during sexual intercourse or with defecation. Cases may be post-traumatic, such as after a fall or childbirth, but may be idiopathic.
- *Examination:* There is usually tenderness of the coccyx on palpation.
- *Investigations:* This is primarily a clinical diagnosis. Imaging may be used to exclude other causes such as sacral radiculopathy.
- *Management:* Non-surgical management with analgesia, activity modification, ergonomic adjustments (such as with pressure-relieving cushions or improving posture) and physiotherapy is often successful. Pelvic floor rehabilitation is key in pain related to pelvic floor muscle dysfunction. Corticosteroid injections around the coccyx and sacrococcygeal ligaments can aid diagnosis and be therapeutic. Surgery in the form of coccygectomy is a last resort.

NEURAL COMPROMISE

Cervical Myelopathy

Cervical myelopathy is a common condition where the cervical spinal cord is compressed. It is often caused by degenerative cervical spondylosis, with osteoarthritis of the posterior facet joints, osteophytes and degenerative intervertebral discs causing narrowing.

- *Presentation:* Usually altered sensation in both hands (numbness, paraesthesia), clumsiness in the hands and gait imbalance. The underlying degenerative process of the cervical spine may cause neck pain and stiffness.
- *Examination:* Abnormal gait pattern (particularly tandem) with loss of balance. A positive Romberg's test indicates dorsal column dysfunction. Hoffman's sign is often positive. Reduced range of cervical movement is consistent with osteoarthritis. Neurological examination may identify motor weakness in the hands and more concerningly, the legs. Sensory function of the dorsal columns (proprioception) as well as the spinothalamic pathways (pinprick sensation) may be abnormal.
- *Investigations:* MRI is the investigation of choice. Plain radiographs may identify degenerative processes (osteophyte formation, disc space narrowing, etc.). However, they will not diagnose myelopathy. MRI will identify effacement of cerebrospinal fluid at the point of stenosis and signal changes (i.e. appear bright on T2 weighted images). Cord signal changes on T1 weighted images are associated with a poorer prognosis.
- *Management:* The aim of management is to stop progression. Exercises and lifestyle modification can help in mild disease with no functional impairment. Otherwise, surgical decompression is the treatment of choice. Reversal of symptoms may not always occur following surgery.

Radicular Back Pain

Radicular back pain is common. The term 'sciatica' suggests pain along the L4-S1 nerve roots, whereas radicular back pain refers to pain from any nerve root compression in the spine. The most common site is in the lumbar spine. Structures that can compress nerve roots include disc protrusions, osteophyte complexes and spondylolisthesis. Depending on severity, nerve root compression can cause pain, numbness, paraesthesia and loss of power. As muscles often receive innervation from multiple nerve roots, loss of muscle power is often a result of a severe radiculopathy.

CLINICAL CONSIDERATIONS

It is important to consider the cause of nerve compression. Disc prolapse is the most common, but often resolves after 6–8 weeks with exercise. It is important to ensure that a sinister cause of nerve compression is not missed and there are specific 'red flag' questions that raise the index of suspicion:

1) Cauda Equina

   a. Severe or progressive bilateral neurological deficit of the legs
   b. Recent-onset urinary retention
   c. Recent-onset faecal incontinence (due to loss of sensation of rectal fullness)
   d. Perianal or perineal sensory loss (saddle anaesthesia or paraesthesia)

2) Spinal Fracture

   a. History of trauma

3) Malignancy

   a. Unexplained weight loss
   b. Night pain
   c. Night sweats

4) Infection

   a. Fever
   b. History of intravenous drug use
   c. History of TB/HIV
   d. Immunocompromised

- *Presentation:* Commonly, acute low back pain with pain radiating down one lower limb. If the nerve root compression is at the upper lumbar levels (L2–4) then radiation typically travels down the anterior thigh.
- *Examination:* There may be altered sensation in a dermatomal area. If significant compression, then reduced power of knee extension, hip adduction and hip flexion may be seen. Compression of the L5 nerve root will cause a radiation of pain down the lateral aspect of the lower limb and weakness of great toe extension and ankle dorsiflexion. S1 compression results in a posterior lower limb distribution of symptoms with a weakness of plantar flexion. If the cause of the radicular back pain is disc protrusion, lumbar flexion will often exacerbate symptoms and extension will ease symptoms. Neural tension tests (e.g. straight leg raise and slump test) will often reproduce symptoms.
- *Investigations:* With neural symptoms, MRI is the modality of choice as it will be able to differentiate between inflammatory, malignant, or discogenic causes. The indications for MRI include radicular symptoms lasting longer than 6–8 weeks, failed conservative management and positive red flags. Nerve conduction studies (NCS) and electromyography (EMG) are accurate only after 3 weeks of persistent symptoms because they depend on fibrillation potentials developing after an acute injury.
- *Management:* Most cases of lumbosacral radiculopathy are self-limiting and will resolve with conservative management. Weight loss advice is often helpful. Simple analgesia can help keep patient's mobile during their acute episode. Gabapentinoids, antiepileptics, oral corticosteroids and benzodiazepines are not recommended for the treatment of acute radicular back pain. Treatment should be focused on self-management and exercise therapy. Tools, such as the Keele STarT Back, can help guide who to refer for physiotherapy and who to advise self-management. According to NICE guidelines, the use of epidural injections for patients with radicular back pain should only be considered if their symptoms are acute (less than 3 months) and severe (NICE, 2020). However, epidural injections are often used prior to decompressive surgery as a diagnostic tool. Should an injection provide no benefit, then decompressive surgery would not be advised.

Spinal Stenosis

Spinal stenosis is a degenerative condition in which there is diminished space available for the neural and vascular spinal structures. Not all patients with spinal narrowing develop symptoms. Spinal stenosis refers to the symptoms of pain and not the narrowing itself. It is a significant cause of disability in the elderly, and is the most significant cause of spinal surgery in patients over 65 years. Spinal stenosis can affect all

Table 7.2 Questionnaire to Diagnose Lumbar Spinal Stenosis (Konno et al., 2007).	
Q1	Numbness and/or pain in the thighs down to the calves and shins.
Q2	Numbness and/or pain increase in intensity after walking for a while, but are relieved by taking a rest.
Q3	Standing for a while brings on numbness and/or pain in the thighs down to the calves and shins.
Q4	Numbness and/or pain are reduced by bending forward.
	Key questions for diagnosis of cauda equina symptoms:
Q5	Numbness is present in both legs.
Q6	Numbness is present in the soles of both feet.
Q7	Numbness arises around the buttocks.
Q8	Numbness is present, but pain is absent.
Q9	A burning sensation arises around the buttocks.
Q10	Walking nearly causes urination.

areas of the spine. It is most commonly seen in the lumbar spine, less commonly seen in the cervical spine and rarely seen in the thoracic spine.

- *Presentation:* Lumbar spinal stenosis presents as low back pain exacerbated by prolonged sitting and ambulation. Lumbar extension further narrows the spinal canal resulting in symptom exacerbation. Compression on exiting nerve roots can result in radicular symptoms. Flexing the spine, by sitting or leaning forwards, opens the spinal canal, eases the compression on neural structures and therefore improves pain. Patients often describe claudication type symptoms (Table 7.2). Upon reaching a certain walking distance the patient will have to sit or lean forward, the pain will ease, and the patient can repeat their previous walking distance.
- *Examination:* There may be positive neurology on examination. It is important to also consider cauda equina symptoms.
- *Investigations:* Up to 20% of individuals with spinal stenosis are asymptomatic. It is therefore important to relate symptoms to any positive radiology finding. MRI is the investigation of choice for

identifying central, lateral recess and foraminal stenosis. However, CT scans have been found to offer similar accuracy for the assessment of central stenosis.

- *Management:* The natural history of spinal stenosis patients treated conservatively is variable. In patients presenting with mild to moderate symptoms, progression can be minimal in up to 50% of patients. However, less is known about the natural history of patients presenting with severe symptoms. Conservative treatment usually focuses on pelvic control and alignment. Lumbar flexion and hip mobilisation exercises are important. Exercises aim to reduce lumbar lordotic posture. Analgesia is recommended and the use of neuropathic painkillers is helpful. Epidural injections are not recommended by NICE for patients with spinal stenosis due to the lack of evidence for short and long-term benefit (NICE, 2020). Should conservative management fail, and the patient feels the symptoms are significantly affecting their life, then surgery (usually decompressive laminectomy) may be performed.

Questionnaires can be used to identify and classify patients with spinal stenosis (Table 7.2).

MULTIPLE CHOICE QUESTION (MCQ) QUESTIONS

1. A 16-year-old male cricketer presents to your clinic with gradually worsening lower back pain. It felt worse after a recent bowling session. You suspect spondylolysis or spondylolisthesis. Which of the following examination findings would you least expect to find?

    A. A limitation of lumbar flexion and extension
    B. Pain with single-leg standing and lumbar extension toward the affected side
    C. A positive straight leg raise test on the affected side
    D. 'Heart-shaped' buttocks on inspection
    E. An abnormal, 'stiff-legged' gait

2. You are performing a neurological examination on a patient with back pain. You move on to reflexes. Which nerve root is the patellar tendon reflex primarily transmitted through?

    A. L2
    B. L3
    C. L4
    D. L5
    E. S1

3. Whilst providing medical cover at a Rugby Union match, you attend to a player with a suspected cervical spine injury. Which of the following fracture types is considered the most stable?

    A. Burst fracture
    B. Flexion teardrop fracture
    C. Clay-shoveler fracture
    D. Extension teardrop fracture
    E. Hangman's fracture

4. A 32-year-old female attends clinic with lower back pain radiating down her left leg. She has an unremarkable past medical history and is also getting paraesthesia at the lateral aspect of her left foot. You suspect radiculopathy. Which of the following aetiologies of radiculopathy is most likely?

    A. Metastatic cancer
    B. Spondylodiscitis
    C. Haemangioblastoma
    D. Osteophytosis
    E. Disc herniation

5. A male footballer comes to see you with a unilateral foot drop. He describes an absence of sensation in his lateral left leg and left foot. On assessment, you notice that he has full power with ankle eversion; however, dorsiflexion and inversion are weak with resisted testing. What is the most likely diagnosis?

    A. Common peroneal palsy
    B. Cervical stenosis
    C. Cauda Equina Syndrome
    D. S1 Radiculopathy
    E. L5 Radiculopathy

MULTIPLE CHOICE QUESTION (MCQ) ANSWERS

1. Answer D

   Although a 'heart-shaped' buttocks is seen due to sacral retroversion, this usually occurs in severe cases of lumbosacral spondylolisthesis and is rare. Answers A, B and E are characteristic findings. Answer C may occur due to hamstring tightness or neural involvement from spondylolisthesis.

2. Answer C

   Although the L2 and L3 nerve roots contribute, L4 is the primary nerve root contributing to the patellar tendon reflex.

3. Answer C

   A Clay-shoveler fracture is a single column fracture that avulses the spinous process, usually after sudden flexion. Although some of the other answers may be stable, they are not always considered stable.

4. Answer E

   In this scenario, there are no red flag features. Disc herniation is the commonest cause of lumbar radiculopathy. Degenerative spondylolisthesis and osteophytosis would be more common causes in an older population.

5. Answer E

   Answers A and E can both present with weakness of dorsiflexion. However, peroneal nerve palsy would present with ankle eversion weakness (the peroneal muscles are affected). L5

radiculopathy usually presents with ankle inversion weakness, as in this case.

REFERENCES AND FURTHER READING

Cleland, J.C., Koppenhaver, S and J, Su. J. (2016). *Netter's Orthopaedic Clinical Examination: An Evidence-Based Approach*. 3rd ed. Philadelphia: Elsevier.

Hay, E., Dunn, K., Hill, J., Lewis, M., Mason, E., Konstantinou, K., Sowden, G., Somerville, S., Vohora, K., Whitehurst, D., Main, C. (2008). A randomised clinical trial of subgrouping and targeted treatment for low back pain compared with best current care: The STarT back trial study protocol. *BMC Musculoskeletal Disorders*, 9, p. 58.

Kalichman, L., Hunter, D.J. (2007). Lumbar facet joint osteoarthritis: A review. *Semin Arthritis Rheum*, 37(2), pp. 69–80.

Konno, S., et al. (2007). A diagnostic support tool for lumbar spinal stenosis: A self-administered, self-reported history questionnaire. *BMC Musculoskelet Disord*, 8, p. 102.

National Institute for Health and Care Excellence (NICE). (2020). Low back pain and sciatica in over 16s: Assessment and management. *NG59*. Available at: www.nice.org.uk/guidance/ng59

Savage, R.A., Whitehouse, G.H and Roberts, N. (1997). The relationship between the magnetic resonance imaging appearance of the lumbar spine and low back pain, age and occupation in males. *Eur Spine*. 6, pp. 106–114.

Paediatric Sport and Exercise Medicine **8**

David Whittaker, Jude McDowell and Kush Joshi

ANATOMICAL AND PHYSIOLOGICAL SPECIFICS OF CHILDREN AND YOUNG PEOPLE RELEVANT TO SPORT AND EXERCISE MEDICINE

The anatomy and physiology of the developing athlete is unique compared to individuals of skeletal maturity, resulting in important considerations for the sports physician. Growth in long bones is primarily by endochondral ossification. Primary ossification centres are present by birth and secondary ossification centres develop throughout childhood, allowing for bone lengthening and maturation.

Between the metaphysis and epiphysis of a skeletally immature bone, lies the physis—the site of bone growth. The physis is made up of several zones: the germinal zone, which is adjacent to the epiphysis; the proliferative zone; the hypertrophic zone and the zone of ossification, which is adjacent to the metaphysis. Damage to the vulnerable physis can have a significant impact on growth.

Developing bones are more elastic than the skeletally mature, and the periosteum is thicker. This can result in bowing and greenstick-type fractures. The healing time of developing bone is faster than in the skeletally mature. Developing cartilage is thicker and at greater risk of injury in the paediatric population.

The bony sites of tendon insertion, known as apophyses, are considerably weaker than in adults. The apophyses are weaker than the attaching tendons, increasing the risk of avulsion injuries and apophysitis (due to repetitive traction). In children, ligaments and tendons are not only stronger than the apophyses,

they are more elastic, hence trauma to these structures is less likely.

Other differences in children include evolving neurodevelopment, skill acquisition, coordination and psychology. One must also consider the relevance of growth spurts, with increases in bone length and muscle mass. These are important when planning rehabilitation and exercise programmes for children.

These anatomical and physiological differences, when compared to skeletally mature athletes, are reflected in the injury patterns seen in the paediatric population. Acute injuries may provoke specific fracture patterns, growth plate injuries, sprains and apophyseal avulsions. Chronic injuries are often a response to repetitive microtrauma, and can present with apophysitis, osteochondrosis and stress fractures.

RED FLAGS IN PAEDIATRIC SEM

An outline of important signs and symptoms is covered in Table 8.1.

Juvenile Idiopathic Arthritis (JIA)

JIA describes an inflammatory arthropathy, defined as arthritis of one or more joints, for 16 or more weeks, in those under 16. There are subsets of JIA that include oligoarticular JIA, polyarticular JIA, and systemic onset JIA. The aetiology is not fully understood, but genetic susceptibility is thought to play a role, with multiple genes implicated. Infections may

DOI: 10.1201/9781003179979-8

PAEDIATRIC SPORT AND EXERCISE MEDICINE

Osteosarcoma

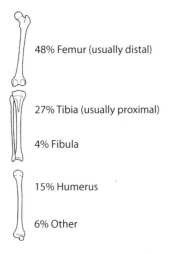

48% Femur (usually distal)

27% Tibia (usually proximal)

4% Fibula

15% Humerus

6% Other

Ewing Sarcoma

 20% Pelvis

 16% Chest wall and ribs

45% Lower limbs (femur most common)
19% Other
85% Bone
15% Soft tissue

Salter-Harris classification for physeal injuries

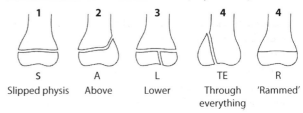

1	2	3	4	4
S	A	L	TE	R
Slipped physis	Above	Lower	Through everything	'Rammed'

Osteochondrosis and Apophysitis

Sinding-Larsen-Johansson disease – inferior pole of patella

Osgood-Schlatter disease – tibial tubercle

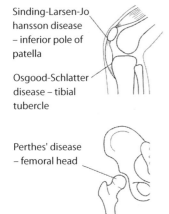

Perthes' disease – femoral head

Freiberg's disease – metatarsal head

Iselin's disease – apophysitis at the base of 5th metatarsal

Kohler's disease – navicular

Sever's disease – calcaneal apophysitis

Traction Apophysitis
- Injury to the cartilage and bony attachment of tendons
- More common in growth spurts (rapid bony growth with a lag in muscle and tendinous growth)
- Usually self-limiting
- Associated with poor flexibility and strength
- Management is usually activity modification

Osteochondrosis
- Self-limiting developmental derangement of normal bone growth, involving necrosis at the epiphyseal ossification centres
- Genetics and repetitive trauma can predispose
- Can be articular, non-articular or physeal
- Management is usually activity modification to prevent additional trauma, secondary deformity
- Surgery may be required to remove loose bodies or realign fixed bony deformities

Figure 8.1 Pictorial overview.

Table 8.1 Red Flag conditions and their associated signs and symptoms

Condition	Signs and Symptoms
Inflammatory arthritis	Motor milestone delay or regression, swollen joints, fever, systemic illness
Inflammatory muscle disease	Myoglobinuria, systemic illness, weakness, motor milestone delay or regression
Fracture	Bone pain, unremitting pain, abnormal loss of function, gait disturbance
NAI	Incongruent history and presentation, bruising, delay/frequency with medical services, inappropriate interactions etc.
Malignancy	Bone pain, systemic illness, malaise, night pain, weight loss, back pain with red flags or neurology, lymphadenopathy
Infection	Fever, systemic illness

be involved in triggering an immune response at the start of disease onset.

Aside from common features of joint pain and swelling, other signs of JIA include early morning joint stiffness, gait disturbance, loss of usual developmental motor milestones, change in behaviour and lack of enjoyment (or avoidance) of activities. Systemic onset JIA may present with rash and fever.

Oligoarticular JIA is commonest and tends to affect large joints. Polyarticular JIA usually affects the small joints of the hands. Management includes urgent referral to a rheumatologist for investigation. Serum ANA is commonly raised. FBC, U&E, LFT, CRP, ESR, anti-CCP and Rheumatoid factor may be requested in the SEM setting.

Infection

Infection, including septic arthritis and osteomyelitis, may present with soft tissue, bony or joint pain and swelling, erythema, fever, and systemic features of inflammation. Urgent management with antibiotics is usually required, with surgical intervention sometimes needed. Osteomyelitis in children is most often due to haematogenous seeding of bacteria to the metaphyseal bone.

Cancer

Bone, soft tissue and joint malignancy should always be considered by the sports physician. Features of concern include atraumatic or non-activity related pain, night pain, limp, reduced joint range of motion or mass. An assessment should also be made of systemic features of malignancy, such as weight loss, appetite change and night sweats. A thorough examination is important, including for lymphadenopathy.

At the time of writing, NICE guidance recommends that an urgent (within 48 hours) plain X-ray should be performed in children and young people with unexplained bony pain or swelling, and an urgent (within 48 hours) ultrasound conducted for unexplained soft tissue lumps. The guidance recommends an appointment with a specialist within 48 hours if these tests are suggestive of bony or soft tissue malignancy. An MRI may be needed to aid diagnosis.

OSTEOSARCOMA

Osteosarcomas are a malignant mass of osteoblasts, and are the most common bony malignancy in children and young adults. They are more common in males than females. The most frequent sites are the distal femur, the tibia and the humerus. High vigilance is needed, as individuals may present months after initial onset of pain and often following trauma (pathological fracture should also be considered).

EWING SARCOMA

Ewing Sarcomas are a malignant mass of neural crest cells, and are the second most common bone malignancy of children and young adults of all ages (but the commonest bone malignancy in those under 10). Males are more commonly affected than females and there is a predominance toward Caucasian populations. Common sites of involvement include the femur, pelvis, upper limb bones, spine and ribs.

Typically, they present with night pain. Because lung metastasis is common, considering respiratory symptoms is also important.

LEUKAEMIA

Leukaemia may present with bone and joint pain. Other features include recurrent infections, bruising, bleeding, fever and fatigue. A blood test will indicate abnormality in the full blood count.

NEUROBLASTOMA

Neuroblastomas arise from the peripheral nervous system and commonly present with abdominal pain, abdominal swelling or mass, or organomegaly. Paraspinal masses can cause radicular features.

SOFT TISSUE SARCOMAS

Examples include rhabdomyosarcoma and synovial sarcoma. The former is more common in children and young people and can be found anywhere on the body; the latter more commonly found in the extremities. They usually present with a rapidly growing mass or soft tissue pain. An urgent ultrasound is normally recommended for further evaluation.

Non-Accidental Injury (NAI)

NAI should be considered for all paediatric presentations, especially those involving injury. A full history and examination are key and it is important to receive the history from the child, not just a parent or guardian. Certain factors such as paediatric developmental delay, chronic medical conditions, disability, prematurity, inappropriate parenting skills and parental mental health issues, alcohol or substance misuse, can increase the risk of NAI.

CLINICAL CONSIDERATIONS

Some features that should alert a clinician to consider NAI include:

- History inconsistent with injuries sustained or examination findings
- Injuries or history inconsistent with a child's developmental age

- History of non-accidental injury or intimate partner violence within the family
- Unusual bruises, bites, burns or abrasions
- Occult rib fractures or spiral fractures
- Delay in seeking medical assistance
- Frequent attendance at medical services
- Inappropriate interaction between child and caregiver

STRESS FRACTURES

Although uncommon, the sports physician should always have a high level of suspicion for stress fractures, particularly in the sporting environment. As with adults, the history will be one of worsening pain with activity. Training loads should be monitored; however, it can be difficult to quantify what a child is doing outside an academy environment. This may be influenced by the expectations of parents and family, and a collateral history is key. Table 8.1 Red Flag conditions and their associated signs and symptoms.

CHILD PROTECTION OVERVIEW

The GMC highlights that all doctors have a responsibility to consider the wellbeing and needs of children and young people and to protect them. Decisions should always be made in the best interests of children and young people and, whilst they have a right to confidentiality, this must not prevent the appropriate sharing of information to protect them.

Healthcare providers should have a clinician named as the safeguarding lead for children, who should be a contact for clinicians concerned of child abuse or neglect.

BONY INJURIES

The bones of children and young people respond to traumatic forces in different ways than in adults, leading to different patterns of injury.

Common Fracture Patterns

BUCKLE

Buckle fractures (also referred to as Torus fractures) are the result of an axial force to a bone, resulting in compression. These are most common at the junction between the diaphysis and metaphysis and produce a characteristic bulging of the bony cortex. In children, the most common site of buckle fracture is the distal radius. These can be managed with a cast.

GREENSTICK

Greenstick fractures are partial thickness bony injuries, with cortical interruption on only one side of the bone and commonly occur in response to a longitudinal force. They occur due to the increased elasticity and thicker periosteum of developing bones. The fracture pattern often shows cortical fracture along the convex side, but an intact cortex on the concave side. Most can be managed with immobilisation; however, some may require open reduction and fixation depending on the level of angulation.

BOWING

Skeletally immature bone may respond to longitudinal force with bowing or bending as opposed to breaking. Sometimes these require manipulation and reduction if the angulation is greater than 20 degrees. The ulna is a commonly affected bone.

PHYSEAL INJURIES

Fractures affecting the growth plate (physis) may have an impact on bony growth, so prompt assessment and management is key. The potential impact on bony growth and the management required is dependent on the position and site of injury. An important aim of management is to reduce the risk of limb shortening or deformity secondary to physeal injury. Because of this, classification of the fracture is important; the most commonly used classification system is the Salter-Harris classification.

Salter-Harris Classification

- Type 1: fracture through the physis only
- Type 2: fracture through the physis and metaphysis
- Type 3: fracture through the physis and epiphysis
- Type 4: fracture through the physis, metaphysis and epiphysis
- Type 5: crushing injury to the physis

These can be more easily remembered using the mnemonic SALTER:

- **S**lipped physis
- **A**bove the physis
- Be**L**ow the physis
- **T**hrough **E**verything
- **R**ammed

Type 1 and 2 fractures do not affect the germinal layer of the physis and, therefore, should not impact bone growth. They should be referred for orthopaedic assessment but can usually be managed with casting. Types 3 and 4 should be referred urgently for orthopaedic assessment due to the risk of growth arrest and are often managed with open reduction and internal fixation. Type 5 injuries are rare and should also be referred urgently.

APOPHYSEAL INJURIES

The apophyses are the cartilaginous tendon attachment sites of developing bones and are prone to avulsion.

Table 8.2 Common Avulsion Sites

Site	Tendon Attachment
Base of fifth metatarsal	Peroneus brevis
Tibial Tubercle	Patellar tendon
Lesser trochanter of femur	Iliopsoas
Greater trochanter of femur	Gluteus medius
Ischial tuberosity	Hamstring
Anterior inferior iliac spine	Rectus femoris
Anterior superior iliac spine	Sartorius
Medial humeral epicondyle	Wrist flexors

Common patterns of avulsion injury seen in children and young people are included in Table 8.2.

These injuries commonly present during activity with acute pain, often after acute eccentric muscle contraction (e.g. from sprinting). Examination may identify tenderness at the insertion/origin site and weakness and pain on resisted muscle testing. A plain X-ray is the first line investigation.

Management may be conservative or surgical, depending on the impact on functional state and degree of displacement. Those with minimal displacement can be managed with initial rest before physiotherapy. This aims to restore range of motion and strength before a graduated return to play. Those with large degrees of displacement, typically with a gap ≥2 cm, require surgical fixation.

HIP PATHOLOGY

Slipped Upper Femoral Epiphysis (SUFE)

SUFE is a condition where there is slipping of the epiphysis in relation to the metaphysis in response to mechanical forces. SUFE most commonly occurs in older children, often between the ages of 12 and 15 years. It is associated with raised body mass index and endocrine disorders such as thyroid dysfunction and is more common in boys.

A slip may occur acutely or can be a more gradual process. It is usually unilateral although it can be bilateral. Presentations include pain in the hip, groin or thigh; however, it may present with knee pain or an isolated limp. Examination may demonstrate an abnormal gait and a shortened and externally rotated leg, with reduced range of hip internal rotation and abduction. During hip flexion the leg may be seen to move into external rotation.

Plain X-rays are the usual first line investigation (a frog-leg view may be included). Klein's line, a line drawn along the superior femoral neck, should intersect the lateral border of the epiphysis in a normal patient—lack of intersection suggests slipping of the epiphysis. Patients with SUFE are at risk of avascular necrosis and management includes prompt orthopaedic assessment for consideration of surgical fixation. In the interim, a period of non-weight bearing should take place to avoid propagation of the slipping.

Perthes' Disease

Perthes' Disease is an osteochondrosis affecting the proximal femoral epiphysis. It occurs most commonly in children aged 4 to 10 and is more common in boys than girls.

Presentations include pain in the hip, thigh, groin and knee, as well as limping. Examination may demonstrate reduced hip abduction and internal rotation and an antalgic or Trendelenburg gait.

Plain radiographs may demonstrate irregularity of the femoral head and medial joint space widening. MRI may be more sensitive at identifying early disease.

Most cases can be managed in a SEM setting, however surgical management is sometimes required. Education is key to explain the condition and highlight the risk of early onset osteoarthritis with poor management. Those under 8 years are often managed with analgesia, activity modification (avoidance of running and jumping) to reduce the risk of progression and physical therapy to restore range of motion. Older patients with lateral pillar collapse may be managed surgically with femoral osteotomy, amongst other techniques.

Transient Synovitis and Septic Hip

Transient synovitis is a diagnosis of exclusion in a limping child. The condition is thought to be in response to a viral infection, as there is often a history of a preceding upper respiratory tract infection. It is most common between the ages of 2 and 8.

Presentation is usually via a limp, hip or knee pain. There may be reduced global hip range of movement. Exclusion of more serious causes of hip pathology involves blood tests (inflammatory markers) and plain radiographs, to evaluate for trauma, SUFE and Perthes' disease. Ultrasound may be required, with consideration of aspiration to differentiate between transient synovitis and septic arthritis.

Septic arthritis requires antibiotic therapy, often alongside surgical washout, whereas transient synovitis normally improves with rest and simple analgesia.

Other

Snapping hip (either external—the iliotibial tract sliding over the greater trochanter—or internal—the iliopsoas tendon sliding over the femoral head, iliopectineal ridge, iliopsoas bursa or an exostosis of the lesser trochanter) is common in adolescent females. Cases usually respond well to activity modification and physiotherapy.

KNEE PATHOLOGY

Osteochondritis Dissecans of the Knee

Osteochondritis Dissecans refers to a process of avascular necrosis of subchondral bone, which can result in osteochondral defects and intra-articular loose bodies. In the lower limb, it most commonly affects the medial femoral condyle of the knee and is thought to be secondary to a vascular event, primary trauma or repetitive trauma. It is associated with jumping sports.

Presentation is with activity related pain. There may be joint line tenderness and swelling on examination. X-ray can be used first line and may demonstrate bony irregularity, fragmentation and loose bodies; however, MRI is generally the investigation of choice and should be used if there is high clinical suspicion.

The condition is usually managed with rest from aggravating activities and physiotherapy. The presence of loose bodies or larger osteochondral lesions with mechanical symptoms should prompt surgical consideration for fixation or removal of loose bodies, the latter placing athletes at increased risk of early-onset osteoarthritis.

Osgood-Schlatter Disease

Osgood-Schlatter Disease is an osteochondritis of the tibial tuberosity growth plate. The pathophysiology is thought to be due to repetitive quadriceps contraction causing traction of the patella tendon at the growth plate. The condition is more common in boys and associated with growth spurts, running and jumping sports. It can be unilateral or bilateral.

The condition commonly presents with activity related anterior knee pain. Examination may reveal tenderness and swelling at the tibial tuberosity and pain with knee extension.

The diagnosis is clinical; however, X-rays are sometimes performed to exclude bony malignancy or other pathology. It is a self-limiting condition and activity modification, but not complete rest, is key. Ice and simple analgesia after activity may provide symptomatic

relief. Education is important to allow patients, parents and coaches to understand the role of load in the condition. Physiotherapy and biomechanical assessment may be useful to correct abnormalities such as excessive pronation and tight quadriceps muscles. With correct management, the individual can continue athletic pursuits with little to no discomfort.

Sinding-Larsen-Johansson Disease

This is an osteochondritis of the patella tendon origin at the inferior pole of the patella. It is commonly seen in adolescent athletes but is less common than Osgood-Schlatter Disease.

It presents with activity-related anterior knee pain, with examination findings of tenderness and swelling at the inferior pole of the patella and pain with knee extension.

Management is similar to that of Osgood-Schlatter Disease, with a focus on education and activity modification. Ice and simple analgesia after activity may provide symptomatic relief.

Other

Patellofemoral pain is an extremely common presentation in the paediatric population. Most often, there is no significant underlying pathology and it is biomechanical in nature or related to overload. This condition is covered in more detail in Chapter 6.

FOOT AND ANKLE

Sever's Disease

Sever's disease is a calcaneal apophysitis thought to be due to repetitive traction of the Achilles tendon at its insertion. It is commonly seen in skeletally immature athletes and has an association with tight gastrocnemius and soleus muscles.

It commonly presents with activity related posterior heel pain. Examination may reveal limited ankle dorsiflexion and tenderness and swelling at the Achilles tendon insertion. The diagnosis is clinical; however, ultrasound or MRI may be useful to exclude other pathology.

Management should consist of an initial period of activity modification followed by gradual increases in training load. Heel raises in shoes, or taping, may help reduce pain, along with ice and simple analgesia. Physiotherapy focusing on posterior calf stretching and plantar flexor strengthening is the mainstay of treatment.

Iselin's Disease

Iselin's disease is an osteochondritis of the base of the fifth metatarsal, thought to be due to repetitive traction from the peroneus brevis tendon on the apophysis. It is commonly seen between the ages of 8 and 14.

The condition often presents with activity related pain in the lateral foot that improves with rest. Examination may reveal tenderness and swelling at the base of the fifth metatarsal, with pain exacerbated by resisted eversion. X-ray is the first line investigation and may demonstrate irregularity at the apophysis with bony fragmentation.

Management involves activity modification and off-loading. Simple analgesia and ice may help with pain acutely. Those that do not respond to conservative management could be considered for a period of off-loading in a walking boot, or referral to an Orthopaedic surgeon in cases of non-union.

Traction Apophysitis at the Navicular

This commonly presents with medial foot pain that is worse with activity and is associated with pes planus and excessive pronation. On examination, there may be pain with resisted foot eversion (as the tibialis posterior tendon provides traction on the navicular).

Management is by off-loading from aggravating activities, before a gradual strengthening programme of the tibialis posterior tendon.

Kohler's Disease

Kohler's disease is an idiopathic osteochondrosis of the navicular. It usually affects those below the age of 8 and is more common in boys than girls. The underlying pathophysiology is not completely understood; however, it may relate to repetitive mechanical forces upon the late ossifying navicular.

Kohler's disease usually presents with midfoot pain and limping. Examination may show tenderness and

swelling over the navicular. Plain radiographs are the first line investigation and may demonstrate flattening, fragmentation and sclerosis of the navicular.

It is a self-limiting disease that resolves with time. A walking boot for 6 weeks can decrease the duration of symptoms.

Freiberg's Disease

Freiberg's Disease is an osteochondrosis of the metatarsal head. It is often seen in the second metatarsal and is thought to be due to infarction and avascular necrosis that can lead to collapse of the metatarsal head. It is regularly seen in dancers and female athletes between 12 and 18 years old.

It usually presents with forefoot pain aggravated by weight bearing. Examination may demonstrate tenderness and swelling at the metatarsal head, with possible reduced range of joint motion. Plain radiographs are the first line investigation and can demonstrate a spectrum from flattening, fragmentation and subchondral sclerosis at the metatarsal head, to collapse and joint space loss. MRI can be useful and is more sensitive.

Early-stage disease can be managed with off-loading, footwear and padding to reduce pressure on the metatarsal heads. A walking cast or boot for 4–6 weeks can help settle symptoms. Intractable cases should be referred to an Orthopaedic surgeon.

Other

Other common conditions include sprains, ankle instability and normal variant walking patterns:

- Leg alignment discrepancy
- Flat feet (pes planus)
- Out-toeing
- In-toeing
- Toe-walking

Toe-walking is conservatively managed with stretching, gait re-education and strengthening. If this fails, serial casting or orthopaedic referral is warranted. In-toeing and out-toeing is also managed conservatively (such as with modified activities and sitting positions), unless external or internal torsions are severe enough to require surgery. Tibial torsion usually corrects with normal growth by six years and femoral anteversion by twelve years. Curved feet (metatarsus adductus), which is associated with in-toeing, usually corrects by walking age.

SHOULDER

Rotator Cuff Injuries

These are much less common in the paediatric population than in adults, though have been reported in throwing athletes and swimmers, who develop rotator cuff instability and subacromial impingement. Management is via rest from aggravating activities and rehabilitation, focusing on scapular and rotator cuff biomechanics and strengthening.

Clavicle Fractures

The clavicle is more commonly fractured than other bones in the shoulder, with the middle third the most likely site. Neurovascular injury is rare and management is usually via immobilisation in a sling for 6–10 weeks. Surgery is necessary for open or significantly displaced fractures, or those with neurovascular complications.

Shoulder Instability

Glenohumeral instability is often secondary to traumatic anterior dislocation, sustained typically with the arm in an abducted and externally rotated position. Recurrent subluxation may also reduce joint stability. Acute dislocation should be managed with reduction and assessment for fracture, neurovascular injury and bony or soft tissue Bankart lesions. Reported recurrence rates in the literature are high, and rehabilitation with physiotherapy is key. Surgical stabilisation may be considered for recurrent instability and in those aged under 25, as they are at high risk of further dislocation.

Atraumatic instability may be seen in upper limb athletes including gymnastics, tennis and throwing sports and may be related to hypermobility, another common presentation seen in the paediatric population. Rehabilitation includes education, refining sport-specific biomechanics and rotator cuff strengthening.

Proximal Humeral Physeal Stress

Little Leaguers' Shoulder, so named after its prevalence amongst young throwing athletes, is a condition of repetitive stress upon the proximal humeral physis, that can result in widening and fragmentation. It is often seen between the ages of 10 and 13 and presents with activity related shoulder pain. Examination can demonstrate reduced range of movement and muscle wasting around the shoulder girdle. Diagnosis is typically clinical; however, X-rays can be valuable and demonstrate a widened physis on AP views. Management is through rest from aggravating activities, limiting throwing activities and correction of throwing biomechanics.

ELBOW AND WRIST

Supracondylar Fractures

Fractures of the supracondylar region are the commonest elbow fracture in children. The usual mechanism of injury is falling onto an outstretched hand. Presentation is with pain and deformity, and neurovascular compromise to the anterior interosseous and radial nerves is possible. Neuropraxia normally spontaneously resolves. X-rays are important but more subtle fractures can be missed. Elevation of the posterior fat pad can indicate underlying fracture and should be looked for on X-ray. Referral to orthopaedics for review is required—non-displaced fractures are usually managed with cast immobilisation for 3–4 weeks; displaced fractures may require closed or open reduction and pinning.

Panner's Disease

Panner's disease is an osteochondrosis of the capitellum. It is most commonly seen between 5 and 10 years of age and may be related to trauma, axial loading of the radio-capitellar joint (e.g. in gymnasts) and repetitive valgus stress during throwing. It is more common in the dominant upper limb.

It presents with activity related elbow pain and elbow stiffness. On examination, effusion may be present along with a reduced range of motion, especially elbow extension. There may be capitellum tenderness.

X-ray is the first line investigation, which commonly demonstrates irregularity of the capitellum, with sclerosis and possible fragmentation. Loose bodies suggest an alternative diagnosis of osteochondritis dissecans of the capitellum. Furthermore, Panner's disease is typically seen in younger children, whereas osteochondritis dissecans is seen in teenagers.

The condition is usually self-limiting and management involves off-loading from aggravating activities, correction of upper limb biomechanics (e.g. avoiding valgus stress when throwing) and range of motion exercises.

Osteochondritis Dissecans of the Capitellum

Osteochondritis Dissecans refers to a process of avascular necrosis of subchondral bone, which can result in osteochondral defects and loose bodies. In the elbow, it is associated with throwing sports and gymnastics and thought to be secondary to repetitive trauma.

Presentation is with activity related pain and restriction of joint range of motion, with localised tenderness and swelling on examination. X-ray is the initial investigation and may demonstrate bony irregularity, fragmentation and loose bodies, however MRI should be used if there is high clinical suspicion in the absence of X-ray changes.

The condition is usually managed with rest from aggravating activities and physiotherapy with a focus on forearm strengthening and biomechanics, however the presence of loose bodies should prompt orthopaedic review.

Traction Apophysitis at the Medial Humeral Epicondyle

This condition is commonly termed 'Little Leaguers' Elbow' due to the prevalence amongst throwing athletes. Repetitive valgus force at the elbow leads to a traction apophysitis of the wrist flexors. It commonly presents with medial elbow pain aggravated by throwing. There may be tenderness and swelling over the medial humeral epicondyle, with pain aggravated by resisted wrist flexion with the elbow held in extension.

Avulsion at this site is possible so an X-ray may be indicated. Management involves resting from aggravating activities, correction of throwing biomechanics and a stretching and strengthening programme for the wrist flexors.

Distal Radius Fractures

These are common in children and may follow a buckle or greenstick pattern. Management is with wrist splinting or casting, with manipulation and/or open reduction required for those with gross displacement or neurovascular compromise. It is important to assess for a Galeazzi fracture pattern—a distal radius fracture with distal physeal disruption and therefore radio-ulnar joint disruption—as these require reduction.

Distal Radius Physeal Stress

Repetitive wrist loading in the skeletally immature athlete (e.g. with gymnastics) can result in stress at the ulnar and radial physes. Presentation is with wrist pain and reduced range of movement, with stiffness and tenderness on examination. Plain X-ray may demonstrate physeal widening with irregular borders and a positive ulnar variance in longstanding cases.

Management is via rest and immobilisation for 3–6 weeks, with education and management of training load.

SPINAL DISORDERS IN CHILDREN

Scheuermann's Disease

Scheuermann's disease is a disorder of the vertebral bodies of the thoracic and lumbar spine that results in wedging of the anterior vertebrae and thoracic kyphosis. It commonly presents with activity related thoracic back pain. On examination there may be thoracic kyphosis, increased lumbar lordosis and reduced range of motion of the hamstrings.

Plain X-rays are first line, with the radiographic diagnostic criteria being vertebral wedging of >5 degrees in 3 or more consecutive vertebrae. Schmorl's nodes and end-plate deformity may also be present.

Management includes physiotherapy, focusing on postural control, hamstring and lumbodorsal fascia flexibility and abdominal strengthening. Kyphosis of greater than 50 degrees should prompt consideration of bracing, and more than 75 degrees (with poor response to conservative treatment) should prompt consideration for.

Spondylosis and Spondylolisthesis

Spondylosis, a defect of the pars interarticularis, is usually second to repetitive lumbar spinal extension and rotation and is associated with sports such as cricket (bowling) and gymnastics. It is usually seen at the fifth lumbar vertebra, followed by the fourth. It can be unilateral or bilateral—the latter predisposing to anterior vertebral slippage (in relation to the vertebra below it), termed spondylolisthesis.

Patients may have asymptomatic spondylosis with radiographic evidence of a stress response, or a symptomatic stress response, or a stress fracture. Previous pars fractures may result in chronic non-union.

The presentation for symptomatic injury is lumbar back pain, possibly radiating toward the buttocks, aggravated by lumbar extension and rotation. Examination may reveal reduced lumbar spinal range of motion and tenderness over the pars interarticularis region.

Plain X-ray may demonstrate a pars interarticularis fracture on oblique views—the so-called 'Scottie Dog Sign.' MRI should be performed first line to assess for stress response and fracture. Bone scans are useful to identify bone stress, whilst CT is more useful to evaluate bone bridging, however the risk of radiation, particularly in the paediatric population, must be considered.

Management involves off-loading from activities and avoidance of lumbar extension and rotation. Physiotherapy is important to strengthen the core, back and hip musculature and to correct postural imbalances such as a posterior pelvic tilt and hamstring tightness. Braces are sometimes used for patients with pain with day-to-day activities. Once asymptomatic with no radiological evidence of bone stress, athletes can begin a return to sport programme, with the likely return to play between 3 and 6 months.

Spondylolisthesis is graded by the degree of slipping of the vertebra in relation to the vertebra below (Table 8.3).

The management involves similar rehabilitation to spondylosis. In young people, slippage may progress

Table 8.3 Spondylolisthesis Grading

Grade	% Slipping
I	0–25
II	25–50
III	50–75
IV	75–100

during growth spurts. Those with a slip of grade III or IV should avoid contact sports and be referred for specialist management, as surgical fixation may be indicated.

Scoliosis

Idiopathic scoliosis is often an incidental finding and is more common in females. It may be managed with bracing in skeletally immature athletes with significant growth remaining and with a curve of >25 degrees, or in those that demonstrate curve progression. The Adams forward-bend test may be helpful and genetic testing can predict curve progression. Plain X-rays are the common investigation to assess curvature. Those that fail to respond, or with curves of >50 degrees, should be referred to a paediatric spinal surgeon for consideration for fixation.

Other

Low back and neck pain in adolescents is becoming more common in an increasingly sedentary population. Excluding other significant pathology is key; however, advice regarding lifestyle modification and exercise is often sufficient.

MEDICO-LEGAL AND ETHICAL CONSIDERATIONS

Consent and Capacity in Children and Young People

The GMC guidance 'Protecting children and young people: the responsibilities of all doctors' states capacity to consent is assumed at the age of 16 years old; however, those under 16 may also have capacity depending on their ability to understand risks and benefits and their maturity. This involves understanding what is involved, why it is being performed and the possible consequences of having or not having the proposed treatment or investigation. They must demonstrate an ability to understand, retain, weigh up the information and explain their decision.

When assessing best interests, it is important to consider the views of the child, parents, those close to the child, other healthcare professionals and cultural, religious or other beliefs.

Confidentiality

The GMC guidance 'Protecting children and young people: the responsibilities of all doctors' advises that appropriate agencies should be informed promptly if you are concerned that a child or young person is at risk or suffering from abuse or neglect. The guidance advises you should ask consent to share information unless there is a compelling reason not to do so, and inform them what information has been shared and why, unless this may put them at risk of harm.

Physical Activity Guidelines

The UK Chief Medical Officer sets physical activity guidelines for all ages. Physical activity is important to promote healthy bone and joint development, maintain a healthy weight and support development of movement and coordination. The current UK physical activity guidelines at the time of publication are summarised below:

UNDER 1 YEAR

A recommended 30 minutes of tummy time per day. As mobility increases this should include a variety of activities such as crawling.

1–5 YEARS

A recommended 180 minutes of activity per day, including activities such as playing, jumping, games, throwing, skipping and walking. The activity should ideally be spread out across the day.

5–18 YEARS

Children and young adults should achieve 60 minutes of physical activity per day. This may include playing, active travel, walking, running, cycling, sports and dance.

MULTIPLE CHOICE QUESTION (MCQ) QUESTIONS

1. An 11-year-old female sprinter attends clinic with right hip pain. The pain came on acutely during sprint training the day before. On examination, the leg length and position is normal. There is full range of motion in the hip but pain with hip flexion. There is focal tenderness around the anterior inferior iliac spine. What is the most likely diagnosis?

   A. Iliopsoas bursitis
   B. Slipped upper femoral epiphysis
   C. Avulsion fracture involving rectus femoris
   D. Avulsion fracture involving sartorius
   E. Osteonecrosis of the femoral neck

2. A 16-year-old male ice skater presents with an 8-week history of right anterior knee pain. There is no history of injury. The athlete identifies the tibial tuberosity as the site of pain. Pain was initially present with activity but now is painful all the time, including at night. The athlete's coach reports the athlete has lost some weight recently and had a loss of appetite. On examination, there is a palpable bony tender mass at the tibial tuberosity. What would your next step be?

   A. Knee X-ray
   B. Knee MRI
   C. Patellar tendon ultrasound
   D. Knee CT
   E. No imaging required

3. A 13-year-old male recreational football player attends with a 6-week history of left hip and groin pain with activity. There is no history of trauma. He has a history of mild asthma and obesity. On examination the patient has an antalgic gait but normal appearance of the hip and groin. Adductor squeeze tests are negative and there is no hernia. When supine, the leg is noted to be in slight external rotation, with reduced internal rotation and abduction noted on examination. You arrange a left hip X-ray. What are the most likely findings?

   A. Joint space narrowing and osteophyte formation
   B. Subchondral sclerosis
   C. Femoral head irregularity and joint space widening

D. Slippage of the upper femoral epiphysis and an abnormal Klein's line

E. Normal findings

4. A 39-year-old lady is referred to your clinic for exercise advice after recently being diagnosed with type 2 diabetes. She has a raised BMI and reports she was bullied as a child for being overweight. She asks about the level of activity her 4-year-old should be aiming for. There is a family history of ischaemic heart disease and raised cholesterol in the maternal grandparents. The child is well and is achieving expected developmental milestones. What should you advise?

A. 30 minutes of physical activity per day

B. 60 minutes of physical activity per day

C. 120 minutes of physical activity per day

D. 180 minutes of physical activity per day

E. 200 minutes of physical activity per day

5. A 4-year-old attends ED in distress following a fall from a climbing frame in a local park. Her parents report she landed heavily on the right arm. She is too distressed to allow you to palpate, but points to her elbow as the source of pain. She is moving her hand, but is unable to flex the interphalangeal joint (IPJ) of the thumb and the index finger distal IPJ to form an "OK" sign. The rest of the neurological examination of the hand and forearm is normal. What is the most likely diagnosis?

A. Supracondylar fracture with anterior interosseous nerve injury

B. Mid shaft humeral fracture with radial nerve injury

C. Lateral humeral condyle fracture with median nerve injury

D. Radial head fracture with ulnar nerve injury

E. Medial humeral condyle fracture with posterior interosseous nerve injury

MULTIPLE CHOICE QUESTION (MCQ) ANSWERS

1. Answer C
The correct diagnosis is avulsion fracture of the rectus femoris, which attaches at the anterior inferior iliac spine. Due to weakness of the apophyses in comparison to the tendons, avulsion at the muscular attachment is likely to have

occurred. SUFE can occur acutely, though is less likely to produce tenderness at the anterior inferior iliac spine.

2. Answer A
Tibial tuberosity pain is not uncommon in young adults and is most commonly caused by Osgood Schlatter's disease. This patient displays red flag symptoms including night pain, weight loss, poor appetite and a bony mass. An urgent knee X-ray to examine for bony malignancy should be arranged. Osgood-Schlatter's disease presents similarly, however the red flag symptoms would be absent.

3. Answer D
This patient has a slipped upper femoral epiphysis (SUFE). This condition is most commonly seen between the ages of 12 and 15, is associated with male gender, raised body mass index and endocrine disorders. Klein's line, drawn along the superior femoral neck, should intersect the lateral border of the epiphysis in a normal patient—lack of intersection suggests slippage of the epiphysis. Joint space narrowing, osteophyte formation and subchondral sclerosis are changes associated with osteoarthritis. Femoral head irregularity and joint space widening are seen with Perthes' diseases, an avascular necrosis of the femoral head. This condition can present similarly to SUFE, however is more common between the ages of 4 and 10.

4. Answer D
The current UK Chief Medical Officer guidelines recommend that children between the ages of 1 and 4 should achieve 180 minutes of physical activity per day.

5. Answer A
This patient's pattern of neurological compromise fits with an anterior interosseous nerve injury, in which patients are unable to form the 'OK sign' with their thumb and index finger. The anterior interosseous nerve is the most commonly injured nerve in supracondylar fractures.

REFERENCES AND FURTHER READING

Armstrong, N and van Mechelen, W. 2017. *Oxford Textbook of Children's Sport and Exercise Medicine.* Oxford University Press, Oxford, UK. Third edition.

Rehabilitation and Disability Sport **9**

David Eastwood and Pippa Bennett

BACKGROUND

A disability is defined by the Equality act 2010 as 'a physical or mental impairment which has a substantial and long-term negative effect on your ability to do normal day-to-day activities.'

Sport for disabled athletes (Parasport) has grown significantly over recent years and the Paralympic Games is now one of the largest international sporting events globally. Physical activity has significant benefits in the disabled population, however the choice of sport or activity may require consideration of the physiological demands, as well as the cognitive and social ability of the participant. The availability of any additional facilities or support must also be considered such as wheelchair provision or extra assistance in moving and handling. Many para athletes have either acquired or congenital comorbidities, making adequate medical provision essential.

APPROACHING REHABILITATION

Rehabilitation is a process where a disabled person is assisted to enhance their functional ability. This may involve addressing physical, social or psychological needs. The rehabilitation process aims to promote ability and participation. Methods to achieve this include reducing disability with environmental or social adaptations or by promoting new skills that may reduce the impact of disability. Skills such as mobilisation using walking aids can be taught and

environments may be improved with adaptations such as stair rails or improved access.

As well as providing functional benefit for the patient, rehabilitation can help to reduce unnecessary complications. For example: if left untreated, incontinence issues may lead to urinary tract infection, sepsis or pressure sores.

Rehabilitation relies on teamwork and involves the coordinated efforts of professionals including doctors, nurses and various therapists. This approach can help coordinate care and improve outcomes. Care should be goal-oriented and roles should be allocated that are specific to the individual members of the team based on their strengths.

DISABILITY TYPES

Spinal Injuries

Spinal disability may be the result of a congenital problem such as neural tube defects, vascular issues such as spinal stroke, infection, tumour, degeneration or trauma. Motor vehicle accidents are the leading cause of spinal injuries. Other traumatic causes include falls, sport and secondary to violence.

The lowest unaffected part of the spinal cord is referred to as the neurological level of injury. Complete injuries are where there is complete paralysis below this level and incomplete injuries occur where there is some motor or sensory function below this level. Tetraplegia or quadriplegia means that arms, trunk, legs and pelvic organs are all affected by the injury,

DOI: 10.1201/9781003179979-9

REHABILITATION AND DISABILITY SPORT

Classification

Paralympic
1) Impaired muscle power
2) Impaired range of movement
3) Limb deficiency
4) Leg length difference
5) Short stature
6) Hypertonia
7) Ataxia
8) Athetosis
9) Vision impairment
10) Intellectual impairment

Amputation
A1 Bilateral above knee
A2 Unilateral above knee
A3 Bilateral below knee
A4 Unilateral below knee
A5 Bilateral above elbow
A6 Unilateral above elbow
A7 Bilateral below elbow
A8 Unilateral below elbow
A9 Combination of upper and lower limb

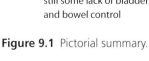

Wheelchairs with camber

Cerebral Palsy
CP1 Quadraplegic – significant spasticity, electric wheelchair users

CP2 Quadraplegic – able to propel wheelchair, better upper body control than **CP1**

CP3 Quadraplegic or severe hemiplegic – wheelchair users, almost full functional strength in dominant upper limb, may be able to transfer or mobilise short distances with assistance

CP4 Diplegic – moderate to severe. Wheelchair users, may be ambulant, upper limbs often have normal strength

CP5 Diplegic – moderate. Triplegic may be present in this class. Ambulant with assistive devices and normal static balance. May be able to run on track

CP6 Athetoid or ataxic – moderate. Ambulatory without assistance. Better lower limb function than **CP5**, may have more upper limb control issues than **CP5**

CP7 Hemiplegic – ambulatory, often have a limp due to lower limb spasticity

CP8 Minimal involvement – suitable for the minimally affected diplegic, hemiplegic, monoplegic, or athetoid/ataxic athlete

Autonomic Dysreflexia
- Usually level of **T6** or above is injured
- Unopposed sympathetic response causes hypertension
- May be used as a method of doping ('Boosting')

Spinal Injury
C1–C4 Tetraplegia/quadriplegia. Typically, paralysis of arms, legs and respiratory muscles. Require breathing support and all personal care

C5–C8 May have some upper limb sensation and function

T1–T5 Paraplegia, arm and hand function is usually normal

T6–T12 Typically, normal upper body movement. Likely to be paraplegic and able to manage manual wheelchair

L1–L5 May be able to walk

S1–S5 Likely to be able to walk, still some lack of bladder and bowel control

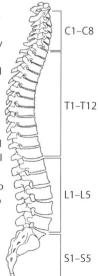

C1–C8

T1–T12

L1–L5

S1–S5

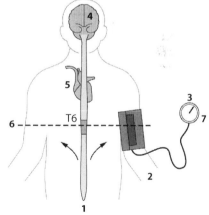

1. Stimulus
2. Sympathetic response = vasoconstriction
3. Hypertension
4. Baroreceptors signal to brain (Cranial nerves IX, X)
5. Heart rate slowed; vasodilation above spinal lesion
6. Inhibitory signals blocked beyond spinal lesion
7. Refractory hypertension

Figure 9.1 Pictorial summary.

whereas paraplegia means paralysis affects all or part of the trunk, legs and pelvic organs. The American Spinal Injury Association (ASIA) impairment scale is commonly used to grade injuries (Roberts et al., 2017). Grade A describes complete sensory or motor loss below the level of injury and at the other end of the scale, grade E denotes normal sensation and motor function.

Spinal injury can cause a number of unique medical problems:

- *Autonomic dysreflexia:* when the level of spinal cord injury is T6 or above, the normal sympathetic 'fight or flight' response can be unopposed. This imbalanced reflex sympathetic discharge can cause significant hypertension, which may be life threatening. As baroreceptors detect hypertension, the vagus nerve is stimulated, leading to bradycardia. Suspicion for this phenomenon, confirmed by hypertension, should prompt an emergency medical assessment. Sitting upright can help reduce blood pressure and anything restrictive should be loosened. Common causes should be identified and addressed promptly (e.g. bladder overdistention from urinary retention or faecal impaction). Antihypertensives may need to be administered.
- *Sensory loss:* increasing the risk of skin problems including pressure injury and infection.
- *Reduced exercise capacity:* in higher spinal lesions, sympathetic stimulation is compromised meaning cardiac contractility can be reduced and maximum heart rate can be limited to approximately 120 bpm, subsequently reducing cardiac output. Motor impairment of respiratory muscles may also adversely limit exercise capacity.
- *Impaired thermoregulation:* increasing the risk of heat illness and potentially impairing performance. This can be caused by the loss of autonomic control described above, impairing sweating and appropriate vasoconstriction or vasodilation.

CLINICAL CONSIDERATIONS

In the context of disability sport, it is important to recognise 'boosting,' or intentionally induced autonomic dysreflexia, as a form of improving performance. In this state, athletes may have a reduced perception of effort whilst exercising. Common methods include blocking catheters (causing bladder distension) and applying tight strapping to limbs. An athlete's pre-event blood pressure may be measured and if exceeding 180 mmHg systolic, they can be removed on the grounds of safety.

Levels of Injury

- C1-C4: Paralysis of the upper limbs, trunk, pelvic organs and lower limbs. The patient may not be able to breathe without support (C3, C4, C5 supply the phrenic nerve, which provides motor innervation of the diaphragm). Speech can be impaired and 24-hour personal care is needed.
- C5-C8: Depending on the level of injury there may be some upper limb function and sensation. This means patients may be able to transfer to and from a wheelchair and self-manage lack of bladder control with special equipment.
- T1-T5: These nerves affect the muscles of the chest, mid-back and abdomen. Patients are paraplegic but arm and hand function is usually normal.
- T6-T12: The patient should have normal upper body movement but is likely to be paraplegic. These nerves affect trunk muscles and depending on the level, there may be good balance in a seated position. They are likely to use a manual wheelchair.
- L1-L5: These injuries usually result in some loss of leg function (requiring a wheelchair). With adequate strength they may be able to use braces to mobilise. They will still have a lack of bowel and bladder control.
- S1-S5: Injury here will usually result in some loss of leg function but patients are likely to be able to walk. They will still have some lack of bowel and bladder control.

Amputees

Amputation is the surgical removal of a limb, but patients may have congenital limb deficiency. Amputation is usually required due to cancer, vascular disease or trauma, such as a road traffic accident.

The majority of sports can be played by below-knee amputees with the aid of prosthesis. Some sports, such as swimming, do not require a prosthesis and other sports, such as cycling, rugby and basketball, can be played with a wheelchair.

Cerebral Palsy

This is a group of permanent disorders of movement and coordination. It is due to damage to the developing brain and can happen before, during or after birth. It is either due to injury, disease or a developmental disorder.

There are three main groups:

1. Spastic: As a result of damage to the motor cortex, this causes stiff muscles, limiting movement. This can affect different limbs to varying degrees. Quadriplegia refers to all limbs involved. Diplegia is when symmetrical parts of the body are involved (legs or arms). Hemiplegia is when one side of the body is affected, triplegia three limbs and monoplegia only one limb.
2. Dyskinetic: As a result of damage to the basal ganglia, this causes involuntary movements.
3. Ataxic: As a result of damage to the cerebellum, muscle tone is reduced and balance is poor.

People with cerebral palsy are also at increased risk of other health problems including epilepsy, visual and hearing impairment and emotional disturbances.

Learning and Intellectual Disabilities

Learning disabilities are variable in their severity and are usually caused when a person's brain development is impaired. This may be caused by many things, such as a chromosomal disorder like Down's syndrome, or the result of a childhood illness such as meningitis. Learning disabilities are processing problems such as with reading (dyslexia), writing (dysgraphia) and mathematics (dyscalculia).

Intellectual disability involves difficulty with reasoning, problem-solving and decision making. People with intellectual disability tend to have a similar injury profile to non-disabled people. However, performance may be affected by difficulties in processing and executive function. Coaching and medical care may require careful communication so that information is understood and retained. The sport physician should also have an increased awareness for safeguarding issues in this vulnerable cohort.

CLINICAL CONSIDERATIONS

Down's syndrome can cause decreased muscle tone and atlantoaxial instability, which in turn can increase the risk of spinal injury. Although risk of atlantoaxial instability and neurological injury in sport is very rare, it is important to be aware of this possible complication, particularly in higher risk sports such as trampolining and diving. Pre-participation screening with radiography in asymptomatic individuals with Down's syndrome is not recommended.

DISABILITY CLASSIFICATION

Classification is a system that allows fair competition between people with different types of disability. It is usually sport specific, as impairments affect performance to a different extent depending on the goal.

In Paralympic classification, there are 10 eligible impairment types:

1. Impaired muscle power
2. Impaired range of movement
3. Limb deficiency
4. Leg length difference
5. Short stature
6. Hypertonia
7. Ataxia
8. Athetosis
9. Vision impairment
10. Intellectual impairment

The numerical figure in Para athletics classification represents the level of impairment. The lower the number, the more severe the impairment. E.g. In athletics track events, T11–13 is the class for visually impaired athletes, prefix 'T' for track, with T11 athletes being the most impaired (running blindfolded with a sighted guide).

Amputee Classification

The International Sports Organisation for the Disabled (ISOD) amputee classification ranges from A1 to A9. A1 to A4 are for people with lower limb amputations (bilateral above-knee, unilateral above-knee, bilateral below-knee and unilateral below-knee), A5 to A8 are for people with upper limb amputations (bilateral above-elbow, unilateral above-elbow, bilateral below-elbow, unilateral below-elbow) and A9 are for people with combinations of both.

Cerebral Palsy Classification

The classification system developed by the Cerebral Palsy International Sport and Recreational Association (CP-ISRA) includes eight classes: CP1-CP8. These classes are grouped into wheelchair and ambulatory classes. They are dependent on the extent of spasticity and athetosis. CP1 is the class for the group most physically affected by their cerebral palsy. CP2, CP3 and CP4 are general wheelchair classes. CP5, CP6, CP7 and CP8 are ambulatory classes.

Visually and Hearing Impaired Disability Classification

Deaf athletes may compete against other deaf competitors or may be integrated into competitions with other disability and non-disability sportspeople.

As outlined by the International Committee of Sports for the deaf, deaf sports people compete against others with a minimal hearing loss of 55 decibels in the better ear.

For visually impaired athletes, classification arises from an ophthalmological assessment of visual acuity and visual fields and can be placed into one of five sight categories. Most sports, including paralympic sports, use B1-B3. Only the British Blind Sport classification system uses B4 and B5.

- B1: From no light perception in either eye to light perception, but an inability to recognise the shape of a hand at any distance or in any direction. Visual acuity is poorer than LogMAR 2.60 with best corrected vision.
- B2: The ability to recognise objects up to a distance of 2 metres. Visual acuity ranges from LogMAR 1.5 to 2.60 (below 2/60) with best corrected vision and/or visual field of less than ten (10) degrees diameter.
- B3: Can recognise contours between 2 and 6 metres away. Visual acuity ranges from LogMAR 1.40-1.0 (2/60-6/60) with best corrected vision and/or visual field of more than ten (10) degrees and less than forty (40) degrees diameter.
- B4: Visual acuity LogMAR 1.0-0.6 (6/60-6/24).
- B5: Visual acuity LogMAR 0.6-0.48 (6/24-6/18).

Les Autres

This is a classification system that includes physical disability that does not fit within the other categories described. People with conditions such as multiple sclerosis, significant arthritis, muscular dystrophies and congenital disorders are included. LAF1, LAF2 and LAF3 are wheelchair classes, whereas LAF4, LAF5 and LAF6 are ambulant. SS1 and SS2 include people with short stature or a disability that is not described in the criteria above.

SPECIAL NEEDS OF DISABLED ATHLETES AND EXERCISERS

Disabled athletes and exercisers are at a similar risk to sport specific injuries that exist in non-disabled athletes. Throwing athletes or tennis players may be at an increased risk of shoulder injuries, for example. It is recognised that lower extremity injuries are more common in walking athletes and upper extremity injuries are more common in wheelchair athletes.

There are also some unique issues. Wheelchair users may be vulnerable to wrist nerve compression or hand injuries. Modification of training volume may need to be considered, with coaching of technical factors such as wheel propulsion being important to avoid unnecessary load. Different sports may also require different types of wheelchair or prosthetics that have their own biomechanical load demands that could predispose to injury.

There is strong evidence that physical activity in disabled adults (with physical and cognitive impairments) increases cardiorespiratory fitness, improves muscular strength, functional skills, psychosocial wellbeing and reduces disease risk. And, although some exercise is better than nothing, higher doses of physical activity are associated with higher levels of cardiovascular and metabolic health. General advice is that disabled adults should engage in 150 minutes of physical activity per week of a moderate to vigorous intensity. This is in line with general adult UK guidelines.

Measuring intensity may be difficult, but the 'talk test' can be a simple means to gauge intensity. Generalising, moderate intensity exercise should allow the participant to talk but not sing, whereas vigorous intensity would allow a person to say a few words but not talk comfortably without taking a breath.

There is no evidence that appropriate intensity exercise is a risk for disabled adults, however, it should be graded, gradually progressing in frequency, duration and intensity—particularly in those with medical comorbidities.

There have been reported issues with orthostatic hypotension and pressure injuries in disabled exercisers, therefore monitoring may be advised to avoid these problems. There is minimal evidence on physical activity for disabled children and adolescents, but it is perceived that the potential significant health benefits remain and being active for at least 60 minutes per day is helpful. Many games for non-disabled children can be modified with larger or softer balls, or decreased distances.

PROSTHETICS AND WHEELCHAIRS

A prosthesis is an artificial device, designed to replace a missing body part. There are multiple sport-specific prostheses available, including those designed for running, water sports and sports requiring rotation, such as golf.

Running

Running prostheses tend to be manufactured from carbon fibre—a lightweight, durable but strong material. The focus of the design is to provide 'spring-like' properties that replicate propulsion from a foot during gait. Prosthetics designed for sprinting events will only include a small surface area for ground contact, eliminating heel strike and mimicking the toe. These blades are not compatible with standing and day-to-day activities.

Water Sport

Prosthetics used in water sports are designed using waterproof materials. Treading can be incorporated in the sole to provide increased friction and safety in wet areas. Some prosthetics can be adjustable, for example ankles and arms can be fixed in varying degrees to aid swimming ergonomics.

Rotation Sports

Prosthetics used in sports such as golf and tennis, may incorporate shock absorbers or fittings that absorb any rotational force that would usually be transmitted through the missing limb. An upper limb amputee can use a terminal device, which connects the prosthesis directly to a sports instrument (e.g. tennis racquet). This can improve grip and power generation.

Design

A conventional prosthetic will require stump measurement, measurement of the body to configure the size of the required limb and then manufacture. The stump model is usually created and then a thermoplastic sheet encompasses the model so that the prosthesis can be tested before the permanent socket is made. The limb is then made from appropriate materials. With some carbon fibre designs, up to 90 sheets of material may be cut and layered before being pressed into the final shape. The weight of the athlete will help determine how much material is used.

Wheelchairs in Sport

The prescription of a wheelchair should involve finding the best possible match to the needs of the wheelchair user. Traditional wheelchair prescription involves selecting an appropriate frame, castors and wheels, footrests, armrests, backrests, height adjustability and rear wheel positioning.

The majority of sport wheelchairs have angled wheels. This introduces a negative camber. If a wheel is perpendicular to the ground, the camber angle is zero. A negative camber has many advantages in sporting activity. It provides more stability (with a wider base), places push rims in a more ergonomic position, reduces shoulder strain by placing wheels in a closer plane to the shoulders and allows quicker turning. The superior part of the wheel is closer to the wheelchair user however, increasing the risk of skin injury. Care also has to be taken for athletes transitioning from traditional wheelchairs to chairs with a negative camber, as the necessary upper limb forces are different and may increase load, resulting in injury.

MULTIPLE CHOICE QUESTION (MCQ) QUESTIONS

1. You are assessing a female patient in order to aid in her musculoskeletal rehabilitation. She has tetraplegia following a motor vehicle accident. She is currently maintaining conversation with up to 10 syllables per breath and has good power in shoulder abduction and elbow flexion. She is unable to extend her elbows or move her wrists. Which level of spinal injury does this best describe?

    A. C2-C3
    B. C4-C5
    C. C5-C6
    D. C6-C7
    E. T1-T2

2. You are a team doctor for a Paralympic athletics team. Prior to setting off to the games, you are having a medical meeting with your colleagues and team management. You discuss autonomic dysreflexia with them. Which one of the following statements is true?

    A. The lacrimal glands are inhibited in an athlete with a C4 spinal lesion
    B. One of the most common causes of autonomic dysreflexia is urinary tract infection
    C. Pre-event hypotension can be a diagnostic sign of autonomic dysreflexia

    D. A common sign is diaphoresis below the level of the spinal injury
    E. This phenomenon does not occur in an athlete with a spinal injury above the level of T6

3. You are delivering a lecture presentation on disability sport at your local medical school. Which of the following statements about disability classification are true?

    A. Classification in disability sport is based on the disability type, not the functional ability of the athlete
    B. Athletes with a B3 or equivalent classification have the least severe visual impairment for Paralympic sport
    C. CP1 is a cerebral palsy classification for ambulatory athletes
    D. An athlete with a hearing loss of 38 Db can compete in competitive sport, according to the International Committee of Sports for the Deaf
    E. The Paralympic games do not use classification in their medal events

4. You are part of the pitch side medical team at an international wheelchair basketball competition. The game has only just started and one of your players is static, on his wheelchair within your team's free throw circle. You know that he is a 21-year-old athlete with a background of asthma, taking a regular steroid inhaler. He travelled by train to the competition yesterday, a few days behind his teammates. Play continues around him for a few moments, but you are quickly invited onto the field of play to assess him. When you get to him, he is not responding to voice, is upright in the chair but slumped forward. You can only hear one breath sound in 10 seconds. He is warm to touch. There is no sweating below the level of his spinal injury. You are unable to feel a radial pulse. What is the most likely diagnosis?

    A. Cardiac arrest
    B. Autonomic dysreflexia
    C. Acute exacerbation of asthma
    D. Epilepsy
    E. Pulmonary embolism

5. You are discussing physical activity with one of your 42-year-old female patients with cerebral palsy. She has mixed cerebral palsy with some upper limb spasticity and ataxia. She is ambulant and has no other comorbidities. She does not take any regular medications. She confesses that she is largely sedentary with 'poor' physical fitness. Which one of the following physical activity plans is most appropriate?

   A. Walking or slow jogging for 20 minutes, three times per week, with a friend
   B. Walking or slow jogging for 35 minutes, four times per week, where she can talk throughout exercise; a mixture of light upper and lower body weights for 20 minutes, twice per week
   C. Running for 30 minutes, four times per week, and a high intensity interval training class for 20 minutes, twice per week, at her local gym
   D. Football, once per week, for 90 minutes; three 10-minute home workouts, including sit ups, press ups and squats
   E. Walking for 30 minutes, four times per week, to a point where she can sing throughout exercise; a mixture of light upper and lower body weights for 20 minutes, twice per week

MULTIPLE CHOICE QUESTION (MCQ) ANSWERS

1. Answer D
   A and B are incorrect as the patient does not require any respiratory support. Because there is some preservation of shoulder abduction and elbow flexion, the level of injury is likely to be below C5 and C6 (making C incorrect). Arm and hand function should be normal if the injured level is T1/T2, leaving D as the correct answer.

2. Answer B
   Urinary tract infection, bladder distension from retention and a blocked catheter are very common causes of autonomic dysreflexia. This phenomenon is most commonly above the level of T6 and is unlikely to develop if the injury is below T10 level. A is incorrect as the lacrimal gland is innervated by the lacrimal nerve (the smallest branch of the ophthalmic nerve and a branch of the trigeminal nerve). Inhibition is a sympathetic response. Pre-event hypertension is a sign of this condition and profuse diaphoresis above the level of the injury is a common sign.

3. Answer B
   B. and B5 categories are only used in the British sport classification and not in the Paralympics. The Paralympics also relies on classification to create a fair platform for competition so E is incorrect. Classification focuses on the functional ability of the athlete, so A is also incorrect. CP1 is a classification for wheelchair cerebral palsy athletes and an athlete needs a hearing loss of at least 41 Db to qualify for 'moderate' hearing loss in the English deaf football leagues.

4. Answer A
   This is a cardiac arrest until proven otherwise. The athlete has suddenly stopped in a non-contact situation, away from play. It is only because he is positioned in his wheelchair that he is not collapsed to the ground. With autonomic dysreflexia you would expect significant hypertension and a stimulus, which is not provided in the question stem. There is no clinical information such as an increased respiratory rate or wheeze to suggest an acute exacerbation of asthma. Although pulmonary embolism is a potential cause of cardiac arrest, this is unlikely in a young and otherwise medically fit disabled athlete, despite a recent long train journey.

5. Answer B
   Answer B most closely follows the UK recommended physical activity guidelines for adults with disabilities: 150 minutes of moderate intensity aerobic activity per week with strength and balance activities at least twice per week. Although having a friend present such as in Answer A, may be useful, particularly with this patient's ataxia, there is no evidence to say that it is unsafe for disabled adults to exercise independently. Answer C is likely to be too intense for this patient. Although Answer E may also be appropriate for this patient, the intensity may be less beneficial as she is able to sing throughout exercise, as opposed to talking in Answer B.

REFERENCES AND FURTHER READING

Equality Act 2010, c.15. Available at: www.legislation.gov.uk/ukpga/2010/15/section/6 [Accessed 1 May 2022].

Paralympics GB, 2023. Paralympics Classification. Available from: https://paralympics.org.uk/footer-pages/classification—This is an overview and guide to the Paralympic classification process.

Roberts, T.T., Leonard, G.R., Cepela, D.J. (2017). Classifications in brief: American Spinal Injury Association (ASIA) impairment scale. *Clin Orthop Relat Res*, 475(5), pp. 1499–1504.

www.activityalliance.org.uk—This is a national charity for disabled people in sport and activity. The website includes a list of inclusion gyms as well as a host of resources on how to begin exercise if you are disabled.

Elite Sport **10**

Rishi Dhand, Sarah Hattee and Jonathan Power

TEAM MEDICINE

Providing medical care in an elite sporting environment can be a challenging, time consuming, but ultimately, rewarding experience. The role involves working closely with athletes and support staff and the relationships that are developed may be much closer than those with a typical patient group. Managing the balance of building rapport whilst maintaining doctor-patient boundaries is a potential challenge. Often, there are a number of variables that can affect day-to-day interactions. For example, a team's on field results can drastically alter team and staff morale. The medical team may experience the highs of promotion or the lows of relegation as well as the potential job instability associated with team success and failure.

The medical team offers multidisciplinary support to the athletes and may be composed of a wide range of practitioners. The number of staff and their time commitment to the organisation can vary between departments and there are often budgetary constraints. Support teams may include roles as diverse as doctors, physiotherapists, sports therapists, rehabilitation coaches, manual therapists, strength and conditioning coaches, osteopaths, chiropractors, podiatrists, psychologists, nutritionists, alongside other allied professionals.

Doctors in sport may have a variety of medical backgrounds. Different knowledge, skills and experience lend themselves to different sports. Doctors may have completed specialist training in Sport and Exercise Medicine or have qualifications in General Practice, Emergency Medicine, Pre-Hospital Care, Orthopaedics or Anaesthetics.

As a Team Doctor it is useful to develop a network of trusted, experienced specialists who are experts in their field, with experience of working alongside athletes. It is common for sporting organisations to have links with cardiologists for advice on cardiac screening and neurology consultants with experience in managing head injury and concussion. Orthopaedic surgeons with special interests in specific injuries are often consulted by the medical teams of injured athletes nationally and internationally.

Internal department structure can vary depending on the skill mix of staff and the needs of the department. A Head of Department may be a doctor, physiotherapist or allied health professional. Their role is not only to lead the department with overall responsibility for medical services and strategy but to provide management and leadership to the whole staff group. A high functioning team requires outstanding leadership. By working toward a common goal with a shared philosophy, the department can consistently perform well despite the pressures of the sporting environment. Staff may have to work long and unsocial hours, spending time away from family and friends. Maintaining staff morale is essential to continued high performance. The Head of Department may develop a close working relationship with the Head Coach and other senior managers to discuss strategy, updates on injured players, training optimisation and recruitment and retention decisions.

IMMEDIATE TRAUMA CARE, TRAINING AND EQUIPMENT

The increasing professionalisation of athletes in sport has been mirrored by the requirement for appropriately trained and qualified medical support staff. Pitchside Immediate Care and Pre-Hospital Care

DOI: 10.1201/9781003179979-10

ELITE SPORT

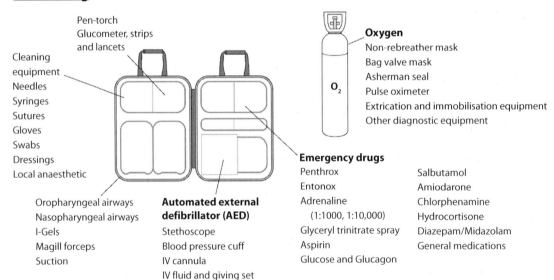

Emergency action plan (EAP)

- Specific roles for trauma and cardiac arrest
- Team leader
- Equipment
- Nearest hospital (trauma and cardiac centre)
- Extrication plans
- Practice
- Contact details of key personnel

Team travel

P – Paperwork (passports, insurance)
A – Athletes (pre-medicals, medications, TUE's)
S – Self
S – Staff

T – Travel (timings, nutrition)
I – Immunisations
L – Location (climate, catering)
T – Talk (education re. hygiene, sexual health etc.)
E – Equipment (EAP in place)
D – Doctor's bag

Safety at venues

- 2000+ spectators → Crowd doctor
- 5000 spectators → Fully equipped ambulance
- 5000-25,000 → 1 Paramedic ambulance, 1 Statutory ambulance officer
- 25,000-45,000 → 1 Paramedic ambulance, 1 Statutory ambulance officer, 1 Major incident equipment vehicle, 1 Control unit
- 45,000+ → Paramedic ambulances, 1 Statutory ambulance officer, 1 Major incident equipment vehicle, 1 Control unit
- 1 First aider / 1000 spectators up to 10,000
- 1 First aider / 2000 spectators up to 10,000

Doctor's bag

Pen-torch
Glucometer, strips and lancets

Cleaning equipment
Needles
Syringes
Sutures
Gloves
Swabs
Dressings
Local anaesthetic

Oropharyngeal airways
Nasopharyngeal airways
I-Gels
Magill forceps
Suction

Automated external defibrillator (AED)
Stethoscope
Blood pressure cuff
IV cannula
IV fluid and giving set

Oxygen
Non-rebreather mask
Bag valve mask
Asherman seal
Pulse oximeter
Extrication and immobilisation equipment
Other diagnostic equipment

O₂

Emergency drugs
Penthrox
Entonox
Adrenaline
  (1:1000, 1:10,000)
Glyceryl trinitrate spray
Aspirin
Glucose and Glucagon

Salbutamol
Amiodarone
Chlorphenamine
Hydrocortisone
Diazepam/Midazolam
General medications

Therapeutic use exemption (TUE)

1) Athletes would experience a significant impairment of health without the substance/method
2) The use of method would not produce a significant enhancement in performance
3) There is no reasonable therapeutic alternative
4) The TUE is not due to prior use of a substance or method which was prohibited at the time of use

Figure 10.1 Pictorial summary.

training is essential and qualification is mandated for medical staff by many governing bodies. Providing cover without necessary qualifications may be seen as acting outside of the clinician's scope of practice. This can be negatively viewed by their regulatory body and invalidate indemnity cover.

Training courses are attended by those providing immediate pitchside support e.g. team doctors, physiotherapists and sports therapists. There are a number of courses that are approved by the Faculty of Pre-Hospital Care (FPHC). They provide medical staff with the required training to allow development and display competency in the management of a wide range of emergencies that may occur in sport. The endorsement by the FPHC is a verification of the curriculum content and quality of education, ensuring that the course meets the required standards. Whilst many governing bodies will run their own pre-hospital course, there is cross recognition for courses that are approved by the FPHC because of the thorough endorsement process. Qualifications may last up to three years; however, many courses will have annual components to refresh knowledge.

In the advanced trauma courses, a number of emergency scenarios are covered. This includes Basic and Advanced Life Support, the initial 'ABCDE' assessment, medical emergencies and major trauma of the head, face, chest, spine, abdomen and musculoskeletal system. The structure of the course may vary, but most commonly there is a pre-course element with reading and questions to be completed prior to attendance. During the course there are skill stations with a final assessment scenario and theory paper. It is best practice to have regular practice on trauma scenarios with the medical team to aid familiarity with emergencies, the trauma kit and understanding staff roles. The role of each team member should be part of the Emergency Action Plan and discussed before each game. Some staff (e.g. paramedics or stretcher bearers) may only be present on matchday so it is important to ensure there is communication on roles. If possible, practice scenarios with all team members present should be arranged.

The contents of the pitchside medical equipment may vary depending on the sport. The list below shows suggested equipment but is not intended to be exhaustive:

- *Airway:* oropharyngeal airways, nasopharyngeal airways, supraglottic airway device, lubricating jelly, Magill's forceps, manual suction device with catheter, cricothyroidotomy set, intubation kit, pulse oximeter, capnograph
- *Breathing:* oxygen cylinder, non-rebreather mask with reservoir bag, bag valve mask device, pocket mask, Asherman seal, thoracic needle decompression kit, stethoscope, pulse oximeter
- *Circulation:* automated external defibrillator with two sets of pads, razor and towel, rapid haemostatic gauze, combat application tourniquet, intravenous and/or intraosseous access kits, intravenous fluid bags and giving sets, pelvic binder, stethoscope, sphygmomanometer
- *Disability:* pen torch, glucometer, strips and lancets
- *Diagnostic and general equipment:* Glasgow coma scale chart, ophthalmoscope and otoscope, tympanic thermometer, rectal thermometer, tongue depressor, urinalysis sticks, tuff cut scissors, pocket concussion recognition tool, crutches, towel, umbrella, ice and ice bags, referral letters, head injury instructions, iSTAT, radios/communication device, prescription pad, musculoskeletal ultrasound
- *Wound management:* sharps box, local anaesthetic, long acting (e.g. bupivacaine) and short acting (e.g. lidocaine), antiseptic e.g. chlorhexidine sachets, alcohol wipes, sterile syringes, hypodermic needles, saline pods, clinical waste bags and bin, hand gel, sterile and non-sterile gloves, nasal tampons, sterile and non-sterile swabs, dressings, bandages. suture material, tissue adhesive glue, steristrips, suture packs, dressing packs, saline ampoules, petroleum jelly, skin staple, staple remover
- *Emergency drugs:* nitrous oxide:oxygen (entonox) or methoxyflurane (penthrox), adrenaline 1:10,000, adrenaline 1:1000 autoinjector, glyceryl trinitrate spray, aspirin 300 mg tablets, dextrose gel, glucagon injection, chlorphenamine 10 mg/1 mL, oral rehydration fluids, hydrocortisone, local anaesthetic, salbutamol nebules and nebuliser, salbutamol inhaler with spacer device, spare oxygen cylinder with high flow mask, amiodarone, buccal midazolam.

- General Medications

  ○ Antibiotics: amoxicillin, clarithromycin, phenoxymethylpenicillin, flucloxacillin, metronidazole, azithromycin, co-amoxiclav, nitrofurantoin, trimethoprim, doxycycline

  ○ Gastrointestinal: gaviscon, lansoprazole, anti-emetic, mebeverine, buscopan, loperamide, docusate sodium

  ○ Ear Nose and Throat: beclometasone nasal spray, saline nasal spray, earcalm, otomize, benzydamine throat spray, bonjela, strepsils, sudafed, olive oil

  ○ Ophthalmology: sodium cromoglycate 2%, chloramphenicol, fluorescein

  ○ Dermatology: hydrocortisone 1%, betnovate, bactroban, clotrimazole 1%, terbinafine (oral and cream) ketoconazole shampoo, daktacort cream, emla cream, Aveeno

  ○ Analgesia: paracetamol (oral and dispersible), NSAIDs (topical, oral, intramuscular and dispersible)

  ○ Allergy: cetirizine, fexofenadine

- *Extrication:* spinal board with triple immobilisation, semi-rigid adjustable cervical collar, split device with adjuncts for immobilisation, basket stretcher, vacuum mattress or equivalent

- *Fracture immobilisation:* triangular bandage, lower limb traction splint (e.g. Kendrick splint), SAM splints, vacuum splints, pelvic splint, box splints, rescue blanket

EVENT MEDICINE

When planning the medical arrangements necessary for a sporting event, a thorough risk assessment should be performed. This can be a complex process, covering multiple factors, which will be bespoke to the individual event. To illustrate this, the example of the factors considered when planning a mass participation marathon are discussed below:

About the Event

It is important to know the course route and layout to plan the appropriate positioning of the medical team. In some events, there may be a **number of races** occurring simultaneously (e.g. there may be staggered start times depending on competitor numbers and ability). Information on the competitors should be obtained, such as the total number, their age, the standard (e.g. elite vs non-elite). Pre-competition medical screening allows identification of higher risk individuals. The **environment** of the event, such as the likely climate and altitude, may indicate if a period of acclimatisation is required beforehand. The terrain encountered may impact potential injury risk.

Additional medical provision will also be required if there is a **crowd** present. The **Location** of the event will enable prior research into nearby hospitals and medical services. It would be sensible to coordinate with the hospital(s) before the event to facilitate a seamless pathway for athletes requiring use of services and to have established points of contact. Services to consider would be provision of a 24-hour Emergency Department, Neurosurgery, Cardiology (including catheterisation lab), Orthopaedics and General surgery. The **budget** available for medical planning will influence many of the factors described. For some events, medical staff will be volunteers, in others there will be paid roles.

Medical Team

Once more information about the race (above) is established, **the number and the skill mix** of members of medical staff required can then be determined. Their **positioning** across the distance of the race should also be planned. The medical team at endurance events will typically be made up of doctors, paramedics, physiotherapists, sports therapists and nurses. It is sensible to make use of a number of **different specialities** within medicine whose skillset is relevant to the potential medical emergencies. For example, many larger marathon events have small intensive care units, staffed by doctors and nurses with critical care experience due to the potential for conditions such as cardiac arrest, hyponatraemia and hypo or hyperthermia. Depending on the event and the risk of injury, it may be worth considering doctors with a background in the above specialities, in addition to sports medicine physicians, general practitioners and orthopaedic surgeons. Medical cover may also be required for athlete accommodation, particularly out of hours. The Chief Medical Officer would have other responsibilities, such as ensuring that the doctors have **indemnity** to perform their roles and have necessary **qualifications**. As medical staff will be spread throughout the event in small teams, appointing a **team leader** for each group allows there to be clarity for decision making and a definite **communication lead** for each team with the chief medical officer. The team leader should assign his team to particular roles within a trauma scenario in accordance with their expertise.

Venue

Having an **Emergency Action Plan** (EAP) is a critical part of event planning. The Emergency Action Plan needs to contain details on how a casualty can be extricated from the field of play for further assessment, either at the venue or in hospital. It is important to consider the **location of your medical assessment area**(s), which should be private, large enough for access of a casualty on a stretcher (plus stretcher bearers) and be easily accessible from the field of play. The **method of transferring a casualty** from the field of play to the medical room and to the ambulance should be decided. Prior to the event, it is essential to run a mock trauma scenario and assign roles to different team members that they will fulfil in the event of an emergency. There may be volunteers assigned to be stretcher bearers. In bigger events, buggies or other transport vehicles may also be required to move athletes longer distances to assessment areas or to ambulances. The location of player and spectator **ambulances** should also be considered for accessibility and proximity to the field of play and medical assessment areas. An ambulance will usually be the mode of transport to more definitive care in a hospital; however, an air ambulance may also need to be considered if the event is remote or a large distance from a major trauma centre. Contact details for key personnel at the event, such as relevant management and medical team leaders, are important parts of the EAP.

Equipment

Most of the equipment that would be required at major sporting events is listed in the 'Team Medicine' section, however it is important to think about the **environment** of the event. Climate, altitude and terrain may affect the **type of medical emergencies** that are likely and the equipment and medication that you carry as a result. Access to trauma bags, oxygen, spinal immobilisation, extrication devices, limb splints, wound care, defibrillator and cardiac drugs is standard for most events. Access to common treatments for hypo or hyperthermia (e.g. blankets or cooling fluids) would be relevant to marathon medicine. Similarly, a point of care analyser for electrolytes (particularly sodium) is needed because of the risk of hyponatraemia from overhydration. **Communication** between the medical team with radio devices is vital. **Documentation** of consultations on formal history sheets is necessary. Athletes may also want to take a copy of this home to give information to their regular practitioners. Documentation should be stored as per information governance regulations. Stocks of medication should be recorded pre-event on an inventory list and updated when medications are used. This can be used to restock bags if they are to be used for future events.

Post Event

After the event, it is essential to debrief medical incidents that have occurred. These can be viewed as learning opportunities in an effort to improve services the next time the event happens. In multi-day events, this may be the very next day. Medical processes and EAPs may be adjusted if there are any significant events or near misses. Feedback from athletes, team managers and other stakeholders may also be useful.

SAFETY AT VENUES

The Sports Ground Safety Authority (SGSA) advises the UK government on safety at sports grounds and its Guide to Safety at Sports Grounds ('Green Guide') is well recognised as an international standard of safety (Sports Ground Safety Authority, 2018). The main objective of the Green Guide is to provide appropriate guidance as to the number of people that can be safely accommodated to watch a particular event. In addition to medical and first aid provision for spectators, it also covers safety planning, fire safety, media provision and communications and control.

The guide outlines the measures that should be taken to prevent a serious incident. A risk assessment should be undertaken outlining physical factors (e.g. the layout and design of the venue) and safety management factors (e.g. safety management structure, staff training and spectator behaviour).

There are set requirements for the first aid room including a minimum size of 15 square metres and space to hold a couch. This increases to 25 square metres and space for an extra couch if the capacity of the venue is greater than 15,000. There are specifications for fittings and facilities of the first aid room including heating, lighting, ventilation, water supply (hot, cold and drinking water) and telephone lines.

The location specifications discuss the importance of accessibility and clear signposting. The management team must ensure that if there is not a defibrillator on site permanently, that the medical or first aid team are supplying one for the event. Storage of medical equipment and inspection of the first aid room is the responsibility of management.

In events expecting more than 2,000 spectators, at least one crowd doctor with pre-hospital immediate care experience should be present prior to arrival of all spectators and until all spectators have left. Minimum ambulance provision is also dependent on attendance figures:

- An event with 5,000 spectators requires one fully equipped ambulance.
- 5,000–25,000 spectators should have one paramedic ambulance and on one statutory ambulance officer.
- 25,000–45,000 requires a paramedic ambulance, statutory ambulance, one major incident equipment vehicle and a one control unit.
- Above 45,000 spectators requires a minimum of two paramedic ambulances, one statutory ambulance officer, one major incident equipment vehicle and a control unit.
- All events should have at least two first aiders. The recommended first aid provision for all seated grounds is 1 first aider per 1,000 spectators (up to 10,000 spectators). After 10,000, one first aider per 2,000 spectators is advised. If there are also standing areas, there should be one first aider per 1,000, up to 20,000 spectators. After 20,000 it is advised for one per 2,000.

TRAVELLING WITH TEAMS

There are a number of aspects of planning when travelling with a team. The acronym 'PASS TILTED' from the FIFA Diploma in Football Medicine is a useful framework to use (FIFA Medical Network, 2021).

Paperwork—ensure that players and staff have valid passports and medical insurance. There should be contact details for next of kin for everyone on the trip. Customs approval documentation will be required for transport of medications in and out of countries. An inventory of medications on the trip will allow a record to be kept of medicines used. Therapeutic Use Exemption (TUE) forms may also be brought in case of requirement.

Athletes—awareness of how many athletes are travelling. A pre-travel medical assessment may be considered, particularly if the athletes are not known to the medical team. Ensure that any TUEs are up to date.

Self—ensure that your own personal health is adequate for travelling abroad and that you have correct medical indemnity. You should ensure that the treatment room is separate from your own room so that you have personal space on the trip.

Staff—ensuring awareness of the medical details, medications and allergy status for all of the travelling party is a vital part of planning and may influence some of the contents of your medical kit. Ensure that all the travelling party has appropriate medical and travel insurance for fitness to travel.

Travel—it is important to liaise with members of staff who are responsible for booking travel to gain details of the route, flight times, any flight transfers and change in time zones. This will enable a more detailed plan for players' sleep and nutrition. Some medications may be required on the journey, such as analgesia, decongestants, throat lozenges and medication for motion sickness, diarrhoea, vomiting and insomnia.

Immunisations—knowledge of the location in advance will allow planning for the administration and timing of any mandatory immunisations required. Some immunisations may be recommended or mandated for entrance into the country. There are numerous online resources that provide this information e.g. NaTHNaC, Masta.

Location—considering climate will inform the need for acclimatisation and preventative measures to avoid overheating (e.g. water breaks, cool towels, training times during cooler periods of the day). Athlete accommodation, catering and venue medical facilities should be inspected prior to travel to ensure that they meet the required standard. Ideally, this should be done in person, by appropriate members of staff. The medical team should ask the hosts for an EAP for training and matchday venues. An EAP may also be formulated for the team accommodation. It is important to know the standard of general healthcare in the country and have contingency plans for significant injuries, including repatriation to the home country.

Talk to all members travelling—prior to travel, all traveling members should be educated about specific matters for the trip, such as hand washing, sexual health, travel and food hygiene.

Equipment: consider the equipment you will need to take, including a trauma bag, laptop and other medical equipment (such as plinths, strappings, etc.). It may be useful to contact your hosts, as they may be able to provide or locally source some equipment which is difficult to transport, such as oxygen cylinders.

Doctor's Bag—ensure that your bag is stocked with supplies of common medications to last the trip. You may need to notify customs regarding some medications that you will be bringing with you.

There are a number of other aspects to consider depending on the location of the trip:

- *Jet lag:* travel across multiple time zones can disrupt circadian rhythm. This cannot be prevented but there are methods available to reduce the impact:

  - Adequate rest and sleep prior to departure
  - Adjusting to the time zone prior to departure e.g. going to bed or waking up one hour earlier/later
  - On departure, synchronising watches to the destination time zone and reverting to their sleep/wake times during the flight
  - Relaxing during the flight and stop overs e.g. utilising airline lounges and business class flights (if possible). This includes limiting alcohol intake, as it may impair sleep quality
  - Direct flights to the destination—reducing stop over and travel time
  - On arrival, adapting to local time—timing bright, natural light exposure and darkness can help to adapt to local time

  - Melatonin can be used as an adjunct to help with time zone adjustment

- Deep vein thrombosis (DVT) prevention— although the risk of DVT is low in those without risk factors, there are measures which can be taken to reduce risk:

  - Avoiding prolonged immobility—undertaking regular walks, stretching of calves and calf muscle exercises
  - Wearing comfortable and loose clothing
  - Staying hydrated, reducing caffeine and alcohol intake
  - Compression stockings or flight socks may be considered

- Heat acclimatisation

  - Pre-departure acclimation may include replicating conditions e.g. with the use of heat chambers, sauna, warm baths after training
  - Acclimation is an intervention involving 4–21 days of repeated exposures to temperatures >30 degrees Celsius and humidity >50%
  - The majority of acclimation can be achieved in 4–6 days
  - Recognising the symptoms of heat illness and ensuring that you have appropriate preparation to help prevent it e.g. hydration, shaded areas, cooling methods such as cooling towels pre- and post-exercise

- Altitude acclimatisation

  - Pre-departure preparation may include exercising in simulated altitude rooms and sleeping in hypoxic conditions
  - If possible, ascending slowly with stops at intermediate altitude
  - Avoiding high intensity exercise within the first few days of arrival
  - Acetazolamide may be used prior to an ascent and after arrival
  - Low flow oxygen may be used at night if sleeping at altitude
  - Medication for High-Altitude Pulmonary Oedema (HAPE) e.g. nifedipine and High-Altitude Cerebral Oedema (HACE) e.g. dexamethasone
  - Emergency action plan for rapid descent should be prepared

- Sunburn

  - Avoiding being in the sun between 11 am and 3 pm where possible
  - Applying high SPF sunscreen before sun exposure and reapplying regularly

- Insect bite avoidance

  - Mosquitos that transmit dengue, zika and malaria bite commonly during the daytime and at dusk. Loose fitting clothing that avoids skin exposure is preferable where possible
  - Insect repellent should be worn day and night. DEET 50% is most effective. DEET reduces the SPF of sunscreen, so it should be applied after sunscreen. A higher SPF sunscreen e.g. SPF30 or 50 should be used to compensate
  - Travellers should be counselled of the risk of these viruses before the trip
  - Malaria prophylaxis should be considered depending on the malarial risk of the area being visited

- Travellers' diarrhoea

- Ensuring that there are high food preparation standards at the accommodation is of paramount importance
  - Those travelling should be educated on food and hand hygiene prior to the trip
  - Regular handwashing after using the toilet and before eating or preparing food
  - Oral rehydration e.g. dioralyte should be part of the medical supplies
  - Consideration should be given to the use of prophylactic antibiotics if travelling to high-risk areas

INJURY REHABILITATION

Generally, injuries can be approached with conservative rehabilitation, active intervention or surgical management. A number of factors should be considered when deciding on management including evidence-based practice, the wishes of the athlete and the short and the long-term health of the athlete.

Active intervention may be used alongside conservative rehabilitation, in some cases as an option before surgical management is considered, or to avoid surgery. For example, injection therapy (steroid, PRP, sclerosant) or adjuncts to rehabilitation e.g. extracorporeal shock wave therapy.

Although rehabilitation programmes differ according to individual injuries, there are some general principles which can be applied to the majority of injuries:

1) *Pre-rehabilitation*

   - Once the extent of the injury is known, it is important to involve the athlete (and their support team, if required e.g. family) and the multidisciplinary team (the medical team, coaching staff, nutritionist, biomechanics, podiatry).
   - Educate the athlete on the injury and likely timescales and rehabilitation stages. It may be useful to introduce goal-setting for certain competitions or matches.
   - Psychological support may be required. It is also important to ensure that the athlete does not feel completely isolated from the team.
   - It is important to consider how cardiovascular fitness will be maintained e.g. swimming, bike, anti-gravity treadmills.

2) *Acute Phase*

   - The priority is to reduce pain and swelling.
   - Apply 'POLICE' principles. Protect and Optimally Load the injury- this may involve a brace or boot or crutches. Ice, Compression, Elevation.

3) *Range of movement*

   - Systematically monitor and review range of movement until optimal range has been restored.

4) *Strength and coordination*

   - Strength training should be done as symptoms allow e.g. isometrics. Consider upper body strength training for lower body injuries and vice versa.
   - Increase repetitions, load and velocity in strength training.
   - Target the affected structure and supporting muscle groups.

5) *Sports-specific movements*

- ○ On-field sessions.
- ○ Gradually increase speed, load and endurance

6) *Prevention of re-injury*

- ○ Ongoing rehabilitation should continue once the player has returned to play, to help reduce the risk of future injury.

ROLE OF THE TEAM PHYSICIAN

A team physician may fulfil a number of diverse roles in their care of athletes (and support staff). As well as musculoskeletal medicine and general practice, the doctor may provide services in fields such as sexual health, psychology, performance optimisation, anti-doping, clinical governance, infectious diseases, travel medicine and pastoral care.

The Faculty of Sports and Exercise Medicine Professional Code outlines the responsibilities and standards for doctors working in Sports Medicine (FSEM, 2016). It encompasses a number of different responsibilities for the team physician:

- *Knowledge, Skills and performance:* ensuring that you have appropriate skills to provide medical care for your patients, maintaining continuing professional development, ensuring appropriate indemnity, providing medical care without discrimination.
- *Communication, partnership and teamwork:* working in the multidisciplinary team, giving explanations to patients in language that they understand, asking patient's consent to discuss their medical diagnosis with others e.g. coaches, management, parents.
- *Maintaining Trust:* the athlete's welfare is your primary concern, even if contracted to your employer. Involvement in safeguarding, maintaining confidentiality and anti-doping.

MEDICOLEGAL ASPECTS

There are numerous medico-legal aspects to consider as a physician in elite sport. Key topics to consider are consent, duty of care, confidentiality, dual responsibility, ethics and professional risk.

Consent can be verbal, written or implied. As in any other medical practice, a physician should have the player's informed consent before proceeding with an investigation or procedure. Whilst consent can be implied in an emergency situation, the treatment involved should still be in the best interests of the patient. The consent of the athlete should be obtained prior to sharing any personal information to coaching staff and directors.

Confidentiality is of paramount importance and an athlete's right to privacy must be respected. It is essential to have an area at the training ground where the physician can speak with athletes and staff in private. For sensitive issues, reassuring the athlete that what they disclose is confidential is crucial. However, patient safety must always be the overriding responsibility—a physician would only have reason to break confidentiality if the athlete is at risk of harming himself, others, or if they were committing a serious crime.

Despite being employed as a doctor by an organisation, there is a duty of care to the athlete and the priority must be the health of the athlete, over the desires of the employer.

There is professional risk working as a sports physician, due to the responsibility for the general health and emergency care of athletes. There have been numerous cases of legal proceedings for clinical negligence brought against physicians, for example in concussion management and player medicals during transfers. It is essential that clinical documentation is thorough and that appropriate indemnity cover is obtained for the relevant scope of practice and the risk attached to it.

PRE-PARTICIPATION SCREENING

Cardiac Screening

In Italy, screening for all young competitive athletes has been mandatory by law since 1982. Whilst some studies suggest that electrocardiogram (ECG) is limited in identifying cardiovascular disease, with high false positive abnormal results and low diagnostic power, Italy has found that the incidence rate of sudden cardiac death has fallen since the introduction of their programme. Prior to the introduction of this law, in athletes aged 12–35 years, there was a death rate of 3.6/100,000 person years. Two decades later, the rate was 0.4/100,000 person years, with the greatest decline in sudden cardiac death related to car-diomyopathy (Corrado et al., 2006).

Research has demonstrated higher than anticipated incidence of cardiac abnormalities and sudden cardiac death in UK professional football (Malhotra et al., 2018). Because there have been cases of death following normal cardiac screening, a number of elite sports have introduced regular (annual) screening programmes. For example, the FA screening programme now includes ECG in the season a player turns 15, 18, 20 and 25 and an ECG and echocardiogram at 16. The Rugby Football Union and Rugby Football League recommend athletes are screened every 2 years with a minimum of a questionnaire and ECG, with particular emphasis on athletes under the age of 20.

The screening questionnaire includes questions on the athlete's past medical history and family history, in particular any sudden (cardiac) death. The athlete will be asked if they have experienced chest pain or tightness, shortness of breath, palpitations, fainting or dizzy spells. If there are any abnormal questions, this should be discussed with the club doctor and/or cardiologist.

Those against cardiac screening of whole populations may reference the false positive ECGs, which may incorrectly exclude athletes from playing sport. There are also cost implications for screening, as well as considering the cascade of further investigations that may be required. Those in favour of cardiac screening make a case for Sudden Cardiac Deaths (SCDs) being highly visible events with loss of numerous years of life. Screening can reduce the number of SCDs and identify at risk family members.

Concussion

The Sport Concussion Assessment Tool 5 (SCAT5) is a multimodal assessment of concussion. It includes assessments of concussive symptoms, cognition, concentration, neurology and balance, alongside details of previous injury and other modifying risk factors. Although concussion screening tools do not predict a risk of concussion, they can form useful baseline information for players, which can be used to map full recovery from subsequent injury. After an injury, a Graduated Return to Play (GRTP) is followed. This ensures the athlete is safe to resume sport. In professional clubs and international teams, regular

specialist medical review, baseline SCAT5 and neuropsychometric testing is possible. Therefore, an enhanced protocol can be followed, allowing the athlete to safely return to play more rapidly than an amateur athlete.

Medical Screening

Pre-season screening can often be a useful time to ensure that personal details for players (including details of their next of kin, address and general practitioner) is obtained, if this had not been done in a pre-signing medical. Assessing past medical history, family history, allergies, regular medications and supplements is vital. Depending on resources, some clubs may perform baseline blood and urine tests to detect any potential abnormalities e.g. full blood count, renal and liver function tests and urine dipstick tests to detect protein, glucose or blood. Immunisation history and status is also mandated by many governing bodies as well as checking for Hepatitis B status.

Musculoskeletal Screening

Periodic health examinations are used by many professional clubs (assessing range of movement, isokinetic strength and functional testing). There is debate as to whether this truly can be used to mitigate injury risk. In the context of hamstring injury there is an association with decreased eccentric strength as a risk factor for injury. However, there are other risk factors including age and previous injury. It can be difficult to establish a 'threshold' that would indicate an individual having a higher injury risk, particularly as there is natural variability in strength measurements between players. Roald Bahr outlined a number of tests that could be used to validate a 'screening' test, including a strong relationship between the baseline marker and injury risk (Bahr, 2016). The intervention programme for 'at risk athletes' should be more beneficial than the same intervention if it was given to all athletes. Nevertheless, periodic health examinations can detect current injuries or symptoms that an athlete may be experiencing. This can be used to gain a baseline strength marker at a healthy state, which can be referred back to if a player were to sustain a relevant injury.

ANTI-DOPING POLICY

The World Anti-Doping Agency (WADA) was formed in 1999. It regulates anti-doping internationally, ensuring that there is consistency for anti-doping rule violations (ADRV) in domestic and international athletes.

UK anti-doping (UKAD) is the national anti-doping organisation for the United Kingdom. It was set up in December 2009 and is an independent body accountable to the Department for Digital, Culture, Media and Sport (DCMS). UKAD works with national governing bodies to provide education, testing and intelligence to protect clean sport in the UK.

Anti-doping rule violations apply to all athletes and many also apply to athlete support staff. It is a common misconception that an athlete has to return a positive test to be sanctioned for an anti-doping offence.

The 11 ADRV's Are

- Presence of a banned substance
- Use or attempted use of a banned substance or method
- Evading, refusing or failing to submit to sample collection
- Whereabouts failure
- Possession of banned equipment or a banned substance
- Administration of a banned substance
- Tampering (or attempted tampering) of part of the testing procedure
- Trafficking of a banned substance
- Complicity—helping someone commit a ADRV or covering up a ADRV
- Prohibited association—athletes associating with athlete support personnel who are currently serving a ban for, or guilty of an offence equivalent to, an ADRV
- Acts by an athlete or other person to discourage or retaliate against reporting to the authorities

CLINICAL CONSIDERATIONS

Medical support staff play an important role in informing athletes and support staff about anti-doping information and the importance of clean sport. Athletes should receive anti-doping education from their National Governing Body and team physician. The key principle of anti-doping for athletes is the premise of 'strict liability,' i.e. all athletes are solely responsible for any banned substance that they use, attempt to use, or found in their system, regardless of how it got there or whether the intention was to cheat or not. Athletes should be encouraged to use the 'Global DRO' app to check any medications they take whilst away from the team environment, or to check with the team physician. This is particularly important if they receive emergency treatment or see their own GP. Only using supplements with an 'Informed Sport' logo, which ensures that they have been batch tested, is a further risk minimisation scheme to reduce the risk of contamination with banned substances.

Athletes are required to input their whereabouts details (if they are part of a registered testing pool) into the Athlete Central app or the Anti-Doping Administration Management System (ADAMS), both of which are overseen by WADA. Athletes must supply contact information, overnight address, regular activities/competitions information and a 60-minute time slot with a location where they must be available for testing. By the WADA code, three whereabouts 'failures' (incorrect whereabouts information or a missed test) within 12 months represents an ADRV, which may bring about a ban.

Therapeutic Use Exemptions (TUEs) are used when an athlete has a medical condition or illness that requires the use of a medication or administration method that is prohibited by WADA. Medications may be prohibited 'In competition' (the period starting at 11:59 pm on the day before the competition, through to the end of the competition) or both in and out of competition (doping control that takes place at any time). National athletes should submit a TUE to their National Anti-Doping Organisation (NADO). For substances banned in and out competition, WADA recommends that a TUE should be submitted at least 30 days prior to the start of the competition, as it may take up to 21 days for a decision to be made. Applications are reviewed by the TUE committee of the NADO and the athlete is informed in writing as to whether their application is successful. Once they have received written confirmation, the athlete may commence their treatment. In the event of treatment needing to be administered in an exceptional emergency, where there is insufficient time or opportunity to submit a TUE, a retroactive TUE should be applied for.

There are four criteria that must be satisfied for a TUE to be approved:

1) The athlete would experience a significant impairment to health without the use of the prohibited substance or method.
2) The use of the prohibited substance or method would not produce a significant enhancement in performance.
3) There is no reasonable therapeutic alternative to the prohibited substance or method.
4) The TUE is not due to prior use of a substance or method which was prohibited at the time of use.

The WADA Prohibited list acts as the international standard for substances banned in competition, out of competition and in specific sports. The list is updated annually and comes into effect on January 1st each year. In recent years, there have been changes to commonly used medications e.g. glucocorticoid administration, beta-2 agonists and cannabinoids. There are also limits on intravenous injections of >100 mL per 12-hour period. It is vital that physicians stay up to date with any changes in the WADA Prohibited list so that they can inform athletes and support staff.

REGULATIONS FOR TRAVELLING WITH MEDICAL EQUIPMENT AND MEDICINES IN SPORT

The regulations of transport of medications across international borders can vary significantly across the globe. It is therefore recommended to carefully check the regulations for the specific countries that you will transit through and your ultimate destination in a timely manner. It is best practice to compile a list of medications that you intend to travel with including name, quantity and strength. This should be submitted in advance to customs for prior authorisation to save time on entering the country. Generally, controlled drugs are prohibited, but if required, it is essential to apply for permission well in advance. It is important to bring enough medical supplies to last for the duration of the tour, as locally sourcing medication can be difficult (especially if you are not a registered medical practitioner in that country). Additionally, some medications

may have different ingredients when sourced abroad, representing a potential doping risk. Medication being brought by team members should have supporting documents including a copy of their prescription and/or a doctor's letter.

GOVERNANCE OF PROVIDING MEDICAL COVER AT SPORTING EVENTS

Doctors have a legal and ethical obligation to have appropriate medical indemnity insurance, whether they are working full time in sport, providing casual matchday cover or volunteering. The GMC advises that all doctors should 'work within the limits of their competence' and, as such, they should have the required skills to be able to perform their role, even if it is unpaid. Indemnity companies will differentiate assisting in a clinical capacity as an event doctor with a 'Good Samaritan Act,' where a doctor may help in an emergency e.g. when attending as a fan. Some sporting organisations or governing bodies will provide indemnity for doctors; however, it is advisable for the individual to confirm with their own indemnity organisation that they are covered by current policy. Indemnity companies will require information regarding the specific role you will be performing, for whom you will be providing cover, your medical training and qualifications including full registration and clinical specialty, income, and, if appropriate, the level of supervision whilst working in sport or at an event.

CLINICAL CONSIDERATIONS

It is essential that an Emergency Action Plan (EAP) is produced. This document provides information for emergency medical arrangements including location of emergency equipment, roles and responsibilities and extrication plans for all venues and activities that athletes undertake e.g. home games, away games, travel, training. Medical staff are required to have training and qualification recognised by the Faculty of Pre-Hospital Care in order to be able to proficiently manage possible medical emergencies. Although these qualifications may be renewed annually, it is advisable to have regular 'in house' training sessions to refresh knowledge and skills in the management of simulated medical emergencies. This process also helps to establish individual roles within the team and emergency scenarios become more familiar and well-practised. Debriefing both practice and real-life clinical scenarios is essential for team learning and fine-tuning the resuscitation and extrication process.

MULTIPLE CHOICE QUESTION (MCQ) QUESTIONS

1. You are asked to arrange crowd ambulance provision for a boxing event with an expected capacity of 12,000 spectators. What is the minimum requirement according to the Sports Ground Safety Authority (SGSA) 'Green Guide'?

   A. One paramedic ambulance only
   B. One paramedic ambulance and one statutory ambulance officer
   C. Two paramedic ambulances and one statutory ambulance officer
   D. One paramedic ambulance, one statutory ambulance officer, one major incident equipment vehicle and a control unit
   E. Two paramedic ambulances, one statutory ambulance officer, one major incident equipment vehicle and a control unit

2. An Athlete requires emergency hospital admission for appendicitis. She is septic and is given 500 mL of IV fluid over two hours. She is concerned about this being a prohibited method and is unsure what to do. What is the most appropriate statement?

   A. This is not a prohibited method so no further action is required.
   B. She does not fulfil the criteria for a TUE and so she should refuse treatment.
   C. She does not fulfil the criteria for a TUE so she only accepts the fluid at a rate of less than 50 mL/6 hours in line with WADA
   D. She fulfils the criteria for a TUE but should await approval from her NADO before accepting treatment
   E. She fulfils the criteria for a TUE but as this is an emergency situation, she can apply for a retroactive TUE after she has received the full treatment

3. When discussing the Emergency Action Plan (EAP) prior to a major event, which of the following is most appropriate?

   A. The EAP is not a necessary aspect of event planning
   B. The EAP is only required for competition venues, not training venues
   C. The EAP should only be completed by a doctor
   D. The EAP should contain details on location of medical areas, ambulances, routes for extrication, nearest hospitals and contact details for key event personnel
   E. The EAP should be written on the day of the event after visiting the venue and completing a practice scenario

4. You have recently completed an accredited pitchside trauma course and have been asked to cover a professional Netball game as a lone doctor for both teams. There will be an ambulance and two paramedics and each team will have a physiotherapist with a pitchside trauma qualification. Your current indemnity policy only allows you to cover sports games with the direct supervision of another doctor present on-site. What do you do?

   A. Advise that you can only cover the event if there is another doctor present to supervise you
   B. Cover the event, arrange for another doctor to be available on the phone as supervision
   C. Cover the event, using the physiotherapist and paramedics as direct supervision to fulfil your indemnity requirements
   D. Cover the event but leave all patient contact to the physiotherapists and paramedics
   E. Cover the event and agree to treat any players as a 'Good Samaritan' Act

5. With regard to pitchside resuscitation, which of the following would NOT be used to directly assist with an airway?

   A. Oropharyngeal airway
   B. Nasopharyngeal airway
   C. Jaw thrust
   D. Bag valve with face mask
   E. Manual suction device with catheter

MULTIPLE CHOICE QUESTION (MCQ) ANSWERS

1. Answer B
    Events with 5,000–25,000 spectators should have one paramedic ambulance and one statutory ambulance officer.

2. Answer E
    Although the IV method is a prohibited method (>50 mL in six hours), she does fulfil the criteria for a TUE. She is septic and so would experience a significant impairment to health without the fluids. Giving fluids would not give a significant enhancement in performance and there is no reasonable alternative to the prohibited method. Given this is an emergency situation, it would be unsafe and unreasonable to wait for a TUE to be approved and so a retroactive TUE would be applied for.

3. Answer D
    An EAP is critical and should be completed for all competition and training venues. It can be done by medical or non-medical personnel and needs to contain details on how a casualty can be transferred from the field of play to a medical room at the venue or hospital. The method of moving a casualty from the field of play to the medical room and/or to the ambulance should be considered. Knowing the location of the nearest hospitals for access to various specialties and contact details for key personnel at the event e.g. relevant management and medical team leaders would be an important part of the EAP. Prior to the event, it is useful to run a mock trauma scenario and assign roles to different team members that they will fulfil in the event of an emergency, however the writing of the EAP does not need to wait for this.

4. Answer A
    The terms of your indemnity policy are absolute as to what cover you are able to give. If they specify that you are indemnified to work under certain conditions e.g. under direct supervision of another doctor onsite, any work you do outside of this scope would not be indemnified and potentially in breach of GMC advice that doctors should 'work within the limits of their competence.' Indemnity companies will differentiate assisting in a clinical capacity as a pitchside doctor with a 'Good Samaritan Act,' where a doctor may help in an emergency e.g. when attending as a fan.

5. Answer D
    A bag valve with face mask provides oxygenation and ventilation to a patient and is therefore not primarily airway related.

REFERENCES AND FURTHER READING

Bahr, R. (2016). Why screening tests to predict injury do not work- and probably never will . . .: A critical review. *British Journal of Sports Medicine*, 50(13), pp. 776–780.

Corrado, D., Basso, C., Pavei, A., Michieli, P., Schiavon, M., Thiene, G. (2006). Trends in sudden cardiovascular death in young competitive athletes after implementation of a preparticipation screening program. *JAMA*, 296(13), p. 1593.

Faculty of Sports and Exercise Medicine. (2016). *Faculty of Sport and Exercise Medicine UK Professional Code.* [online] Fsem.ac.uk. Available at: www.fsem.ac.uk/wp-content/uploads/2017/05/FSEM-Flipbook.pdf [Accessed 2 March 2022].

FIFA Medical Network. (2021). *FIFA Medical Network.* [online] Fifamedicalnetwork.com. Available at: www.fifamedicalnetwork.com/courses/diploma?so=1&deeplinkHash=id%2F620d93fc6647fd6a56977cc0#object/1960 [Accessed 2 March 2022].

Malhotra, A., Dhutia, H., Finocchiaro, G., Gati, S., Beasley, I., Clift, P., Cowie, C., Kenny, A., Mayet, J., Oxborough, D., Patel, K., Pieles, G., Rakhit, D., Ramsdale, D., Shapiro, L., Somauroo, J., Stuart, G., Varnava, A., Walsh, J., Yousef, Z., Tome, M., Papadakis, M., Sharma, S. (2018). Outcomes of cardiac screening in adolescent soccer players. *New England Journal of Medicine*, 379(6), pp. 524–534.

Sports Ground Safety Authority. (2018). *Guide to Safety at Sports Grounds Worked Example.* London: Sports Ground Safety Authority.

Cardiology 11

Amit Verma and Robert Cooper

THE ATHLETE'S HEART

The heart makes subtle electrical, structural and functional adaptations to high training loads. These changes augment diastolic filling, allowing an increased stroke volume to supply more blood and oxygen to exercising tissue. The modifications that can be seen in the elite athlete are important to understand when considering possible overlap with pathology. We can expect to see electrical changes on the electrocardiogram such as bradycardia, repolarisation anomalies and left ventricular hypertrophy. The structural changes seen on scans such as echocardiogram include an increased left ventricular (LV) chamber size and increased LV wall thickness. Pre-existing abnormalities of the heart can be associated with increased risk of arrhythmia.

CARDIAC PHYSIOLOGY

In order to understand the physiological changes of exercise on the cardiovascular system, it is important to consider the physiology at rest.

For the body to function effectively, the heart must pump oxygenated blood at a sufficient rate to meet the continuous demands of the brain and vital organs. The cardiovascular system provides the link between pulmonary ventilation and oxygen usage at cellular level. Cardiac output describes the amount of blood pumped out by the heart each minute, which is the product of the amount of blood pumped per beat (stroke volume) and the number of times the heart beats every minute (heart rate). During exercise, efficient delivery of oxygen to working skeletal and cardiac muscles is vital for maintenance of ATP production by aerobic mechanisms.

A healthy heart with a normal cardiac output pumps around five to six litres of blood every minute at rest. The cardiovascular response to exercise contributes largely to the 35-fold increase in oxygen uptake during submaximal exercise. Cardiac output during exercise increases greatly owing to the high heart rates that are achieved during exercise. Heart rate increases proportionately with workload until approaching maximal values.

It is remarkable that exercise heart rates up to five times resting values are not associated with a fall in stroke volume. The body increases venous return along with other adaptations, such as splenic contraction and increased myocardial contractility, to increase cardiac output at such high demands. Despite the great changes in cardiac output, increases in blood pressure during exercise are maintained within relatively small parameters, as both pulmonary and systemic vascular resistance to blood flow is reduced. Redistribution of blood flow to the working muscles during exercise also contributes greatly to the efficient delivery of oxygen to sites of greatest need.

Training enables more efficient oxygen delivery to working muscle. This adaptation is evidenced by the ability to achieve higher work rates and increased oxygen uptake at sub-maximal heart rates after training. Such adaptations involve increased blood flow or arteriovenous oxygen content difference.

Improvements in blood haemoglobin concentrations during exercise because of training adaptations are recognised but, at maximal exercise, hypoxaemia may reduce arterial oxygen content. More effective redistribution of cardiac output to muscles by increased capillarisation and more efficient oxygen diffusion to cells may also be important means of increasing oxygen uptake after training.

DOI: 10.1201/9781003179979-11

CARDIOLOGY

Athlete's Heart

- Left ventricular (LV) hypertrophy and dilation, increased LV wall thickness
- Right ventricular (RV) dilation and atrial enlargement
- Reversible
- ECG:
  - Sinus bradycardia/arrhythmia
  - Incomplete RBBB
  - ↑ QRS voltage
  - Early repolarisation
  - 1° AV block, 2° AV block (Mobitz 1)
  - Ectopic atrial or junctional rhythm
  - TW ↓ V1-V4 in black athletes
  - TW ↓ V1-V3 if <16 years old

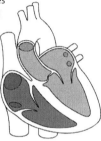

Hypertrophic cardiomyopathy (HCM)

- Usually familial (Autosomal dominant)
- Most common cause of sudden cardiac death if <35 years old
- Asymmetric septal hypertrophy
- Diagnosed with LV wall thickness ≥ 15mm in adults in the absence of abnormal loading conditions
- Usually:
  - ↓ LV chamber size
  - ↓ Diastolic function
  - Hyperdynamic systolic function
  - LV outflow tract obstruction (LVOTO)
  Cardiac MRI gold standard – can show late gadolinium enhancement (indicates fibrosis)
- ECG :
  - TW ↓ (inferolateral leads in apical and concentric HCM)
  - LVH

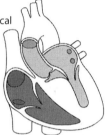

Arrhythmogenic ventricular cardiomyopathy (AVC)

- Usually familial
- Ventricular dilation and dyskinesia (can be right, left or both)
- Systolic dysfunction
- Cardiac MRI is the gold standard test for measuring ventricular volume, function and for assessment of myocardial inflammation and fibrosis
- Echocardiography can show regional wall motion abnormalities of either the right or left ventricle.
- ECG:
  - TW ↓ (usually V1-V3, inferolateral if LV involvement)
  - Epsilon waves

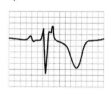

Wolff-Parkinson-White Syndrome

- An accessory pathway between the atria and ventricles
- Re-entrant supraventricular arrhythmias common
- Can lead to sudden cardiac death
- Usually asymptomatic
- ECG:
  - Short PR (<0.12 seconds)
  - Wide QRS
  - Delta waves

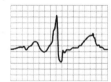

Figure 11.1 Pictorial summary.

CARDIAC SCREENING

The role of cardiac screening is to identify athletes with undiagnosed cardiac conditions that may predispose them to premature cardiac disease including sudden cardiac death (SCD). It does not completely prevent this occurring and may be best thought of as a risk assessment tool, to allow identification of pathology, so that the athlete can be managed and risk reduced.

The discussions about the importance of cardiac screening are often galvanised by an in-competition cardiac arrest, or worse yet, an athlete's death. There have been many high-profile incidents which may come to mind, where athletes have suddenly collapsed without warning. Although this stimulates discussion amongst the public and parliamentary debate, it is important to note that cardiac screening is not directly funded by the government. It may therefore rely on the wealth of a club, a sport or individual, or the presence of a screening charity.

The process of assessing risk is carried out by cardiologists with an understanding of the athlete's heart and expertise in sport-related cardiology. Basic cardiac screening includes a clinical and family history, and a physical examination. The addition of an ECG to screening has a high yield for identification of cardiac abnormalities; its high availability and low cost mean it is part of most screening processes. An echocardiogram has some incremental value in screening for conditions such as valvular abnormalities or aberrant coronary artery origins that will display a normal ECG. There are a number of follow-on investigations that can be triggered if one or more components of clinical history, ECG and echocardiogram are abnormal. These may include:

- Ambulatory ECG
- Exercise testing (exercise ECG or cardiopulmonary exercise test)
- Cardiac MRI
- Signal-averaged ECG

Less common investigations that can be used to understand an athlete's phenotype include:

- Genetic testing
- Blood tests such as cardiac troponin
- Cardiac CT
- Pharmacological provocation
- Electrophysiology study

SCREENING PROTOCOLS

A screening protocol consisting of just clinical history and examination may be cheap and easy to perform but will have poor sensitivity and specificity, with 80% of sudden cardiac death victims asymptomatic. Physical examination identifies few disorders and is often performed by under-qualified individuals. The approach endorsed by governing bodies such as the European Society of Cardiology (ESC), International Olympic Committee (IOC) and International Federation of Association Football (FIFA) includes clinical assessment and ECG. This has been in operation by legislation for >25 years and involves annual screening for individuals undertaking competitive sport.

Pre-participation screening must be considered in terms of advantages and disadvantages. Ultimately, the process is aimed at identifying athletes with pathological adaptation that may increase the risk of SCD or other adverse cardiac outcomes such as syncope, non-life-threatening arrhythmia and premature heart failure. SCD is a highly visible event with a potential loss of numerous years of life and is often perceived by the general public as having an association with exercise. Screening may allow management of cardiac disease to minimise this risk and, in rare circumstances, advice to stop activity. If cardiac conditions with a genetic underpinning are identified it can also prompt screening of at-risk family members.

The disadvantage of screening is predominantly related to cost. SCD incidence within children and young adults amongst the general population is rare (1/20,000) and within sport is even less frequent (1/80,000–100,000), where screening has a cost. The diversity of disorders is such that one single test will not pick up every condition, and changes can evolve over an athlete's career such that pathology will only be identified with repeated screening, incurring more cost. False positives can occur, though these have been minimised with adaptation of screening programmes and modification of what is deemed abnormal (Drezner et al., 2017). Usually, these false positive changes on screening can be clarified with further cardiac testing. False negatives can also occur in which all parameters on clinical review, ECG and echocardiogram appear normal but cardiac arrest still occurs (Malhotra et al., 2018). In 2006, Corrado et al. compared the mortality data of over 40,000 athletes before screening; when it was introduced there was a reduction from 3.6 to 0.4/100,000 person years. They removed 879/42386 (2%) participants from play as a consequence of screening, therefore, for every life saved, approximately 560 athletes were excluded from playing.

A more cost-effective measure in preventing SCD in sport may be greater provision of Automated External Defibrillators (AEDs) in public places. It is impractical to consider cardiac screening in all amateur athletes due to the prohibitive cost associated, but the provision and utility of AEDs may allow better outcomes for those who do suffer cardiac arrest. The survival rate may be as high as 64% with early defibrillation (Drezner et al., 2009).

CLINICAL CONSIDERATIONS

There have been high profile elite level sport players who have survived a cardiac arrest because of this measure. The early recognition of cardiac arrest to prompt early intervention is the cornerstone of every pitch-side course. The principles of basic life support require minimal training amongst the general population for a life-saving measure, and the use of AEDs should be encouraged. Use can be successful with instruction given by the AED console, requiring no training.

THE ECG

Normal ECG Findings in Athletes

Regular and long-term participation in intensive exercise (minimum of 4 hours per week) is associated with physiological adaptations that can manifest as ECG changes.

Isolated left ventricular hypertrophy by voltage criteria is very common in athletes and is present without other ECG change in <2% patients with Hypertrophic Cardiomyopathy (HCM). Right ventricular hypertrophy without other ECG change is also seen in 13% of athletes and does not represent pathology in isolation.

Early repolarisation—elevation of QRS-ST junction (J-point) by >0.1 mV, often associated with a late QRS slurring or notching (J wave) affecting inferior and/or lateral leads—is common in healthy populations

(2–44%). It is more prevalent in athletes, young individuals, males and those of black ethnicity.

Black athletes may demonstrate a normal repolarisation variant ST elevation in V1-4 followed by T wave inversion (TWI) in the absence of other clinical/ECG features. This is more prevalent in black athletes and athletes of mixed race versus a white population, where TWI in V4 is deemed pathological.

Anterior biphasic T-wave inversion in adolescents <16 years is considered normal in a single lead from V1-3.

Sinus bradycardia and sinus arrhythmia are very common, reported to be related to increased vagal tone. Junctional or ectopic atrial rhythms can also be observed with lower frequency. First degree atrioventricular (AV) block, and Mobitz Type 1 2nd AV Block (Wenckebach phenomenon) are also observed, more commonly in athletes with higher training volumes. Partial right bundle branch block (RBBB) can also be observed in up to a third of highly trained athletes.

Borderline ECG Findings

ECG findings previously characterised as abnormal may represent normal variants associated with physiological remodelling. These are considered borderline when observed in isolation. The presence of two or more of these changes should prompt consideration of further investigation (Figure 11.2).

Large studies demonstrated that isolated left or right axis deviation or atrial enlargement in athletes did not correlate with cardiac pathology on echocardiogram. Trained athletes could also have isolated complete RBBB.

Abnormal ECG Findings in Athletes

These are not recognised features of athletic training and warrant further investigation to assess for cardiac pathology.

Abnormal T-wave inversion ≥1 mm in contiguous leads (excluding aVR, III and V1), in anterior, lateral, inferolateral or inferior territory should prompt further investigations (usually echocardiogram). In particular, with lateral or inferolateral T-wave inversion, further investigation with cardiac MRI is usually warranted for a more focused review of possible hypertrophic or arrhythmogenic cardiomyopathy, even if the

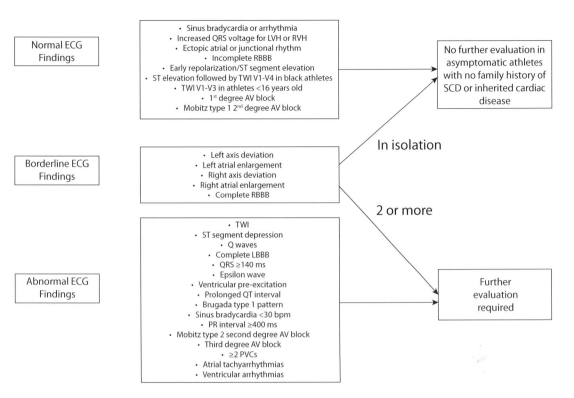

Figure 11.2 ECG findings in athletes.

Source: Adapted from Kumar et al. (2017).

echocardiogram is reported as normal. In the absence of pathology on imaging, serial cardiac imaging should be used to monitor for progression to LVH or myocardial fibrosis, as ECG can precede visible structural change in cardiomyopathy.

ST segment depression is not associated with training and is common among patients with cardiomyopathy and therefore should be evaluated with cardiac MRI.

Pathological Q waves are traditionally associated with myocardial infarction but can be seen in HCM, Arrhythmogenic Ventricular Cardiomyopathy (AVC), infiltrative myocardial disease or accessory pathways.

Complete LBBB (>120 msec) is associated with cardiomyopathy and coronary artery disease (CAD) and should be investigated further. Any QRS complexes ≥140 msec in duration, regardless of the morphology, is also deemed pathological.

Ventricular pre-excitation may be recognised with a short PR interval and delta wave in Wolff-Parkinson-White. Late QRS fractionation associated with

abnormal depolarisation in AVC can sometimes be seen as an Epsilon wave; this is easiest to see in lead V1.

A prolonged QT interval is potentially related to abnormal repolarisation and can predispose to ventricular arrhythmia syndrome. In order to identify those at greatest risk of pathological Long QT syndrome, cut-offs of QTc ≥470 ms in males or QTc ≥480 ms in females should be used for further assessment.

Brugada type 1 pattern has a typical ECG appearance of a coved ST-segment elevation ≥2 mm in an sRs' pattern with inversion of T waves in V1, V2 and V3. This is an inherited primary electrical disease, which predisposes ventricular tachyarrhythmias and sudden death during states of enhanced vagal tone.

Sinus bradycardia and moderate prolongation of the PR interval are recognised as possible athletic adaptation; however, a resting HR ≥30 bpm or PR interval ≥400 ms should prompt investigation for conduction disease.

Although 1ˢᵗ degree heart block and Mobitz type I may be seen in athletes, high grade AV block such as Mobitz type II and 3rd degree (complete) should be evaluated by exercise testing and ambulatory ECG monitoring.

Multiple premature ventricular contractions (PVCs) are uncommon. ≥ 2 ventricular ectopics on a standard 12 lead ECG should warrant further investigation. Supraventricular and ventricular tachyarrhythmias should always warrant further investigation.

Echocardiogram

The availability and non-invasive nature of echocardiography makes it the most commonly used imaging technique in sports cardiology. Echocardiography uses ultrasound and the variable natures and speeds of structures and blood in the heart to create images. It not only demonstrates anatomy but provides a continuous display of the functioning heart throughout its cycle. There are various methods used within an echocardiogram:

M-MODE (MOTION MODE)

- A single-dimension (time) image with high temporal resolution.

2-DIMENSIONAL (REAL TIME)

- A 2D, fan-shaped image of a segment of the heart is produced. Multiple views can be acquired to cover most areas of the heart to assess myocardium and valve movement and function.

3D ECHOCARDIOGRAPHY

- Matrix array probes provide enhanced assessment of systolic function and cardiac volumes.

DOPPLER AND COLOUR-FLOW DOPPLER

- Used to assess speed and direction of blood flow in the heart assessing valves and diastolic function.

TISSUE DOPPLER IMAGING

- This employs Doppler ultrasound to measure the velocity of myocardial segments over the cardiac cycle. This is useful for assessing longitudinal function.

STRAIN IMAGING

Provides deformation analysis of myocardium to assess systolic movement and function and is used for assessment of the LV in clinical environments including sports cardiology. Assessment of right ventricular (RV) and left atrial function is also under investigation.

EXERCISE STRESS ECHOCARDIOGRAPHY

This evaluates ventricular function in athletes; specifically, contractile reserve if resting LV ejection fraction or strain values are reduced. If these values are low at rest due to athletic adaptation there should be an improvement with an appropriate level of exercise.

Echocardiographic Changes Seen in Athletes

High levels of both strength and aerobic training result in increased ventricular volumes and LV mass, key physiological adaptations seen in the athlete's heart.

LV cavity size: Normal LV internal diameter in diastole in a non-athletic population by British Society of Echocardiography guidance is up to 56 mm in males and 51 mm in females. In the athletic or trained population, this can measure up to 64 mm in males and 57 mm in females and be within normal parameters (Harkness et al., 2020).

LV wall thickness: The LV wall is most often thickest at the interventricular septum. In a non-athletic population, this is normal when measured as ≤ 12 mm. In the male athletic population, this can be up to =13 mm; in the female population, LVH is less commonly observed, so the acceptable cut-off is 11 mm (Oxborough et al., 2018). Pathological hypertrophy is usually associated with abnormal diastolic function, with reduced efficiency of LV filling and reduced movement of myocardium on tissue Doppler imaging.

LV geometry: It is more accurate to interpret the LV cavity size and myocardial mass in relation to each other rather than in isolation. In response to training, a physiological adaptation in athletes involves LV cavity size increasing whilst LV muscle mass increases proportionately. If there is LVH but a small LV cavity, this can indicate pathology rather than physiology. A relative wall thickness as a simple measurement from echocardiography can help to clarify:

(Septal wall thickness + posterior wall thickness)/ LV internal diameter, in diastole. A relative wall thickness of <0.42 suggests physiology whereas >0.42 suggests pathology.

Right ventricular size and function: RV size and function is more accurately described by cardiac MRI. Due to the natural geometry of the RV, this is difficult to capture in one plane of imaging. Localised areas of weakness (hypokinesia) are abnormal and suggest a pathological process. Reduced function, as assessed by RV fractional area change of <35% (this is not the same as ejection fraction), can also suggest pathology, as can reduced longitudinal function and movement of the tricuspid valve (Tricuspid Annular Plane Systolic Excursion (TAPSE) on RV tissue Doppler imaging). Dilated RV by single measurements should be clarified with cardiac MRI.

Cardiac MRI

Cardiac MRI offers an excellent insight into cardiac morphology, function, blood flow patterns and myocardial composition. It has lower availability than echocardiogram, takes longer to complete and is more expensive. Therefore, it is reserved for onward investigation after echocardiogram. MRI does not use ionising radiation and reactions to contrast agents are extremely rare, making it a safe test.

Cardiac MRI is performed in most athletes where a possibility of cardiomyopathy has been raised or significant arrhythmia has been observed. Due to its ability to provide an insight into myocardial composition, it is used in conjunction with echocardiography.

STATIC AXIAL IMAGING

- Black blood (HASTE) or white blood (TRUFI).
- To assess thoracic anatomy including venous and arterial connections.

BALANCED STEADY-STATE FREE PRECESSION (BSSFP) CINES

- This provides an accurate assessment of volumes and systolic function of both ventricles

and is generally accepted to be more sensitive than echocardiogram, particularly for the right ventricle. It also offers clear definition of maximum wall width dimensions when considering HCM.

PARAMETRIC MAPPING

- *T1 mapping:* used to assess extracellular volume; this can show interstitial fibrosis as an early stage of a cardiomyopathy.
- *T2 mapping:* used to assess for active myocardial inflammation (myocarditis).

T2 STIR

- Used to assess for myocardial inflammation.

PHASE CONTRAST FLOW SEQUENCES

- Used to assess for total blood volume flow and regurgitant volumes in valve disease.

EARLY GADOLINIUM ENHANCEMENT

- Used to assess masses in the heart and intracardiac thrombus.

LATE GADOLINIUM ENHANCEMENT

- Gold standard for assessment of myocardial fibrosis and infarction. Presence, pattern and extent of fibrosis are important factors in assessing presence and severity of cardiomyopathy, including SCD risk.

Other sequences such as stress perfusion can be used to assess for coronary insufficiency in those with anginal chest pain or other features of CAD. Coronary origins and aberrant anatomy can also be assessed accurately with cardiac MRI.

Cardiac MRI offers information above what is possible from echocardiography, namely assessment of myocardial composition. Assessment of myocardial fibrosis is accurately performed with late gadolinium sequences and recent developments in parametric mapping can allow insights into interstitial fibrosis using T1 mapping sequences.

SUDDEN CARDIAC DEATH (SCD)

Sharma et al. (1997) defined sudden cardiac death as 'Non-traumatic, non-violent, unexpected, and resulting from sudden cardiac arrest within six hours of previously witnessed normal health.' The prevalence in sport of around 1 in 80,000–100,000 may be relatively low, but the after effects are often seen through huge outpourings of grief. This is a catastrophic event in healthy role models and sporting icons, where the resulting psychological and emotional effects are not only felt by their loved ones but also the general public, making headlines across the world.

SCD in Athletes with Abnormal Heart Structure

- Hypertrophic cardiomyopathy (HCM)
- Arrhythmogenic ventricular cardiomyopathy (AVC)
- Coronary artery anomalies
- Premature coronary artery disease
- Other (Marfan syndrome)

SCD in Athletes with Structurally Normal Hearts

- Long QT syndrome (LQTS)
- Brugada syndrome
- Catecholaminergic polymorphic VT (CPVT)
- Wolff-Parkinson-White syndrome
- Commotio cordis
- Drugs
- Electrolyte disturbances/heat stroke

History

Clinicians should pay particular attention to cardiac symptoms that can be the sentinel signs of a dangerous cardiac event (Figure 11.3). These include palpitations, pre-syncope and chest pain with exertion. True syncope should be reviewed clinically with a full history, examination and further cardiac assessment. Disproportionate breathlessness should be taken seriously, with cardiac and respiratory causes considered. There may also be a history of epilepsy or prior cardiac disease.

It is important to ascertain family history as there may be potential for an inherited cardiac condition

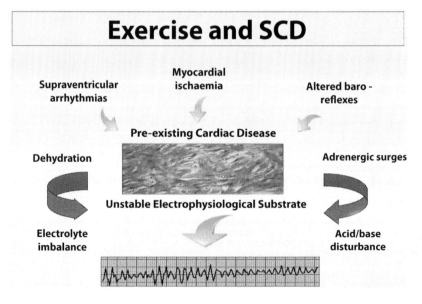

Figure 11.3 Exercise and SCD.

such as cardiomyopathy or channelopathy, or even premature coronary artery disease (in those under 50). Clinicians should also ask about family members who have suffered sudden cardiac death, epilepsy and unexplained drowning or road traffic collisions, as these events may be related to SCD.

Sudden death may be the first presentation in 75–80% of cases.

Hypertrophic Cardiomyopathy (HCM)

HCM is a genetically determined heart muscle disease characterised by thickening or hypertrophy of the myocardium in the absence of abnormal loading conditions (e.g. hypertension, aortic valve disease). The clinical prevalence of this condition is estimated to be one in 200-500. This is usually familial with autosomal dominant inheritance patterns, but isolated cases within families are increasingly recognised. Pathological variants in genes encoding sarcomeric proteins can be found in 30–50% of cases. At a microscopic level, the disease is characterised by myocyte disarray (Figure 11.4), which can lead to interruption of normal electrical conduction and contribute to ventricular arrhythmia (and ultimately SCD).

Left ventricular outflow tract obstruction (LVOT—as in Hypertrophic Obstructive Cardiomyopathy) is

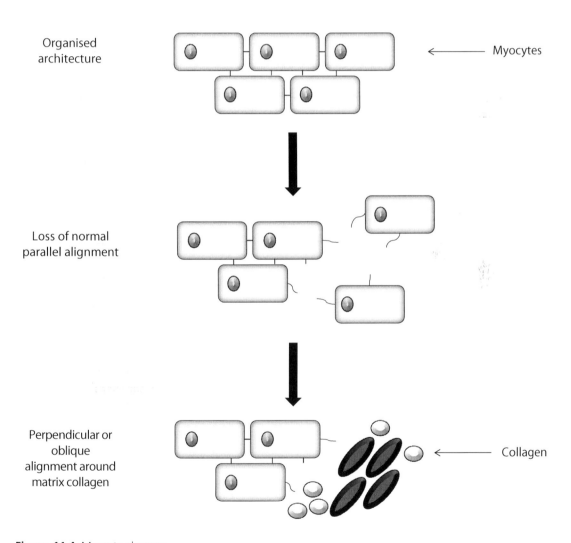

Figure 11.4 Myocyte changes.

reported in up to 70% of patients under clinical care and is associated with a higher symptom burden of dyspnoea and chest pain. Outflow tract obstruction is rarely seen in elite athletes due to the limitations it can place on cardiac output and, therefore, ability to perform at high activity levels. Other morphologies of hypertrophy are more commonly seen in athletes such as apical HCM or concentric LVH. These morphologies are associated with more efficient blood flow patterns in the heart and usually higher cardiac output. The extent of LVH can vary, with a normal wall width generally stated to be ≤12 mm in clinical guidelines. The ESC HCM guidelines suggest a diagnosis when wall width is ≥15 mm in the absence of abnormal loading conditions. High training loads can be associated with mild LVH in a normal heart, which is usually seen in combination with an increased LV chamber size. In HCM, mild LVH is seen in association with a reduced LV chamber size.

CLINICAL FEATURES

Most athletes with HCM are likely to have a mild phenotype (mild hypertrophy with no outflow tract obstruction) and are likely to be asymptomatic. There may be a mild exercise restriction at peak exercise. Most commonly, there will be no clinical signs on examination. An ejection systolic murmur can only be heard when there is outflow tract obstruction. Those with syndromic HCM are unlikely to have the cardiac, mitochondrial and peripheral muscle efficiency to perform as elite athletes.

Investigations

The ECG is abnormal in up to 90% of patients. This can include some changes that are also associated with athletic adaptation (such as LVH by voltage criteria) and intermediate changes (such as left atrial enlargement with P wave inversion in lead V1 and left axis deviation). Inferolateral T wave inversion is often seen in apical and concentric HCM.

Echocardiography may show a hypertrophied non-dilated left ventricle with no predisposing cause for LVH (e.g. aortic stenosis), often with a reduced chamber size. The relative wall thickness (representing the ratio of wall thickness to internal diameter) is often elevated. The myocardium width at the apex of

the normal heart is usually 5–7 mm and tapers from wider measurements seen in the base of the heart (often the septum). In apical HCM, this myocardium may be relatively hypertrophied at 10–11 mm versus what is usually observed, but does not reach the standard limits for true 'hypertrophy' at >12 or >15 mm.

Although systolic function (as assessed by ejection fraction) is preserved until late in the disease process, subtle changes in strain indices can be observed in mild phenotypes. Diastolic filling can be impaired early in the process due to stiffness in the LV. This can often be detected on echocardiograms. LVOT obstruction is diagnosed on echocardiogram with increased velocity of blood out of the heart on Doppler imaging. The extent of this is assessed at rest and with provocation such as valsalva manoeuvre. This is rarely seen in the elite athlete.

Management

Management of athletes with HCM is focused primarily on accurate risk assessment and management of symptoms that may affect performance.

Many clinical factors are incorporated into the ESC SCD risk assessment calculator, including maximal wall width, left atrial size, LVOT obstruction, history of syncope, history of observed non-sustained ventricular tachycardia, family history of sudden cardiac death and age. Other factors that help process SCD risk include level of myocardial fibrosis (scar) as assessed by cardiac MRI and blood pressure response to exercise. All athletes with HCM should undergo at least annual assessment, including cardiac imaging, ambulatory ECG monitoring and exercise testing to assess for arrhythmia and blood pressure response. An accurate assessment of risk can then be conveyed to the athlete and sporting body medical representatives to inform decisions regarding continuation of play. Generally, any features identified that indicate a high risk of SCD lead to a recommendation to cease competitive play and revert to type 1A (low intensity) sports activities.

Arrhythmogenic Ventricular Cardiomyopathy (AVC)

AVC is predominantly a genetic disorder of the myocardium predisposing patients to a high risk of arrhythmia ('arrhythmogenic'). Historically, the condition was believed to affect only the right ventricle, hence the term arrhythmogenic right ventricular cardiomyopathy, but it is now recognised to be predominantly a condition of both left and right ventricles. It is also accepted that there is an overlap with the phenotype of dilated cardiomyopathy, with some shared features such as arrhythmogenesis and weakening of systolic function. This is related to some shared underlying genetic aetiologies.

In some circumstances, this cardiomyopathy is associated with a weakening of connection between myocytes. When exposed to higher strains and myocardial stretch, it can lead to myocyte detachment. This subsequently causes inflammation of the myocardium (myocarditis) and fibro-fatty replacement of cardiomyocytes with irregular muscle disruption. This can lead to malignant re-entrant ventricular tachyarrhythmias.

Clinical Features

Athletes are often asymptomatic. Symptoms of palpitations may be reported as the condition is associated with a high ectopic burden. Syncope can be a dangerous sentinel symptom indicating self-terminating ventricular arrhythmia.

Investigations

ECG can show inverted T waves beyond V3 in the right ventricular phenotype, and inferolateral T wave inversion if there is left ventricular involvement. Ventricular ectopic beats are relatively common and may even be seen on the 12-lead ECG.

Echocardiography can show regional wall motion abnormalities of either the right or left ventricle. This is usually apparent in a reasonably advanced phenotype and may be associated with reduction in overall systolic function.

Cardiac MRI is the gold standard test for measuring ventricular volume and function (part of the diagnostic criteria) and, importantly, for assessment of myocardial inflammation and fibrosis. This cannot be done accurately on echocardiography. Exercise testing can be performed to understand ventricular ectopy and arrhythmia burden on exercise.

Management

Assessment of SCD risk is important and implantable cardioverter defibrillators (ICDs) are commonly used in these patients. Management of arrhythmia with medication is also common, with beta blockers used first-line before considering other medication classes.

It is recognised that intense exercise can pose a significant risk to patients with AVC. The acute period of intense exercise increases the risk of SCD at the time of activity due to myocardial stretch and adrenaline surges. Recurrent physical activity can accelerate the underlying cardiomyopathy and myocardial dysfunction. It is generally recommended that once a diagnosis is made, all intense activity should cease and patients are recommended to keep total activity down to less than 30 MET hours over 7 days.

CORONARY ARTERY DISEASE (CAD)

Coronary artery disease is a common cause of SCD in those >35 yrs and is diagnosed on post-mortem examination where death has occurred during physical activity. The risk factors for CAD are often present, including family history of atherosclerosis, hypertension, abnormal glucose metabolism and dyslipidaemia.

Clinical Features

There may be symptoms suggestive of coronary insufficiency, including anginal chest discomfort on exertion or excessive dyspnoea. High performing athletes may report an unexplained reduction in performance as the first sign of coronary insufficiency but, often, the CAD is asymptomatic, especially in masters athletes.

Investigations

Resting ECG is often normal. If there has been previous myocardial infarction there may be pathological Q waves and T wave inversion. If there is resting ischaemia, there may be ST segment changes. This is rare and usually associated with symptoms of myocardial infarction.

Exercise stress testing may uncover dynamic ST segment ECG changes and recreate anginal chest discomfort. The gold standard test for assessing the presence of CAD is now CT coronary angiography. Invasive angiogram is usually reserved for cases in which revascularisation may be performed with percutaneous coronary intervention at the same procedure.

Echocardiogram may be needed for assessment of LV function and the myocardium may show previous healed infarction.

Management

Risk factor modification and education concerning warning symptoms of chest pain, palpitations, or syncope is recommended. Cessation of high intensity activity whilst symptoms are investigated is advised. If CAD is observed, then medications such as statins and antiplatelets can be considered, along with assessment for revascularisation.

In subjects with structural abnormalities, including valvular disease or congenital lesions (operated or not), advice on exercise participation will be directed by the classification of the activity and consultation with a sports cardiologist.

CORONARY ARTERY ANOMALIES

A coronary artery anomaly (CAA) is a defect in one or more of the coronary arteries of the heart. These can relate to the origin or location of the artery. Coronary arteries originating from the wrong aortic sinus occur in 0.64% of all births.

The most common anomaly associated with exercise-related death is the main left coronary arising from the right coronary cusp, maintaining an acute angle with the aorta. Aortic dilatation on exercise causes obstruction to flow. Other anomalies may include the absence, or under-development, of major coronary branches.

Clinical Features

This is often asymptomatic until SCD, although may present with chest pain or unheralded syncope.

Investigations

A resting ECG is often normal. Echocardiography can see the origins and early course of the coronary arteries in most athletes. Non-invasive imaging using cardiac MRI or CT may detail the origins and course of the coronaries. Exercise testing may show evidence of exercise-induced reversible ischaemia.

Management

Surgical correction, if there is high risk anatomy or symptoms.

MARFAN SYNDROME

Marfan syndrome is a disorder of the body's connective tissues. These patients can have weak major arteries (aorta) and heart valves. The connective tissue abnormality is usually related to a defect in the Fibrillin gene (gene on the long arm of chromosome 15). This is an autosomal dominant condition with variable penetrance, although approximately 15% of cases are sporadic.

Clinical Features

The patient may have a tall and thin body, with pectus excavatum, scoliosis, flat feet and hypermobile joints. Occular abnormalities may include lens dislocation and near-sightedness. There may be a predisposition to pneumothorax and cardiac valve abnormalities, in particular aortic root dilatation.

Investigations

Echocardiography can assess aortic root and cardiac valves. Mitral valve prolapse is a common association. MRI can assess for aortopathy beyond the aortic root and dilation in the ascending aorta that may predispose to aortic dissection.

Management

Medical therapy including beta-blockers and angiotensin converting enzyme inhibitors/angiotensin 2 receptor antagonists can slow aortic dilatation.

If aortic root dilatation is more than 4.5 cm, prophylactic valve-sparing surgery is considered.

VIRAL MYOCARDITIS

A rare, acquired cause of SCD, this is a variable illness associated with symptoms of viral infection. Myocardial lymphocytic infiltration with focal necrosis can lead to cardiac dysfunction and conduction system problems. Myocardial inflammation can also act as a trigger for ventricular arrhythmia. In recent years, precautions have been taken following COVID-19 and the potential risks to the athlete, which has required post infection cardiac screening across various sports.

Clinical Features

Non-specific cold or flu-like symptoms can be reported. There may be tachycardia, supraventricular or ventricular extrasystoles. Rarely, this may progress to cardiomegaly and frank cardiac failure.

Investigations

A serum cardiac troponin is often elevated in myocarditis. ECG may be abnormal with ST-T wave changes, arrhythmias, heart block or other non-specific changes.

Echocardiogram may show systolic dysfunction in severe cases. A cardiac MRI is the gold standard for assessment of myocardial inflammation and fibrosis.

Exercise testing may be indicated to assess for arrhythmia on return to activity.

Management

There is a broad spectrum of severity. Cardiac failure and arrhythmias should be pharmacologically treated. If myocarditis is diagnosed, a period of abstinence from high level activity is recommended for 3–6 months. A graduated return to training following this period of abstinence is indicated. An updated assessment with ECG, cardiac MRI, serum troponin and exercise testing should confirm myocardial inflammation has settled and there is no increased arrhythmia burden.

LONG QT SYNDROME (LQTS)

LQTS affects the repolarisation electrical activity in the heart and is characterised by prolongation of the QT interval and T wave changes on the ECG. LQTS is predominantly an autosomal dominant genetic disorder leading to abnormalities of the sodium and potassium channels, with variable penetrance. It can be exacerbated by certain medications, serum electrolyte disorders and adrenaline surges.

The prolonged QT interval increases the risk of ventricular arrhythmia, with 'R on T' phenomenon leading to polymorphic VT.

Clinical Features

LQTS can be an asymptomatic observation on an ECG. A personal history of syncope is important, as is family history of SCD. SCD when turning off alarm clocks in the morning has been reported, related to a relaxed background state and subsequent stimulus producing an early ventricular ectopic.

Investigations

ECG demonstrates a corrected QT prolongation (corrected for HR) to more than 440 ms in males and 460 ms in females. The QTc is observed to be longer in trained athletes, with acceptable values of <470 msec in males and <480 msec in females. Bradyarrhythmias are common on ECG monitoring and T wave alternans may be induced by emotion.

Exercise testing and adrenaline provocation testing can display frequent ventricular ectopy, non-sustained or sustained ventricular arrhythmia.

Echocardiogram demonstrates the heart is structurally normal.

Management

Avoid medications known to prolong QTc (see crediblemeds.com). Beta blockers are very effective in treating LQTS—specifically, the most common genetic subtype LQT1. ICDs are suggested in high-risk cases, with family screening. Comprehensive evaluation with a sports cardiologist should guide continuation of sporting activity.

BRUGADA SYNDROME (BrS)

BrS is an inherited cardiac disorder, characterised by a typical ECG pattern and an increased risk of arrhythmias and sudden cardiac death (SCD). BrS is a complex disease at a genetic and molecular level, with a strong association with abnormalities of the sodium channel. It is predominantly a genetic disease with autosomal dominant inheritance. It is seen more commonly in males and in certain Asian populations.

BrS can be associated with SCD and risk assessment for this is complex. Avoidance of triggers such as fevers and provoking medications is important (www. brugadadrugs.org/).

Clinical Features

Commonly, no symptoms are reported but syncope may be present. In athletes, it can be associated with SCD soon after exercise.

Investigations

ECG may show a characteristic pattern of down-sloping ST segment elevation in leads V1-V3 with RBBB pattern, which is influenced by autonomic balance and exercise.

Provocation testing with ajmaline or flecainide may exacerbate the ECG changes.

Management

This consists of the avoidance of certain drugs and competitive sport. An ICD is required in high-risk cases, such as for ventricular arrhythmias, polymorphic ventricular tachycardia, or ventricular fibrillation.

WOLFF-PARKINSON-WHITE SYNDROME

An accessory pathway between the atria and ventricles gives a predilection to re-entrant supraventricular arrhythmias. There is a prevalence of 1.5/1000 and approximately 30% have arrhythmias. The presence of a conducting pathway between the atria and ventricles, without the regulation that the atrioventricular node offers, can predispose to dangerous arrhythmia. If atrial arrhythmia occurs, this may conduct directly to the ventricles—if the accessory pathway can conduct at high rates. SCD is a recognised complication, related to 1:1 conduction of atrial arrhythmia.

Clinical Features

Commonly asymptomatic. Athletes can report palpitations or, rarely, syncope.

Investigation

ECG can show a short PR interval (<0.12s) and a wide QRS complex with a delta wave, and initial slurring to the QRS complex (this represents electrical activity in the accessory pathway).

Exercise ECG, to assess for the presence of accessory pathways on surface ECG (delta wave) at high heart rates, can aid risk assessment for rapid atrial arrhythmia conduction (and therefore ventricular arrhythmia).

If symptomatic, an assessment of the accessory pathway should be undertaken. This can include electrophysiology study, which can also offer the possibility of ablation treatment at the same procedure.

Management

If there are rapid ventricular rates as a result of re-entrant SVT, then acute management may include the Valsalva manoeuvre or carotid sinus massage. A careful selection of drug therapy, to avoid retrograde excitation by blockade of the AV node, may be considered. Electrophysiological studies will be used to identify the accessory pathway in order to consider an ablation.

COMMOTIO CORDIS

This is a very rare phenomenon in which the initiation of VT/VF occurs after being struck in the precordium. It has been seen in the USA, with deaths occurring during ice hockey and baseball. There is no structural damage to the heart at post-mortem. Animal studies reveal that low energy blows during repolarisation caused VF.

PULMONARY EMBOLISM

Symptoms can include sudden onset of dyspnoea, pleuritic chest pain and a productive (pink and frothy sputum) cough. It can be associated with environmental hypercoagulable states, such as dehydration and sepsis, and can also be associated with family history of thrombosis or embolus.

Sinus tachycardia is the commonest ECG finding. There may be Right Axis Deviation (RAD), RBBB and right ventricular strain pattern: dominant R wave and T wave inversion/ST depression in V1 and V2; leads II, III and aVF may show similar changes. Rarely, the 'S I Q III T III' pattern occurs: deep S waves in I, pathological Q waves in III, inverted T waves in III.

Early recognition prompts investigation; a normal CXR is commonly seen prior to a CT pulmonary angiogram, which confirms embolus within a pulmonary artery.

Treatment includes subcutaneous low molecular weight heparin for a small PE. In life-threatening cases, i.e. deteriorating symptoms with severe right ventricular strain, thrombolysis or thrombectomy may be indicated.

ROLE OF AUTOMATED EXTERNAL DEFIBRILLATORS (AEDS) IN SPORT

There are 12 SCD events in people under 35 years every week in the UK, and a total of over 30,000 out of hospital cardiac arrests. The chances of survival will reduce by approximately 10% for every minute the patient remains in cardiac arrest. The survival from a sudden cardiac arrest is up to 50% if shocked within two to three minutes and dramatically decreases to less than 10% after ten minutes. Rapid defibrillation is a core component of successful resuscitation.

Basic life support is important in maintaining some cardiac output whilst advanced resuscitation is initiated. Training is available through multiple in-person and online modules and should be encouraged for all.

AEDs are potentially lifesaving equipment. There is a good case for every sporting venue to have one available on site. Their use increases survival chances and no training is required. Each box is simple and includes instructions in written form, along with verbalised instructions as the device is turned on. The presenting rhythm in cardiac arrest in most young athletes will be shockable (ventricular fibrillation or ventricular tachycardia). AEDs are therefore imperative in prompt appropriate treatment.

Many sporting events will arrange for full resuscitation teams to be on site during competition. This allows Advanced Life Support qualified clinicians to facilitate resuscitation, including airway management and use of medications as part of cardiac arrest care. It is important to consider post cardiac arrest care as part of standard operating policies, including handover to onward emergency care, whether or not there has been return of spontaneous circulation.

MULTIPLE CHOICE QUESTION (MCQ) QUESTIONS

1. A 44-year-old marathon runner suffers from sudden cardiac death (SCD) whilst exercising. You are not aware of any relevant past medical or family history. What is the most likely cause of SCD in this patient?

   A. Coronary artery disease
   B. Hypertrophic cardiomyopathy
   C. Arrhythmogenic ventricular cardiomyopathy
   D. Viral myocarditis
   E. Brugada syndrome

2. You discuss exercise with an elderly female patient and how cardiac function changes with age. Which of the following best explains why maximum heart rate decreases with age?

   A. Increased left ventricular stiffness
   B. Decreased electrical activity of sinoatrial node myocytes
   C. Increased acetylcholine release from the parasympathetic nervous system
   D. Decreased myocardial contractility
   E. Decreased stroke volume

3. You are arranging annual cardiac screening at your local football club. A black athlete has an ECG. Which of the following is the most concerning finding?

   A. T wave inversion in leads V1-V3 with preceding ST elevations
   B. Sinus bradycardia of 40 bpm
   C. T wave inversion in leads V4-V6
   D. Complete right bundle branch block
   E. 2nd degree AV block (Mobitz type I)

4. An elite level tennis player is undergoing cardiac screening. She is asymptomatic and has a normal clinical examination. Her grandfather died by drowning when he was 32 years old. ECG reveals LVH by voltage criteria, left atrial enlargement with P wave inversion in lead V1 and left axis deviation. What is the most likely diagnosis?

   A. Coronary artery abnormality
   B. Hypertrophic cardiomyopathy
   C. Arrhythmogenic ventricular cardiomyopathy
   D. Marfan's syndrome
   E. Brugada syndrome

5. The same player undergoes an echocardiogram. Which one of the following features would be most suggestive of the diagnosis?

   A. Reduced systolic function
   B. Regional wall motion abnormalities of either the right or left ventricle
   C. Aortic root dilatation and mitral valve prolapse
   D. Left ventricular wall width ≥11 mm in the absence of abnormal loading conditions
   E. Left ventricular wall width ≥15 mm in the absence of abnormal loading conditions

MULTIPLE CHOICE QUESTION (MCQ) ANSWERS

1. Answer A

   Coronary artery disease is the most common cause of SCD, particularly in older populations.

2. Answer B

   Although decreased responsiveness to adrenergic stimulation is thought to play a role in lower maximal heart rates, the key feature is the reduced intrinsic heart rate caused by reduced sinoatrial node activity with ageing.

3. Answer C

   T wave inversion in anterolateral leads such as this case, should prompt further investigation for structural abnormalities. Although some of the other answers are borderline, in isolation, they may be considered normal.

4. Answer B

   This history paired with ECG findings should raise the suspicion of hypertrophic cardiomyopathy as a diagnosis.

5. Answer E

   The ESC HCM guidelines suggest a diagnosis of hypertrophic cardiomyopathy when there is increased LV wall thickness ≥15 mm in the absence of abnormal loading conditions.

REFERENCES AND FURTHER READING

Drezner, J.A., Rao, A.L., Heistand, J., Bloomingdale, M.K., Harmon, K.G. (2009). Effectiveness of emergency response planning for sudden cardiac arrest in United States high schools with automated external defibrillators. *Circulatio*, 11, 120(6), pp. 518–525.

Drezner, J.A., Sharma, S., Baggish, A., et al. (2017). International criteria for electrocardiographic interpretation in athletes: Consensus statement. *British Journal of Sports Medicine*, 51, pp. 704–731.

Harkness, A., Ring, L., Augustine, D.X., Oxborough, D., Robinson, S., Sharma, V., the Education Committee of the British Society of Echocardiography. (2020). Normal reference intervals for cardiac dimensions and function for use in echocardiographic practice: A guideline from the British Society of Echocardiography. *Echo Research and Practice*, 7(1).

Kumar, S., Kalman, J.M., La Gerche, A. (2017). New international guidelines for the interpretation of the electrocardiograph in athletes: A "traffic light" tool for maximising diagnostic specificity. *Heart, Lung & Circulation*, 26(11), pp. 1119–1122.

Malhotra, A., Dhutia, H., Finocchiaro, G., Gati, S., Beasley, I., Clift, P., Cowie, C., Kenny, A., Mayet, J., Oxborough, D., Patel, K., Pieles, G., Rakhit, D., Ramsdale, D., Shapiro, L., Somauroo, J., Stuart, G., Varnava, A., Walsh, J., Yousef, Z., Tome, M., Papadakis, M., Sharma, S. (2018). Outcomes of cardiac screening in adolescent soccer players. *N Engl J Med*, 9;379(6), pp. 524–534.

Oxborough, D., Augustine, D., Gati, S., George, K., Harkness, A., Mathew, T., Papadakis, M., Ring, L., Robinson, S., Sandoval, J., Sarwar, R., Sharma, S., Sharma, V., Sheikh, N., Somauroo, J., Stout, M., Willis, J., Zaidi. (2018). A guideline update for the practice of echocardiography in the cardiac screening of sports participants: A joint policy statement from the British Society of Echocardiography and Cardiac Risk in the Young. *Endocrine-Related Cancer*, 5(1), G1–G10.

Sharma, S., Whyte, G., McKenna, W.J. (1997). Sudden death from cardiovascular disease in young athletes: Fact or fiction? *Br J Sports Med*, 31(4), pp. 269–276.

Respiratory 12

Daniel Fitzpatrick, David Eastwood and James Hull

INTRODUCTION

SEM clinicians should be aware, and promote the value of, exercise and physical activity in the management of several chronic lung diseases affecting the general population, including asthma and chronic obstructive pulmonary disease (COPD). In the context of COPD, pulmonary rehabilitation is now firmly established as a key non-pharmacological intervention and is recommended by several international guideline committees and the British Thoracic Society (BTS) (Bolton et al., 2013). It should be supervised, comprising two to three sessions each week, and involve aerobic and resistance exercise.

In the athletic population, respiratory problems are common. At the 2016 Olympic Games, 47% of all athlete illnesses affected the respiratory system. A recent British Olympic screening programme found 80% of athletes required assessment for a respiratory complaint.

Asthma is the most prevalent chronic medical condition in athletes, with allergies and sinonasal issues also often encountered. Respiratory tract infections are the most common acute condition requiring medical attention at sporting events and, if recurrent, can result in lost training time. It is therefore important that clinicians working with athletes have a good working knowledge of respiratory issues and are competent in the assessment and management of these issues.

RESPIRATORY PHYSIOLOGY

In order to understand the effects that exercise has on respiratory physiology, it is important to understand the physiology at rest.

Ventilation

Inspiration occurs as the volume of the thoracic cavity increases, reducing intrathoracic pressure and drawing air in through the upper airways. At rest, this is achieved through contraction of the diaphragm and the intercostal muscles. As the diaphragm contracts, it flattens. Intercostal muscle contraction simultaneously pulls the ribcage upwards and, together, this increases the intrathoracic volume.

Expiration at rest is a passive process. The diaphragm and intercostal muscles relax and the elastic recoil of the lungs themselves mean the thoracic cavity returns to its original size, expelling the air drawn in during inspiration.

The volume of air that moves in and out of the lungs at rest is referred to as the tidal volume. Although this varies depending on the size of the individual, a normal tidal volume is around 7 mL/kg of air.

This process of inspiration and expiration occurs 12 to 14 times per minute in healthy individuals at rest. The number of breaths per minute is referred to as the respiratory rate. Amount of air inspired and expired in a minute is called the minute volume and can be calculated as the Respiratory Rate × Tidal Volume (McArdle et al., 2010).

Gaseous Exchange

Once the air is in the lungs, gaseous exchange can occur. This is the process whereby oxygen is transferred to the blood, ready to return to the heart, and carbon dioxide (CO_2) is removed to be expired into the atmosphere. This happens in the alveoli, the terminal air sacs in the lungs, where the air is drawn alongside

DOI: 10.1201/9781003179979-12

RESPIRATORY

Exercise-induced bronchoconstriction (EIB)
- May be present in those with asthma
- Symptoms typically worsen immediately after cessation of exercise
- Spirometry with ↓ FEV1 post exercise challenge can confirm diagnosis
- Indirect bronchoprovocation testing may be needed e.g. eucapnic voluntary hyperventilation (EVH)

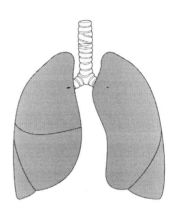

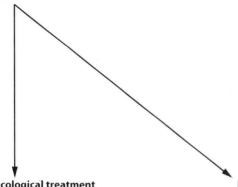

Non-pharmacological treatment
- Warm up 10-15 mins before exercise
- Avoid pollution/smoke
- Face covering/mask in cold air
- Optimise diet e.g. trial Omega-3, low salt diet, increased caffeine intake and Vitamin C

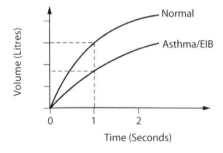

Pharmacological treatment
- Asthma care plan
- Annual influenza vaccination
- If needs B2-agonist >2 times/week:
  - PRN Budesonide/Formoterol

  OR
  - Regular inhaled corticosteroid twice daily +/- Bronchodilator

  OR
  - Oral Montelukast once daily +/- pre-exercise bronchodilator
- If EIB symptoms continue, consider mast cell stabilising drug (e.g. cromoglicate) or inhaled anti-cholinergic 10-15 mins before exercise

Exercise-induced laryngeal obstruction (EILO)
- Occurs during exercise and improves at cessation
- Noisy breathing and upper airway discomfort
- Video may be helpful in diagnosis
- Gold standard is Continuous laryngoscopy in exercise (CLE) testing
- Management: Treating comorbidities and breathing pattern re-training
- Teaching EILO-biphasic inspiratory breathing techniques may be useful
- Laser supraglottoplasty may be suitable in severe cases

Breathing pattern disorder (BPD)
- Excessive breathlessness disproportionate to exercise intensity
- Normal investigations
- Core stability assessment key to ensure adequate diaphragmatic recruitment
- Can co-exist with EIB and EILO
- Management: Treating comorbidities, breathing education and re-training

Figure 12.1 Pictorial summary.

capillaries. Both gases diffuse along concentration gradients across the capillary membrane. A high partial pressure (or amount) of oxygen (pO_2) encourages haemoglobin to bind to it, and the concentration gradient is maintained by blood flow. Meanwhile, a higher carbon dioxide concentration in blood than in air leads to diffusion of CO_2 out of the capillaries, and the concentration gradient is maintained by expiration.

Control of Respiration

In healthy individuals, the partial pressure of carbon dioxide (pCO_2) is the main driver of ventilation. Chemoreceptors for carbon dioxide are located in the medulla oblongata in the brainstem. When they detect an increase in the pCO_2, they stimulate an increase in the Respiration Rate and Tidal Volume. This results in an increase in Minute Volume and a subsequent reduction in the pCO_2.

There are also chemoreceptors for pO_2, located peripherally in the carotid and aortic bodies, that feedback to the medulla oblongata via the glossopharyngeal and vagus nerves. They respond in a similar way, causing the medulla oblongata to affect changes in respiratory rate and tidal volume. This is a secondary mechanism to the central detection of changes in pCO_2 in the majority of healthy individuals. In the absence of chronic respiratory disease, most individuals will tolerate a degree of hypoxia without a change in respiration or symptoms.

ACUTE RESPIRATORY RESPONSE TO EXERCISE

During exercise, increased muscle activity and consumption of ATP means both oxygen demands and CO_2 production increase. This results in changes to respiratory physiology that ultimately increases the total ventilation to meet these demands: first, Tidal Volume increases, followed by an increase in Respiratory Rate.

Increased ventilation occurs within a few seconds when exercising. This time frame is too short for changes in either pCO_2 or pO_2 to be responsible for the increase in ventilation; the major stimulus is via the motor cortex activating the respiratory centre in the medulla oblongata, occurring simultaneously to skeletal muscle activation.

In fact, pO_2 should not fall during exercise as, in healthy individuals, ventilation will respond to allow for oxygen to be absorbed to a greater degree than can be consumed. The arterial pO_2 will remain consistent at the alveolar level and, at moderate exercise intensities, this is also true for pCO_2. At higher exercise intensities (anaerobic respiration), increased lactate production and its subsequent buffering to CO_2 and hydrogen ions, does cause a transient increase in pCO_2, thus increasing ventilation.

This increase in respiratory drive increases both the rate and depth of breathing. Respiratory Rate increases to 35-45 breaths per minute and Tidal Volumes to around 2000 mL. In turn, the Minute Volume rises to around 18 times its resting value. Increases in Tidal Volume require the use of accessory muscles of ventilation for both inspiration and expiration. Inspiration is assisted by the scalenes, sternocleidomastoid, serratus anterior, pectoralis major and minor muscles and latissimus dorsi. The muscles of the anterior abdominal wall and the internal intercostals are responsible for active expiration.

Gaseous exchange also increases during exercise due to greater cardiac output and pulmonary blood flow. Reduced pulmonary vascular resistance allows a greater volume of deoxygenated blood to reach the alveoli before it returns, oxygenated, to the left atrium.

APPROACHING RESPIRATORY SYMPTOMS IN THE ATHLETIC POPULATION

History and Examination

When assessing any medical presentation, a systematic history and examination is essential. Respiratory symptoms including cough, wheeze and shortness of breath should be quantified, and clinical conditions that are more likely in the non-athletic population (e.g. COPD, fibrotic lung disease, anaemia, etc.) should not be disregarded.

Cough is frequently reported in exercising individuals. For many, there may not be an underlying pathological cause, such as asthma or other lung disease. Exercising in dry, cold air is known to increase the frequency of cough, due to irritation of the airways when they lose heat and moisture. It is likely, in some individuals, that the hyperpnoea mandated by exercise may trigger a cough response. Mucosal drying is also thought to lead to mechanical and chemical activation of nerve endings in the airways, promoting inflammatory mediator release. Exercise in air with chemical irritants (e.g. environmental pollutants or the chlorine rich air of an indoor swimming pool) may also promote this response.

An acute history of cough may relate to viral or bacterial infection, possibly requiring anti-microbial treatment. If coughing persists despite appropriate treatment, it is important to exclude alternative underlying pathologies and consider the need for investigations such as a chest X-ray.

Wheeze is both a symptom patients may complain of, and a clinical sign heard on auscultation of the chest. Often patients will present complaining of wheeze, mistaking their noisy breathing for this. Common causes of noisy breathing in an athletic population are Exercise-induced Bronchoconstriction (EIB), asthma and Exercise-induced Laryngeal Obstruction (EILO).

An underlying cause may be determinable by the history alone. An expiratory noise is more likely to be a wheeze, whilst inspiratory sounds may represent stridor. A monophonic wheeze, that is permanent, should raise concern for a fixed structural cause such as a bronchial tumour, whilst a variable wheeze, occurring following exercise, is more suggestive of EIB. A history of other atopic features may point towards asthma or EIB.

Exercise associated with shortness of breath is a common presenting complaint in athletes. EIB, EILO and Breathing Pattern Disorder (BPD) are the three most common causes and are discussed in detail below. Otherwise, there are numerous differential diagnoses for shortness of breath, including cardiac disease (myocarditis or cardiomyopathy being more common in the athletic population), anaemia or overtraining.

Red flag Symptoms

Red flag signs and symptoms may indicate respiratory conditions such as lung malignancy, atypical infections (tuberculosis), pulmonary embolism and pneumothorax. A number of symptoms warrant immediate investigation.

Haemoptysis may signal cancer or a pulmonary embolism. A rare cause is swimming-induced pulmonary oedema (SIPE), whereby circulating blood rapidly centralises due to cold water immersion, horizontal orientation and constrictive clothing. This increases pulmonary vascular pressure, leading to pulmonary oedema. Management includes extricating the athlete from water, removing any constricting clothing (e.g. wetsuits) and warming. Oxygen, diuretics and beta-2 agonists may be considered. A chest X-ray in the acute setting might confirm pulmonary oedema.

A recurrent productive cough should also be investigated, particularly in individuals with a smoking history. Sharp, pleuritic chest pain can be a sign of a pulmonary embolism or pneumothorax. Any person with respiratory symptoms associated with fever, weight loss or night sweats should be investigated for tuberculosis and malignancy.

Shortness of breath with syncope or palpitations are also 'red flag' and cardiac causes must be considered.

The onward investigation of these symptoms is beyond the scope of this chapter but may include same day emergency assessment or imaging performed within a 2-week period, as appropriate.

EXERCISE-INDUCED BRONCHOCONSTRICTION

EIB describes the condition whereby intense exercise causes acute small airways narrowing. It is now preferred over exercise-induced asthma, as exercise does not cause asthma, and EIB can occur in individuals without any other features of asthma. It is, however, seen more often in individuals who do have asthma, in particular in those whose asthma is not well controlled.

Those with EIB have impaired ventilation due to narrowing of their bronchioles (bronchospasm), which is caused by bronchiolar hyper-responsiveness. Triggers include exercise, cold air, dry air, allergens and viral infections, so athletes exercising outdoors in winter may be particularly susceptible. Additionally, there is evidence that swimmers may be at increased risk of EIB due to chronic exposure to chlorine rich atmospheres, which also causes airway inflammation. Exercise in polluted air can also be a trigger.

Presentation

Individuals with EIB present with shortness of breath or reduced exercise tolerance, chest tightness, wheeze or a dry cough. Symptoms are typically worse immediately following intense exercise bouts but some individuals report symptoms at the very start of exercise. Symptoms are usually associated with certain triggers such as exercising in cold, dry air or in environments with noxious airway stimuli such as high ozone, or particulates. It can be worse at certain times of year, e.g. when pollen counts are high. Some individuals present with symptoms following the use of non-steroidal anti-inflammatory drugs or aspirin.

A past medical history including asthma, eczema, hay fever or other allergies supports the diagnosis, as does a family history of atopic conditions. Individuals with concurrent asthma may have a diurnal pattern of symptoms.

Examination of an individual presenting with EIB may depend on the time of day and severity of symptoms. Examination findings will likely be normal at rest but, if an individual is assessed after a provocative activity, then a widespread polyphonic expiratory wheeze may be heard.

Investigations

Whilst some individuals' diagnosis may be based on clinical grounds, it is considered best practice to use objective measures to confirm a diagnosis and to ensure appropriate treatment (Hull et al., 2022). This can be especially important in athletes subject to anti-doping regulations, where robust evidence of diagnosis is required to apply for a therapeutic use exemption (TUE) for certain medications. The world anti-doping agency (WADA) advises that in competitive athletes, the diagnosis should be made with objective measures of variable airways obstruction. They also advise that if a pre-adolescent diagnosis of EIB is present, this should be proved again in adulthood (WADA, 2021a).

An initial investigation in most athletes with respiratory symptoms will be spirometry. This test is widely available and should conform to accepted standards, including repeated testing following the use of a bronchodilator if airflow obstruction has

been demonstrated. In spirometry, the Forced Vital Capacity (FVC) is the maximal volume of air that can be expired as quickly as possible in one breath, following a forced full inspiration. The volume of air expired in the first second is referred to as the Forced Expiratory Volume (FEV1). Once these are measured, the FEV1:FVC ratio can be calculated, which describes the proportion of the FVC that can be expired in one second. A value of less than 70% is considered an obstructive pattern. To investigate further, a bronchodilator (typically a B2-agonist such as salbutamol) is given and the test is repeated. A bronchodilator response > 10% relative to the predicted value for FEV1 or FVC indicates a positive response. An over-reliance on strict cut offs for bronchodilator response should be avoided (Stanojevic et al., 2021).

Peak expiratory flow rate (PEFR) has also been used historically to diagnose asthma. It can be impacted by multiple factors however, including the inspiratory flow and motivation to take a good inspiratory effort. Accordingly, it is recommended that spirometry is undertaken to ensure a reliable diagnosis of EIB.

Fractional exhaled nitrous oxide (FeNO) testing, if available, can detect airway inflammation that may be present in EIB and eosinophilic asthma. In this test, the individual expires at a steady rate into a machine that detects the concentration of nitrous oxide in the expired air. A concentration greater than 40 parts per billion is considered positive. Foods high in nitrates such as beetroot (often used for perceived ergogenic benefits in athletes) can impact the accuracy of this test.

If there is uncertainty, or the clinical history is indicative of EIB but initial investigations are negative, bronchoprovocation testing can be diagnostic. This will always require a referral to secondary care and access to 'gold-standard' indirect bronchoprovocation testing may be limited. Direct methodologies include using a stimulus (e.g. methacholine) that has a direct action on airway smooth muscle. Indirect testing (Eucapnic voluntary hyperventilation test (EVH) or Mannitol provocation test) involves using a stimulus that triggers an inflammatory response, which then acts on airway smooth muscle.

The EVH test is performed as below:

- Baseline maximum minute ventilation (MMV) is calculated by multiplying the baseline FEV1 by 30 or 35 (depending on the protocol used)

- During the test, the athlete will breathe a gas with 21% oxygen and 5% carbon dioxide (normal room air is 0.04% carbon dioxide). This maintains eucapnia (otherwise, hyperventilation would result in hypocapnia)
- The patient then breathes at 85% their calculated MMV for six minutes
- FEV1 is then measured at 1, 5, 10, 15 and 20 minutes after the challenge
- A reduction of >10% FEV1 from baseline within 20 minutes is considered a positive test

Management

Management of EIB should be multimodal including both pharmacological and non-pharmacological measures.

Clinicians should be familiar with the most up-to-date versions of guidelines and international guidance statements available for the management of asthma e.g. BTS/SIGN (2019) and the Global Initiative for Asthma (2022). Because EIB can be a feature of poorly controlled asthma, optimising pharmacological management of asthma must be considered in these individuals, including annual influenza vaccination and review of inhaler technique. Features of inflammatory chronic airway disease (e.g. eosinophilia) may be useful in identifying individuals with co-existing asthma.

Although using an inhaled short-acting B-agonist 10–15 minutes prior to exercise can be beneficial; tachyphylaxis can develop when it is used for frequent exercise (more than twice weekly). Therefore, using an inhaled corticosteroid/fast-acting long-acting B-agonist (e.g. budesonide/formoterol) before exercise, or on demand, is recommended. This is as effective as the alternative of regular twice daily inhaled corticosteroid +/– bronchodilator use before exercise.

Daily leukotriene receptor antagonists (e.g. monteleukast) can also be therapeutic in EIB. It should be taken at least 2 hours prior to exercise for maximal effect and may be an option for some athletes.

Further escalation can include mast cell stabilising medications such as cromoglicate. If further medications are required then onward referral to a respiratory specialist should be made.

Non-pharmacological measures to try and prevent symptoms of EIB include mitigation of triggers. If symptoms occur during cold conditions, a 'snood' (a cloth scarf covering the nose and mouth) can be worn. Wearing this during training can warm and humidify the air prior to inhalation, making it less provocative.

Some athletes have found that including short sprint efforts in warm-ups can prevent exacerbation. This causes an endogenous adrenergic response; which, in turn, causes bronchodilation and can reduce the need for pharmacological intervention. This needs to be at an intensity near to maximum heart rate and may provide a refractory period of two hours.

There is some evidence for dietary modification including omega 3 and vitamin C supplementation or a low-salt diet.

It is also recommended that concurrent allergy, sinus and upper airway disease should be treated to optimise airway health, especially given they commonly coexist.

CLINICAL CONSIDERATIONS

For athletes subject to anti-doping controls, the majority of asthma medications are permitted. Currently, the choice of beta-2-agonist that can be used without a TUE is limited to salbutamol, formoterol and salmeterol, each of which have a maximum daily use. It should be emphasised that the health of the athlete is the primary aim, rather than compliance with anti-doping regulations. If needed, a TUE should be obtained in order to provide optimal management and the latest WADA guidelines should be consulted.

This includes an acute asthma exacerbation when systemic anti-inflammatory medication (e.g. oral corticosteroids) may be required. Clinicians should clearly document in a medical emergency, including all relevant clinical features and results (e.g. peak flow measurements). This will aid retroactive TUE application.

EXERCISE INDUCED LARYNGEAL OBSTRUCTION (EILO)

EILO, also described by some clinicians as exercise-induced vocal cord dysfunction (VCD), is an important cause of breathlessness during exercise. It is a condition whereby structures in the larynx transitorily narrow during high intensity exercise, obstructing the upper airway and therefore limiting inspiration. In most cases, the arytenoid cartilages or aryepiglottic folds (the supra-glottic laryngeal level) narrow at peak exercise, causing symptoms. Those with EILO will often have been treated unsuccessfully for other conditions prior to diagnosis—it is a diagnosis often overlooked.

Presentation

The majority, around 70%, of those with EILO are female and the average age at diagnosis is 24 years. Symptoms associated with EILO are predominantly shortness of breath, noisy breathing and cough. In contrast to EIB, they occur at the peak of exercise intensity rather than afterwards. Symptoms associated with EILO also tend to resolve more quickly, after around five minutes, compared to thirty minutes in EIB. The patient with EILO may have tried beta-2 agonists, with limited success. EILO can exist alongside EIB and has been found in up to 1/3 of athletes with wheeze and cough.

It may be difficult to examine a patient with EILO, as symptoms occur during peak exercise, but an inspiratory stridor, rather than wheeze, is often present and is often audible to others in close proximity. There is likely to be an absence of clinical signs at rest.

Investigations

Currently, diagnosis is made by a respiratory specialist with an interest in unexplained breathlessness. The Gold Standard investigation is Continuous Laryngeal Endoscopy (CLE) (Griffin et al., 2018). CLE would likely be performed in addition to cardiopulmonary exercise testing (CPET) and spirometry. This is important, as it is possible the patient may have asthma, reflux or another contributing cause of symptoms.

CLE allows visualisation of the larynx to see if the supraglottic laryngeal structures or vocal cords (glottis) adduct during peak exercise, and whether this corresponds to symptoms. It is an exercise test conducted typically on a stationary bike or treadmill. Before the test begins, a flexible nasoendoscope is passed posteriorly through the nose and positioned with a view of the larynx from above, with the tip resting in the oropharynx. The endoscope is secured in place using a head-mounted harness and remains in situ for the test. The patient then performs a ramp

protocol on the bike or treadmill to maximum intensity, or to when symptoms occur. Throughout this, the images from the endoscope are reviewed. A positive test is when the supraglottic laryngeal structures or vocal cords adduct, with associated symptom onset.

It may be difficult to access CLE readily and so other means of gathering information can be considered. Showing athletes a video of the noisy breathing features present in EILO may be useful, or the athlete may provide a video of themselves whilst symptomatic. This should be recorded at peak exercise and examined for stridor and breathing patterns.

Management

The treatment approach to EILO is different to EIB, which is one of the key reasons diagnosis is so important. There have not been any randomised control trials on the best treatment options, but international consensus suggests a multi-disciplinary approach. Most, if not all, patients will receive speech and language therapy or respiratory physiotherapy. This may focus on rescue breathing techniques and EILO-biphasic inspiratory breathing techniques to relax the affected structures during exercise. It is also important to treat comorbidities identified such as asthma, allergy or GORD, that may cause upper airway irritation. In some cases, resistant to therapy and with significant symptoms, surgery with laser supraglottoplasty can be considered.

BREATHING PATTERN DISORDER

BPD is defined as any change in the normal biomechanical pattern of breathing that causes an impact on daily activities or athletic performance. The term has previously been used interchangeably with dysfunctional breathing or hyperventilation syndrome. It can occur on its own or in conjunction with any other respiratory condition.

Presentation

Individuals with BPD complain of shortness of breath out of proportion with exercise intensity, difficulty in taking deep breaths and a feeling of throat tightness. Symptoms tend to occur at peak exercise but can be associated with less strenuous activity. They may be related to times of increased stress or anxiety.

Investigations

Assessment should be undertaken at rest and during exercise. Individuals should be observed for abnormal breathing patterns such as: disproportionate breathlessness, excessive mouth breathing, predominant apical chest movement, increased respiratory rate disproportionate to metabolic demands, increased accessory muscle use, slumped posture and audible breathing excessive to the level of exercise intensity.

Management

There is a lack of high-quality randomised evidence on the best treatment; however, breathing pattern retraining physiotherapy is the current mainstay. This should be sport-specific and aim to involve other members of the multidisciplinary team. It is also important to address concurrent issues such as EIB, EILO or symptoms of anxiety.

ALLERGY

Allergic upper airways disease, along with other presentation of allergy such as conjunctivitis and dermatitis, may occur in athletes. Several studies have shown a higher prevalence of allergic rhinitis (up to 29%) in athletes compared to the general population. There have been many reasons suggested for this, including outdoor training with greater exposure to environmental allergens, subjection to chlorinated air in swimmers and training in cold weather. Low temperatures may exacerbate symptoms due to nasal vasoconstriction and a preference to oral breathing, which increases airways exposure to allergens.

There is a spectrum of allergic upper airways disease from rhinitis to sinusitis and obstructive nasal polyps. Nasal polyps are thought to occur as a result of mucosal proliferation and can cause nasal and sinus obstruction due to their size.

Presentation

Symptoms will vary depending on exposure to seasonal or perennial allergens. Typically, tree pollen tends to be released in spring, whereas grass pollen is more prevalent in the summer months. Therefore, a careful history of timing of symptom onset may be sufficient to establish the likely causative allergen.

Symptoms of allergic rhinitis include sneezing, nasal congestion, rhinorrhoea and nasal itch. Both nostrils are usually affected. Sometimes eye symptoms, such as itch or discharge, are present.

Nasal polyps may present with nasal obstruction, nasal discharge, frequent episodes of sinusitis due to obstruction, headache or snoring. Whilst symptoms will likely be exacerbated with exposure to allergens, if the polyps are large enough, there may be constant background symptoms.

Individuals with allergic rhinitis are likely to have other atopic conditions such as asthma or eczema, or a family history of atopy.

Examination can show a swollen nasal septum with telangiectasia. Polyps are sometimes visible on anterior examination of the nose. A unilateral nasal polyp should raise suspicion of malignancy and an urgent referral to an ENT specialist should be made.

Investigations

For many, this diagnosis can be made clinically. However, as with asthma, a number of treatments may require a TUE and other investigations should be sought for objective evidence.

An ENT specialist may perform a more detailed examination using a flexible nasal-endoscope to visualise parts of the nose not visible on anterior rhinoscopy. A peak nasal inspiratory flow can be performed to quantify the degree of nasal obstruction. A CT scan of the sinuses can help to visualise polyps.

In terms of identifying the causative allergen, skin prick testing can be performed in allergy clinics. If this is not suitable, blood tests looking for IgE for specific allergens can be taken.

Management

Where possible, management should include avoidance of the allergen. However, this may be unavoidable and symptomatic treatment should be considered. In those who are known to have seasonal exacerbations, anticipatory treatment can be initiated.

In patients not subject to anti-doping controls, the first line for mild to moderate, intermittent symptoms are either intranasal antihistamines or an oral antihistamine on an as-required basis. They are both equally effective, although the nasal route tends to have a faster onset. More severe or persistent symptoms can be treated with regular intranasal corticosteroids. If that does not control symptoms, or if they are severe, then a short course of oral corticosteroids such as prednisolone can be used for 5–10 days.

Nasal and oral decongestants containing phenylephrine or pseudoephedrine can be helpful in dilating the nasal passages. However, these frequently cause tachyphylaxis and so should be used sparingly. If symptoms persist, an intranasal corticosteroid is preferred.

A number of treatments are prohibited without a TUE for athletes subject to anti-doping controls (WADA, 2021b). Oral and intranasal antihistamines, intranasal corticosteroids and some intranasal decongestants are permitted. Oral decongestants containing pseudoephedrine are prohibited, as are all other routes of corticosteroid administration including oral and injected.

If symptoms are poorly controlled with these measures, referral to an allergy specialist is recommended. Other treatments include allergen immunotherapy (AIT) via subcutaneous (SCIT) or sublingual routes (SLIT).

Nasal polyps can be treated with the above measures but, if this is not successful, surgery may be needed. This is usually functional endoscopic sinus surgery (FESS), performed by an ENT surgeon, and involves resecting the polyps under endoscopic guidance.

MULTIPLE CHOICE QUESTION (MCQ) QUESTIONS

1. You are performing a pre-signing medical for a football player and are asked to complete an assessment of the player's respiratory function. When considering measurement of respiratory volumes, minute volume is calculated by which of the following equations?

   A. Respiratory Rate × Forced Vital Capacity
   B. Respiratory Rate × Tidal Volume
   C. Forced Vital Capacity × 60
   D. Forced Expiratory Volume in 1 second / Forced Vital Capacity
   E. Peak Expiratory Flow Rate × 60

2. A healthy 24-year-old rower begins a 2000 m race. Within the first 100 m their respiratory rate increases from 12 to 30 and they are noted to be breathing more deeply. What is the main mechanism that causes this increase in tidal volume?

   A. Conscious control by the athlete in anticipation of the increased effort
   B. Reduction in arterial oxygen concentration
   C. Motor cortex feedback to the medulla oblongata
   D. Lactate production as a result of anaerobic respiration in the muscles
   E. Increased arterial carbon dioxide concentration

3. You are the doctor for a professional cycling team. One of the cyclists sees you in the off season and complains of intermittent chest tightness, cough and shortness of breath that occurs in the mornings and shortly after completing a race. They have a history of eczema. You suspect a diagnosis of asthma, what is the best initial management plan?

   A. Peak expiratory flow rate diary for 2 weeks and review
   B. Trial of low dose inhaled corticosteroid inhaler
   C. Spirometry with bronchodilator reversibility challenge
   D. Chest X-ray
   E. Trial of short acting bronchodilator such as salbutamol

4. Whilst working as the doctor for the national athletics squad, you refer one of the athletes for a eucapnic voluntary hyperventilation test. The test result confirms your clinical suspicion of exercise

induced bronchoconstriction (EIB). She is currently training most days of the week. What is the most appropriate initial management?

A. Salbutamol inhaler to use as required and 10–15 minutes prior to exercise
B. Low dose inhaled corticosteroid regularly twice daily with salbutamol inhaler to use as required after exercise
C. Low dose inhaled corticosteroid/long acting B-agonist to take 10–15 minutes prior to exercise
D. Oral prednisolone for 1 week with salbutamol inhaler to use as required
E. Trial of leukotriene antagonist to take once daily, 1 hour prior to exercise

5. You are working on a new referral programme for the pulmonary rehabilitation service in a general hospital. Which of the following criteria should result in a referral for pulmonary rehabilitation?

A. Using three or more medications
B. An exercise tolerance of less than 500 metres
C. Referral to a palliative care specialist
D. MRC Dyspnoea score of two
E. Admission to hospital with an exacerbation of COPD

MULTIPLE CHOICE QUESTION (MCQ) ANSWERS

1. Answer B
    Minute Volume = Respiratory Rate × Tidal Volume. Apart from D, which is a measure of airways obstruction, the other options are not routinely used metrics.
2. Answer C
    The initial increase in tidal volume does not occur as a result of any biochemical changes. It is a learnt response and caused by cortical increases in motor activity. This is not a conscious process (A). The increase in respiration means the PO_2 will likely increase during exercise and not decrease (B). Although lactate buffering to carbon dioxide (D and E) would stimulate an increased respiratory rate

through medulla oblongata chemoreceptors, this is not the mechanism for the initial increase.

3. Answer C
    This patient has a history suggestive of asthma. High quality objective evidence of asthma will mean appropriate treatment for the patient and may be required for TUE authorisation later on. A peak flow diary (A) may be helpful in identifying triggers, but not in diagnosis and trials of treatment (A and E) may provide some idea if this is an airways disease but are not diagnostic. An X-ray (D) would not be indicated at this stage without any other clinical details.

4. Answer C
    Low dose inhaled corticosteroid/long acting B-agonist to take 10–15 minutes prior to exercise or on demand is an effective first line treatment in EIB. Answer A is likely to lead to tachyphylaxis as the athlete exercises frequently. Low dose inhaled corticosteroid regularly twice daily with salbutamol inhaler used prior to exercise, and not after, is an appropriate alternative (B). Similarly, a trial of a daily leukotriene antagonist may be appropriate but it is most effective taken at least 2 hours prior to exercise (E). Oral steroids are not appropriate first line and would require a TUE (D).

5. Answer E
    Following admission, it is recommended that patients be referred for pulmonary rehabilitation. Medications (A) or distance of exercise tolerance (B) are not referral criteria. Someone who has been referred for palliative care (C) may still be suitable as this does not necessarily mean they are at the end of their life and they may benefit. However, it is not a referral criterion. An MRC dyspnoea score of three or above would warrant referral (D).

REFERENCES AND FURTHER READING

Bolton, C.E., Bevan-Smith, E.F., Blakey, J.D., et al. (2013). BTS guidelines on pulmonary rehabilitation. *Thorax*, 68, pp. ii1–ii30.

BTS/SIGN. (2019). *British Guideline for the Management of Asthma*. SIGN 158.

Global Initiative for Asthma. (2022). *Global Strategy for Asthma Management and Prevention*. Available at: www.ginasthma.org

Griffin, S.A., Walsted, E.S., Hull, J.H. (2018). Breathless athlete: Exercise-induced laryngeal obstruction. *British Journal of Sports Medicine*, 52, pp. 1211–1212.

Hull, J.H., Burns, P., Carre, J., et al. (2022). BTS clinical statement for the assessment and management of respiratory problems in athletic individuals. *Thorax*, 77, pp. 540–551.

McArdle, W., Frank I. Katch, Victor L. Katch. (2010). *Exercise Physiology: Energy, Nutrition and Human Performance*. 7th ed. Baltimore: Wolters Kluwer.

Stanojevic, S., Kaminsky, D.A., Miller, M., et al. (2021). ERS/ATS technical standard on interpretive strategies for routine lung function tests. *Eur Respir J 2022 Jul 13*; 60(1), p. 2101499.

WADA. (2021a). *TUE Physician Guidelines—Asthma*.

WADA. (2021b). *TUE Physician Guidelines—Sinusitis/Rhinosinusitis*.

Endocrinology **13**

Anoop Raghavan, Rebecca Robinson and Nicky Keay

RELATIVE ENERGY DEFICIENCY IN SPORT (RED-S)

Relative energy deficiency describes the issues related to low energy availability. This is of particular concern to athletes where there is a mismatch between dietary energy intake and exercise energy output. This leads to an impairment in physiology affecting a wide spectrum of body systems and athletic performance.

The International Olympic Committee defines energy availability as:

$$\frac{\text{Energy intake (kcal)} - \text{Exercise energy expenditure (kcal)}}{\text{Fat free mass (FFM) (kg)}}$$

In healthy adults this equates to around 45 kcal/kg FFM/day.

Historically, the outcomes of low energy availability were described by the "female athlete triad" which included disordered eating, low bone mineral density and menstrual disorders. However, there has been a necessary shift in nomenclature in favour of understanding a broader condition, which affects both sexes. A range of body systems including endocrine, bone, cardiac and psychological can be affected.

The endocrine system is complex and highly sensitive to interruptions in dietary intake. The hypothalamic release of gonadotropin releasing hormone is reduced, thus preventing the normal anterior pituitary release of gonadotropins. A fall in circulation of follicle-stimulating hormone (FSH), luteinising hormone (LH) and subsequent sex steroid hormone production reduces fertility and impacts bone health,

in addition to disturbing other functions crucial for athletic performance. Substrate utilisation is also impaired and a reduction in energy availability can reduce muscle protein synthesis. The lower availability of carbohydrates reduces metabolic rate, reflected in down-regulation of thyroid hormones, and the body utilises fat stores. In turn, this can cause reduced insulin, ghrelin and leptin (thus further disordering dietary intake).

The reduced production of oestrogen and testosterone (androgens) negatively affects bone health. This occurs directly in females and indirectly—through testosterone conversion—in males via aromatisation. With reduced androgens, osteoclasts are stimulated, reducing bone mineral density (BMD) and increasing fracture risk. Additionally, the raised cortisol and catecholamines in RED-S patients reduce BMD further, thus increasing lifelong fracture risk, poor injury recovery and impaired biomechanics. Bone density peaks at 25, so identifying young athletes and managing them proactively, with a multidisciplinary team, can optimise short term bone health and reduce the long term osteoporosis risk. There is a higher risk in females with delayed menarche, as there has been less time for bone to be accrued with oestrogen (Elhakeem, et al., 2019). In these cases—no menarche by 15 years with secondary sexual characteristics or no menarche by 13 years without secondary sexual characteristics—referral for specialist investigation should be sought. Bone health screening with dual X-ray absorptiometry (DEXA) can be used, with athletes expected to have an increased BMD compared to the general population (Figure 13.2).

DOI: 10.1201/9781003179979-13

ENDOCRINOLOGY

Obesity

$$Body\ mass\ index = \frac{Weight\ (kg)}{Height\ (m)^2}$$

Underweight	<18.5
Healthy	18.5–24.9
Overweight	25–29.9
Obesity 1	30-34.9
Obesity 2	35–39.9
Obesity 3	≥ 40

Lungs
↓ Tidal volume
↓ Chest wall compliance
↑ Respiratory rate
↑ O_2 consumption with exercise

Gastrointestinal / endocrine
Fatty liver disease
Insulin resistance
Hyperlipidaemia

Cardiac
↑ Peripheral vascular resistance
↑ Blood volume
RV hypertrophy and dysfunction
LV hypertrophy, diastolic and systolic dysfunction

Relative Energy Deficiency in Sport (RED-S)

- Clinical syndrome involving adverse health and performance
- Can affect exercisers of any age, level or sex
- Driven by low energy availability
- Endocrine dysfunction can cause:
  - ↓ Fat and muscle
  - ↓ Bone formation and Bone mineral density
  - ↑ Cortisol
  - ↓ GnRH, LH, Leptin, T3 and IGF-1
  - Menstrual dysfunction in females

- Management with a multidisciplinary approach
- Transdermal oestrogen + cyclical oral progesterone hormone replacement therapy may be appropriate in females with amenorrhea and poor bone health

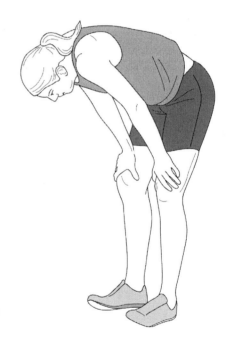

Osteoporosis

Normal	T ≥ – 1.0
Osteopenia	–2.5 < T < – 1.0
Osteoporosis	T ≤ –2 .5
Established Osteoporosis	T ≤ –2 .5 + one or more fragility fractures

↓ Bone density
Deterioration of microarchitecture of the bone

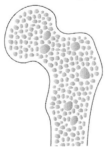

Figure 13.1 Pictorial summary.

A T-score is presented relative to a young, healthy adult, whereas a Z-score compares to someone of the same age. A T-score above -1 is normal. Between −1 and −2.5 is defined as osteopenia and at or below −2.5 is osteoporotic.

Fertility is negatively affected via functional hypothalamic amenorrhoea (FHA). The reduced circulating gonadotropins can manifest as primary and secondary amenorrhoea. Additionally, subtle changes occur including menstrual irregularity and spotting, reducing the chances of pregnancy. FHA must be confirmed via a workup to exclude other causes and so full fertility history, pelvic examination, blood tests (including FBC, gonadotrophins, TFTs) and pelvic ultrasound, may be useful.

CLINICAL CONSIDERATIONS

The psychological impact of RED-S is often overlooked. Healthy relationships with food and exercise are difficult to promote, even with a trusted MDT. Physical changes can be acute, but behaviours are often more chronic. Team physicians should be wary of both overt disorders (anorexia nervosa, bulimia) and subtle changes (binge-purge, fasting, strict diets). Feelings of low self-worth, obsessiveness and poor concentration are common and can often be a cultural norm amongst athletic populations. These can contribute to reduced performance via poor decision making and judgement. Education is vital in overcoming these barriers.

Addressing the cause of RED-S is the mainstay of treatment. This generally comes through increasing nutritious energy intake (carbohydrate and protein rich meals) or reducing expenditure. Treatment seeks to reduce both short- and long-term medical sequelae and involves an MDT with a sports physician, dietitian and psychologist. It is important to remember that there is no concrete guideline, so an open approach and dynamic monitoring is required for appropriate medical care.

In females with FHA and poor bone health (suggested by a Z-score <-1 (lumbar spine) and/or 1+ stress fractures), transdermal oestrogen with cyclical oral progesterone hormone replacement therapy may be appropriate for short term use. The prescription of combined oral contraceptives is not recommended and may mask the return of menses (Mountjoy et al., 2018).

THYROID DISEASE IN ATHLETES

The thyroid gland is situated in the lower, anterior neck and controls various processes. Principally, these can be classified under metabolic, cardiac, muscular and bone health.

The thyroid gland aims to maintain a state of optimal thyroid hormone (T3 and T4) levels. An often vague clinical presentation means a high index of suspicion is required in thyroid disease, especially within the sporting population.

THYROID FUNCTION

The hypothalamic-pituitary-thyroid axis is crucial in regulating thyroid hormone in healthy individuals.

- The hypothalamus secretes thyrotropin-releasing hormone (TRH).
- This acts on the anterior pituitary gland which secretes thyroid-stimulating hormone (TSH).
- TSH stimulates the follicular cells of the thyroid, which release the thyroid hormones: Triiodothyronine (T3) and Thyroxine (T4).

When thyroid hormone levels are sufficiently high, there begins a process of negative feedback to maintain homeostasis: TRH drops, which reduces TSH production and in turn reduces T3 and T4 production. T4 is released at a much higher ratio than T3 (14:1) and this is converted in peripheral tissue by deiodinases to its more active form, T3. The states of thyroid function exist on a spectrum ranging from hypothyroid, euthyroid and hyperthyroid.

HYPOTHYROIDISM

There is a prevalence of about 0.5–5% of the UK population, with a large subclinical group. It is defined by the National Institute of Clinical Excellence (NICE) using clinical findings with TSH >10 mU/L and below-normal free T4. There are multiple causes with the most common being primary thyroid gland failure due to autoimmune response. Other causes include medication (carbimazole, lithium, amiodarone), thyroid/anterior neck surgery and, globally, the leading cause remains dietary

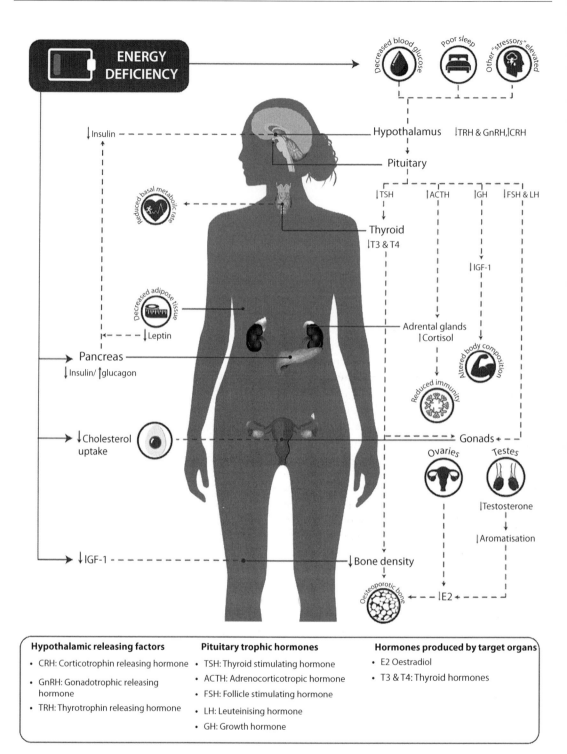

ENERGY DEFICIENCY

Decreased blood glucose
Poor sleep
Other "stressors" elevated

↓Insulin

Hypothalamus ↓TRH & GnRH,↑CRH

Pituitary

Reduced basal metabolic rate

↓TSH   ↓ACTH   ↓GH   ↓FSH & LH

Thyroid
↓T3 & T4

↓IGF-1

Decreased adipose tissue

↓Leptin

Adrenal glands
↑Cortisol

Altered body composition

Pancreas
↓Insulin/↑glucagon

Reduced immunity

↓Cholesterol uptake

Gonads

Ovaries   Testes

↓Testosterone

↓Aromatisation

↓IGF-1

↓Bone density

Oesteoporotic bone

↓E2

Hypothalamic releasing factors

- CRH: Corticotrophin releasing hormone
- GnRH: Gonadotrophic releasing hormone
- TRH: Thyrotrophin releasing hormone

Pituitary trophic hormones

- TSH: Thyroid stimulating hormone
- ACTH: Adrenocorticotropic hormone
- FSH: Follicle stimulating hormone
- LH: Leuteinising hormone
- GH: Growth hormone

Hormones produced by target organs

- E2 Oestradiol
- T3 & T4: Thyroid hormones

Figure 13.2 The endocrine changes associated with RED-S.

Source: www.health4performance.co.uk

insufficiency of iodine. Although the classic presentation is well documented—including cold intolerance, lethargy, dry hair and nails and weight gain, amongst others—the true effects of disease can be more subtle.

Hypothyroidism can affect athletic performance by a reduction in physiological function. Firstly, substrate utilisation is impaired via reduced protein synthesis and carbohydrate metabolism. This can decrease the overall basal metabolic rate (BMR) and increase body weight, reduce muscle mass and increase body fat. Secondly, disruption of metabolism can slow muscle contraction and power output.

The cardiovascular system is also affected. Athletic physiological bradycardia is a well-known topic but can be exacerbated in hypothyroidism. A lack of T3 reduces myocardial contractility, diastolic function and potentiates premature vascular stiffening. ECG can be useful and can demonstrate a triad of bradycardia, flat/inverted T waves and low voltage QRS complexes. This can cause heart blocks, arrhythmias and atherosclerotic disease.

Musculoskeletal health is also compromised. There is slowed bone turnover, causing weakness and increased long term fracture risk. Recognition and monitoring of these patient groups is key through serial imaging (DEXA) and early calcium supplementation. Muscular weakness is caused by changing muscle fibre type from 1 to 2 and reduced power outputs. The change in fibre type leads to pseudohypertrophy and local muscle fibre swelling. Proximal myopathy can co-exist and can present with weakness and fatigue, with associated reduced tendon reflexes.

Treatment comes with levothyroxine and this must be considered carefully among athletes due to its potential for abuse. Competitive advantages can be gained through its metabolic effects in controlling weight. However, the risks from iatrogenic hyperthyroidism: hyperthermia, arrhythmia and muscle dysfunction can be overlooked by athletes.

Subclinical hypothyroidism is defined as TSH >5 mU/L + normal free T4. Clinical findings of hypothyroidism are usually absent. There is a relatively low overall risk of progression to overt hypothyroidism (5%) but impaired thyroid function has issues regardless. There is an association with iron deficiency anaemia, Type 2 diabetes and coeliac disease.

CLINICAL CONSIDERATIONS

Subclinical hypothyroidism may be seen in athletes who have been overtraining or had inadequate recovery time. Therefore, a blood profile suggestive of subclinical hypothyroidism should prompt an assessment of training status and nutrition. A repeated blood sample should then be taken when these are addressed (Nicoll et al., 2013).

HYPERTHYROIDISM

With a prevalence of 1–2%, this is defined as excessive thyroid hormones in peripheral tissue with TSH <0.4 mU/L and raised T3 and/or T4. It is recommended to repeat the blood test after 3 months along with an ESR and thyroid peroxidase antibodies. An USS should be done for all patients with a palpable goitre. This may present with weight loss, heat intolerance, exophthalmos, and tremor. The main causes are Grave's disease (autoimmune), thyroid adenoma, thyroiditis and medications (levothyroxine and iodine being most common). Early endocrinology specialist advice should be sought for management with carbimazole.

There are several implications on athlete health and performance. BMR is inappropriately raised with increased caloric expenditure, weight loss and weakness. This also increases the risk of exercise-induced hyperthermia as well as fatigue from depleted glycogen stores. The cardiac risks come with athletic physiological bradycardia masking the tachycardia from thyroid hormone adrenergic stimulation. This both increases diagnostic difficulty and risks exacerbating arrhythmias, atrial fibrillation and flutter.

The musculoskeletal system is also compromised. Muscle function is impaired with atrophy and fat infiltration. Bones are similarly affected with greater stimulation of osteoclasts leading to weakness of the architecture of both cortical and trabecular bones. This reduced BMD increases fracture risk, especially in those with poorly controlled disease, inadequate nutrition or recovery and high training.

Subclinical hyperthyroidism is defined as low TSH with raised or normal T3/T4. If TSH <0.1 mU/L there is a risk to overt progression of around 1–2%. Though there is a reduced risk of the same complications as overt disease (impaired cardiac, musculoskeletal and bone health), this must be recognised and monitored appropriately.

OBESITY

Obesity is the excessive storage of fat tissue. It is a significant health burden globally, with prevalence continuing to rise in the UK. It places a significant burden on both mortality and morbidity and there is a significant socio-economic and UK geographic disparity, with northern areas experiencing far higher rates of disease.

The classification of weight comes from body mass index (BMI), calculated as:

$$\frac{\text{weight (kg)}}{\text{height (m)}^2}$$

The categories are:

- Underweight: BMI <18.5
- Healthy weight: BMI 18.5–24.9
- Overweight: BMI 25–29.9
- Obesity 1: BMI 30–34.9
- Obesity 2: BMI 35–39.9
- Obesity 3: BMI >40

CLINICAL CONSIDERATIONS

BMI may lead to inaccuracy in the classification of athletes. Some athletes may have a high body weight due to greater lean body mass.

Causes

Obesity is a growing issue and evidence regarding its health impacts are evolving. Life expectancy is reduced by two to four years in persons with a BMI of 30–35 kg/m² and by eight to ten years in persons with a BMI of 40–50 kg/m². Being overweight or obese is associated with an increased risk of developing type 2 diabetes, coronary heart disease, hypertension, stroke and cancers, amongst many other chronic diseases.

There are multiple causes but, principally, there is a mismatch between energy availability and expenditure. This has been attributed to societal factors, with high calorie food choices becoming cheaper and more accessible, busier work schedules, reduced exercise participation and a shift in cultural norms. Medical issues—such as PCOS, hypothyroidism and Cushing's disease—increase fat storage, as do medications—including insulin, oral hypoglycaemics and anti-epileptic drugs.

Physiology

Obesity disrupts various physiological mechanisms. Not only do adipocytes store fat as energy, but they also serve an endocrine function. Adipokines (cell signallers from fat tissue) produce proteohormones, which, along with insulin, regulate fat storage and satiety. These hormones become reduced and insensitive in obesity. Fat tissue also causes inflammation. Tumour necrosis factors, interleukins and cytokines have both local and systemic effects, notably in vessels, contributing to atherosclerotic disease. Additionally, adipokines stimulate the renin angiotensin system, which is intensified in obesity. This exacerbates hypertension and makes its management more challenging.

Fat deposition is another important factor in the manifestation of disease. Buttock fat is less endocrinologically active than visceral fat, acting as a primary energy store. Central obesity stimulates more adipokines, responsible for metabolic syndrome (obesity, hypertension and type 2 diabetes) and abdominal circumference is important when stratifying disease: i.e. greater circumference increases risk. This applies to all ethnicities and genders.

Management

Management strategies are complex, with no universal singular treatment. Open, non-judgmental medical communication is an effective tool. Many obese patients are unaware of their health status, as well as of the host of related comorbidities. Even modest weight loss (5–10%) yields great improvement in many outcomes (HbA1c, blood pressure, insulin sensitivity, joint health and biomechanics). Dieting is the most cost-effective treatment, posing least risk, but has high rates of rebound. Behavioural change can be a useful strategy for clinicians to facilitate this.

Medications can be used, where appropriate, but should not be used in isolation. Orlistat is a lipase inhibitor that reduces absorption of dietary fat and is available to those with a BMI > 30 and risk of metabolic disease. However, abdominal pain and diarrhoea are common side effects and the medication must be stopped if 5% weight loss is not achieved by 12 weeks. Liraglutide is a GLP-1 agonist which increases insulin, reduces glucagon and slows gastric emptying. This has the same g

DIABETES

Diabetes mellitus is a condition of poor blood sugar control, divided into types 1 and 2, and manifests as deficiencies in insulin production, sensitivity or a combination of both. The causes are multifactorial, including both genetic and environmental.

- Type 1 (T1DM), or insulin-dependent diabetes, is where the pancreas produces too little, or no, insulin.
- Type 2 (T2DM) occurs with insulin deficiency and insulin de-sensitivity, due to chronic hyperglycaemia.

With a global prevalence of 8.5%, approximately 4 million people in the UK are diagnosed with diabetes. 90% suffer with type 2, with the incidence continuing to rise. The estimated cost of treating disease and complications is £15 billion annually. Roughly 1/6 hospital inpatients have diabetes, which contributes to, and complicates, a number of medical issues.

Type 1 diabetes is caused by a destruction of pancreatic beta islet cells, which are responsible for producing insulin. Genetic factors include major histocompatibility complex alleles. These form autoantigens that activate T-helper cells, triggering a series of reactions, resulting in the autoantibody destruction of islet cells. This begins as an inflammatory process, mediated through lymphocytes, and progresses to beta cell atrophy. Environmental factors can also trigger the same process, with enteroviruses, H pylori and vitamin D deficiency all implicated. The destruction is severe with roughly 80–90% of cells destroyed over months to years before presentation. There are serious medical issues, with Diabetic Ketoacidosis (DKA) being a common and dangerous initial presentation. Hyperglycaemia and poor peripheral utilisation of glucose lead to

glucagon, cortisol and growth hormone production. These trigger glycogenolysis, gluconeogenesis and ketogenesis, causing a high glucose acidosis.

Type 2 diabetes is characterised by insulin deficiency, peripheral insulin resistance and poor compensatory mechanisms. The risk factors are multifactorial, with both non-modifiable (genetic, family history) and modifiable (diet, activity, weight) implicated. The strongest risk is obesity, due to its interplay with metabolic syndrome. The same processes causing inflammation promote insulin resistance at an organ, tissue and cellular level. Western diets contribute to this and are becoming more globalised. Heavy in carbohydrates and fat complexes, glucose and triglycerides are raised systemically, leading to a rise in reactive oxidative species, causing inflammation. A sedentary lifestyle also promotes pro-inflammatory markers, such as tumour necrosis factor (TNF) and interleukins, which contribute to the destruction of beta islet cells. Regular exercise reduces this inflammation by producing the responsible inflammatory antagonists required to prevent disease progression. The production of glutathione, for example, is an antioxidant responsible for reducing free fatty acids. Higher rates of skeletal muscle contraction also improve local muscle blood flow, improving uptake and utilisation of glucose.

EXERCISE IN DIABETES

Exercise is a key component of improving health. Diabetes is a disease whereby regular activity is proven to reduce weight and blood pressure, while improving glucose and lipid utilisation. Both aerobic and strength-based training are vital components for change. There are various metabolic and psychological changes integral in managing diabetic outcomes.

In normal physiology, raised glucose stimulates insulin release, which increases GLUT-4 proteins. These uptake glucose into tissue but this process is impaired in T2DM. One of the main benefits of activity is the improvement in substrate use. Peripheral insulin resistance is a hallmark feature in T2DM and is improved through both aerobic and strength-based exercise. At rest, energy is predominantly obtained from free fatty acids, whilst in exercise, circulating glucose, fats and glycogen stores are utilised. This is dependent on several factors including anaerobic or aerobic activity, intensity, duration and diet. As substrates are consumed in activity, peripheral glucose and lipids are taken up more readily by cells for metabolism. GLUT-4 proteins are stimulated by muscle contractions in order to replace stores of glycogen to meet demand. This improved muscular uptake can last hours after exercise and is another adaptation that displays the benefits of exercise.

Exercise is prescribed to utilise these mechanisms and supplement or replace medications. This comes with the benefits of reduced cost, side effects and improved self-esteem. Exercise compliance is the most important factor in achieving change and is attained through finding both stimulating and enjoyable forms.

Strength training increases muscle contractions, which improves cellular uptake of glucose, increases capillary networks for transporting and storing nutrients and improves glucose control. Incremental training effects also change body composition, with greater muscle mass and reduced fat (especially visceral), therefore reducing metabolic disease risk.

For those exercising with Type 1 diabetes, insulin management should be adjusted with a view to the type and duration of exercise. To avoid hypoglycaemia, bolus insulin may need to be reduced by 25-75% at the meal before exercise (when exercise takes place within 2 hours of this dose). Typically, mild intensity aerobic exercise requires reduction by 25%, moderate by 50% and vigorous by 75% (Riddell et al., 2017). For longer duration activity, basal insulin adjustment may also be necessary. When exercise is planned to start more than 2 hours after the meal, the regular bolus dose should be given to prevent excessive hyperglycaemia (Adolfsson et al., 2022). For the first meal consumed after exercise, 1.0–1.2 g/kg of carbohydrates and a 50% reduction in bolus insulin should be considered.

DIABETIC EMERGENCIES

Medical emergencies associated with diabetes can lead to serious morbidity and mortality if not appropriately diagnosed and managed. The two most severe include hypo and hyperglycaemia, both of which may have vague presentations. This makes management more difficult, particularly when sport and exercise can exacerbate illness.

Those with insulin-dependent diabetes face the greatest risk with having too little glucose available. Hypoglycaemia occurs when blood glucose levels fall too low to supply metabolic processes. It is defined as a blood glucose level <4 mmol/L. As glucose is the primary fuel for the brain's metabolic function, even a temporary interruption in supply can manifest with rapid and dangerous consequences. Neurological function is impaired, ranging from subtle disturbances such as altered mood and behaviour to lethargy, drowsiness, coma, seizure and death. In normal physiology, this is prevented by homeostatic mechanisms when low blood glucose levels are detected. This includes reduced insulin production (detected via pancreatic islet cells), glycogenolysis of hepatic and muscle stores and gluconeogenesis from proteins and lipids. As this is impaired in diabetes, extra steps are required to try and prevent this arising. There is a difficult balance; if administered insulin is too low, glucose remains free and is not appropriately stored. Exercising tissue does not obtain sufficient glucose and performance decreases. Additionally, this promotes the risk of hyperglycaemia. If administered insulin is too high there is a risk of hypoglycaemia. To achieve this balance, a systematic evaluation is required involving:

- *A history:* including age, past disease, medications, family history, diet, alcohol intake and compliance with diabetic management.
- *Assessment of baseline disease:* including blood pressure, HbA1c, lipid profile, renal function, retinopathy and neuropathy status.
- Planning and communication of training and competition requirements involving exercise type, intensity and duration.
- Available sugary snacks/emergency glucagon kit to counter rapidly falling glucose levels. Recognition of falling glucose levels in the athlete is vital.
- Post-exercise carbohydrate meal to prevent latent hypoglycaemia. This can occur even several hours after exercise completion and should not be overlooked.

Hyperglycaemia occurs when blood glucose levels are too high. This is defined as a value of >7 mmol/L fasting and >9 mmol/L 2 hours postprandial. Thirst, urinary frequency and abdominal pain may be present as well as sweating, dizziness, palpitations and tremor (elicited through sympathetic nervous stimulation). It can often be masked by exercise.

The main two effects are diabetic ketoacidosis (DKA) and Hyperosmolar Hyperglycaemic State (HHS). They both exist on a spectrum of low insulin and high glucose but the degree to which the body is affected is varied. DKA is more severe and typically affects T1DM patients, although can be induced in T2DM with severe stress, infection or injury. The metabolic demand for glucose is raised and there is insufficient insulin to transport it to metabolising tissue. Catabolism occurs with amino-acids and triglycerides broken down from muscle and adipose stores. The subsequent ketone bodies promote an acidotic state and the combination causes a dangerous osmotic diuresis, which can lead to severe dehydration and death. Treatment is with hydration (fluids), insulin, sodium-bicarbonate and potassium.

HHS also involves a high osmotic effect from hyperglycaemia but with enough circulating insulin to prevent the ketogenic-acidotic effects. This protects against the severity of catabolism and diuresis is reduced. However, it is still a dangerous medical emergency and levels of dehydration can exceed 6 L in an adult. Prompt hydration therapy is required via hospital admission.

FEMALE HORMONES AND THE MENSTRUAL CYCLE

The menstrual cycle involves a sequence of several hormonal and physical processes and usually lasts around 28 days (22–35 days is considered normal). A cycle is termed based on the days between the start of one bleed and the start of the next. An interplay between hormones, physiology and psychology can affect athletic performance, and understanding the demands of the menstrual cycle is important in managing female patients. Bleeding can be uncomfortable, impractical and may lead to anaemia, reducing performance. Pain from uterine cramping can be debilitating, which is often overlooked. Other common problems involve lethargy, bloating and constipation. Evidence of the effects on athletic performance by the menstrual cycle is varied: strength may be slightly impaired in the follicular phase; the luteal phase is associated with increased thermoregulatory and cardiovascular strain.

The menstrual cycle is divided into:

1. Follicular phase: from menstruation to the start of ovulation
2. Ovulation
3. Luteal phase: from ovulation to the next menstruation

This process is coordinated principally by four hormones:

- FSH is secreted by the pituitary gland, which begins maturation of the egg. This usually occurs at day 14—halfway in the cycle.
- A surge in FSH and LH cause rupture and release of the mature egg (ovulation) for fertilisation.
- Oestrogen and progesterone increase, stimulating the uterine lining. The egg can be fertilised by a spermatozoon as it travels through the fallopian tube (a few days) before it implants into the endometrium. The ruptured follicle produces oestrogen and progesterone to facilitate this. If successful, the placenta develops and sustains an embryo. If unsuccessful, the lining falls away, resulting in bleeding (a new cycle begins).

CLINICAL CONSIDERATIONS

Menstruation reduces haemoglobin concentrations, decreasing availability for the lungs and tissues. This can result in reduced performance and increased respiratory rate as a compensatory effect, and should be considered in the sport and exercise medicine clinician.

As well as local effects on menstruation and fertility, these hormones have widespread systemic effects. Oestrogen dilates blood vessels and has an atheroprotective effect by inhibiting smooth muscle proliferation. However, it increases coagulation factors, increasing the risk of thromboembolism.

The musculoskeletal effects involve bone metabolism, playing a significant role in homeostasis of bone resorption and remodelling. Positively, oestrogen also enhances muscle mass and strength, as well as bone (Lowe et al., 2010). Deficiencies promote a pro-resorptive state and increase the risk of osteoporosis, particularly in post-menopausal and oophorectomy patients.

Progesterone generally works concomitantly with oestrogen. In addition to its key role in maintaining a thick uterine lining, it thickens vaginal and cervical mucus to prevent both further sperm entry and infection. It promotes osteoblast formation, helping to form a complete bone matrix.

CONTRACEPTION

There are several female contraceptive options. Factors affecting choice include: preference, effectiveness, side effects, plans for future pregnancy and medical conditions. A few common methods include:

- The intrauterine device (IUD) is 99.7% effective, safe, long term and reversible. This small, T-shaped copper device is non-hormonal and functions via local secretion of a copper toxic environment, which has a spermicidal effect. Benefits include immediate effect from fitting, longevity (five to ten years), prompt return to fertility on removal, no hormonal side effects and no issues with compliance. Risks include infection risk at insertion, menorrhagia, dysmenorrhoea, displacement and risk of ectopic pregnancy.
- The intrauterine system (IUS) is a small T-shaped plastic rod which lasts three to five years. It is progesterone-based, thereby thickening cervical mucus (a barrier to sperm entry), thinning the uterine lining (preventing implantation) and, in some women, preventing ovulation. Benefits include efficacy >99%, return to fertility on removal and use in women for whom oestrogen-based contraceptives are contraindicated. Side effects include irregular or absent periods, mastalgia, headaches and acne. It can cause small, but painful, ovarian cysts. Insertion infection is a risk, as is uterine rupture (1/500) and ectopic pregnancy. It can be fitted at any time but only gives immediate cover from days 1 to 7 of the cycle—after this, barrier methods are advised for 7 days.
- The contraceptive implant is a small flexible plastic tube, approximately 4 cm long, fitted in the subdermal tissue of the upper arm. Like the IUS, it releases systemic progesterone to prevent fertilisation and has similar risks and benefits. It is > 99% effective and lasts up to 3 years. It must be fitted in the first 5 days of the cycle for contraceptive cover.

- The depot injection is progesterone-based and administered every 8 or 13 weeks (depending on type). It has a similar function to other progesterone-based options, as well as similar benefits and risks. However, it can reduce bone mineral density and takes up to a year for fertility to return to normal.
- The progesterone-only pill (POP) is taken daily and has a similar function to other progesterone-based methods. Its main benefit is that it is not invasive. There are two main types: a three hour (must be taken within three hours of the same daily time) and a 12 hour (within 12 hours) option—planning and regularity are crucial to ensure effectiveness of > 99%. An additional pill should be taken if vomiting occurs within two hours of ingestion or, if pills are taken outside of their three- or 12-hour window, barrier methods should be used for 2 days.
- The combined pill (COCP) contains both oestrogen and progesterone. It acts by suppressing gonadotropins and ovulation, in addition to the actions of progesterone. The monophasic formulation is taken daily for 21 days with a 7-day break, while the everyday formulation contains seven placebo pills to aid compliance. The phasic type has varying quantities of hormones and must be taken in order (colour coding can aid this). A breakthrough bleed may occur with every type. Benefits include regulating periods and improving menorrhagia, dysmenorrhoea and acne. Risks involve venous thromboembolism and must be weighed against comorbidity, weight and blood pressure. The COCP is contraindicated for those with a history of migraine with aura.

PREGNANCY AND POSTPARTUM

The physiological and anatomical changes of pregnancy predispose to health issues. The production of the hormones relaxin and oestrogen help remodel connective tissue and increase laxity in preparation for childbirth. This, alongside increased soft tissue oedema, contribute to musculoskeletal symptoms.

Symphysis pubis dysfunction (SPD) or Pregnancy-related pelvic girdle pain (PGP) causes pain and impacts mobility. Exercises to strengthen the pelvic floor and other core muscles is the mainstay of treatment. Analgesia and equipment, such as pelvic support belts, may be helpful. SPD resolves for most women in the weeks after delivery; however, it can persist and is associated with other pelvic issues, including pelvic prolapse, incontinence, diastasis recti and low back pain.

Carpal tunnel syndrome and De Quervain's tenosynovitis are also common in pregnancy and the postpartum period.

MENOPAUSE

Menopause occurs when menstruation ceases permanently due to the loss of ovarian follicular activity. In the UK, the average age of onset is 51 years. It is usually a clinical diagnosis, defined by 12 months of amenorrhoea.

As well as vasomotor, urogenital, cognitive and mood symptoms; menopause can adversely influence musculoskeletal health. Due to oestrogen deficiency, there is a link with osteoporosis, sarcopenia and osteoarthritis. These conditions may contribute to increased falls risk and associated morbidity and mortality.

Physical activity, weight loss and an optimal diet may help. Hormone replacement therapy (HRT) is suitable for many individuals. The risks e.g. venous thromboembolism and breast cancer (with combined preparations) should be considered. HRT does not significantly increase the incidence of cardiovascular disease when started before 60 (and may reduce it). HRT can also reduce fracture risk and there is emerging evidence of its benefits for musculoskeletal symptoms, such as joint pain.

METABOLIC DISEASES

Metabolic diseases disrupt the processing of substrates used to derive energy, including carbohydrates, proteins and fats. They can be caused by genetic or congenital factors and present in early life.

Diagnosis remains a high priority and UK guidance states a mandatory 5-day heel prick test for screening in all children. This tests for nine rare disorders:

- Cystic fibrosis (CF) is caused by a mutation of proteins responsible for secretions in multiple systems including skin, the digestive tract and the respiratory tract. There is decreased muco-ciliary clearance causing repeated inflammation and chronic infection. Viscous pancreatic secretions result in exocrine insufficiency; pancreatic ducts become blocked, leading to pancreatitis and fibrosis. Reduced production of digestive enzymes, fat soluble vitamins (A, D, E and K) and biliary duct blockage contribute to liver failure. Moreover, endocrine pancreatic synthesis of insulin is impaired manifesting as CF-related diabetes, Malabsorption of vitamin D and calcium can cause osteoporosis. Management depends on the various manifestations of disease: use of prophylactic antibiotics; nutritional support (Creon); chest physio; etc.
- Familial hypercholesterolaemia: an autosomal dominant condition affecting around 1/250 people, though very few (8%) are currently identified in the UK. Impaired low-density lipoproteins (LDL) clearance results in early onset atherosclerosis and cardiovascular disease. Widespread fatty deposits in the form of tendon xanthoma, corneal arcus and xanthelasma may feature but many patients can be asymptomatic. Management includes statins, which stimulate LDL receptors to clear it from the blood.
- Sickle cell disease: an inherited condition, common in African and Caribbean populations, where abnormally shaped red blood cells are produced. This can cause anaemia, increased infection risk and 'sickle cell crises'—characterised by acute pain.
- Congenital hypothyroidism: an absent or underdeveloped thyroid gland.
- Phenylketonuria (PKU): an autosomal recessive disorder of protein metabolism (phenylalanine). Toxic accumulation in the brain causes seizures, microcephaly, motor and cognitive impairment. Strict control of phenylalanine is required— enough to ensure vital growth, but restricted to prevent toxicity. Sources include egg whites, chicken breast, turkey and tuna.
- Medium-chain Acyl-CoA dehydrogenase deficiency (MCADD): an autosomal recessive disorder of medium-chain fatty acid metabolism, which

often presents as hypoglycaemia following fasting, dehydration or infection. Seizures, coma and liver disease are common. Treatment involves avoiding exacerbation of metabolic decompensation and adding simple carbohydrates during illness to prevent catabolism.

The following rare genetic conditions involve the inability to metabolise certain amino acids:

- Maple syrup urine disease (MSUD)
- Isovaleric acidaemia (IVA)
- Glutaric aciduria type 1 (GA1)
- Homocystinuria (HCU)

MULTIPLE CHOICE QUESTION (MCQ) QUESTIONS

1. A footballer with type 1 diabetes plans on starting additional running sessions in preparation for the new season. He currently takes long-acting insulin twice daily and rapid-acting bolus insulin before meals. He plans on performing an extra 2 hour running session of moderate intensity after breakfast. How would you advise him to manage his insulin?

   A. Make no changes
   B. Take an additional rapid-acting carbohydrate before exercise
   C. Reduce morning rapid-acting insulin by 25%
   D. Reduce morning rapid-acting insulin by 50%
   E. Reduce both long-acting and rapid-acting insulin prior to exercise by 50%

2. You are reviewing a 29-year-old male marathon runner who has been suffering from fatigue and reduced performance for 6 months. He has a number of symptoms including low mood, irritability, erectile dysfunction and impaired judgement in races. You are suspicious of a diagnosis of RED-S. Which one of the following results would best support this diagnosis?

   A. Low serum LH levels
   B. High serum Leptin levels
   C. High serum C Reactive Protein
   D. ECG with high voltage QRS complexes in sinus tachycardia
   E. DEXA with an overall T-score of -0.9

3. The same runner has an injury in training. He has a low energy fall and sustains a distal radius fracture. You arrange a DEXA scan to assess his bone density. Which of the following suggests a diagnosis of osteoporosis?

   A. T score <-1.5
   B. Z score >5.0
   C. T score <-2.6
   D. T score <-2.5
   E. Z score >-1.5

4. You are discussing contraception options with a female athlete of reproductive age. You discuss the advantages and disadvantages of each option. Which one of the following contraceptive options is most likely to reduce bone mineral density?

   A. Levonorgestrel Intrauterine system
   B. Ethinylestradiol 30 micrograms, Drospirenone 30 mg tablets
   C. Desogestrel 75 micrograms tablets
   D. Medroxyprogesterone acetate injections
   E. Etonogestrel implant

5. You are reviewing a 67-year-old female with lower back pain in your musculoskeletal clinic. She has been taking 125 micrograms of levothyroxine daily for twenty years. You check her medical record and see that her last thyroid function tests were completed 5 years ago. Her pain was sudden onset whilst going to kneel at church and has dulled to a 'mild ache' since. Neurological examination appears normal. What is the most likely diagnosis?

   A. Metastatic cancer
   B. Paget's disease
   C. Osteoporosis
   D. Hyperparathyroidism
   E. Osteomalacia

MULTIPLE CHOICE QUESTION (MCQ) ANSWERS

1. **Answer D**

   As per consensus guidelines, prolonged moderate intensity exercise for up to four hours should prompt a reduction of morning rapid-acting insulin by 50%. Answers A, B and C are at increased risk of resulting in exercise-related hypoglycaemia. Answer E may be appropriate for intense exercise lasting a longer duration.

2. **Answer A**

   In RED-S, the physiological response to low energy availability is to increase cortisol, which reduces Leptin (B) and then reduces GnRH and LH from the pituitary, making A the correct answer. Although CRP may be raised, this is not a hallmark of RED-S. Characteristic ECG changes show low-voltage bradycardia (D). Although the DEXA result in E is almost within the osteopenic range, a low LH level is more supportive of the diagnosis.

3. **Answer D**

   A T-score between –1 and –2.5 suggests osteopenia. A T-score of –2.5 or lower indicates osteoporosis (D). T-scores are a comparison of bone density compared to a healthy 30-year-old of the same sex. A Z-score is a comparison of bone density to an average person of the same age and sex.

4. **Answer D**

   There is evidence that medroxyprogesterone acetate injections (D) decrease bone density by inhibiting endogenous oestrogen production. Oestrogen deficiency leads to a negative balance between bone production and bone resorption, resulting in bone loss. Therefore, COCP use may confer a protective effect by providing a continuous exposure to exogenous oestrogen, but evidence is limited. The evidence for other progesterone only contraceptives significantly affecting bone mineral density is also limited.

5. **Answer C**

   This patient has not had her thyroid function tests checked in some time. Overreplacement with levothyroxine is associated with osteoporosis, the most likely diagnosis in this scenario.

REFERENCES AND FURTHER READING

Adolfsson, P., Taplin, C.E., Zaharieva, D.P., Pemberton, J., Davis, E.A., Riddell, M.C., McGavock, J., Moser, O., Szadkowska, A., Lopez, P., Santiprabhob, J., Frattolin, E., Griffiths, G and DiMeglio, L.A. 2022. ISPAD Clinical Practice Consensus Guidelines 2022—Exercise in children and adolescents with diabetes. *Pediatric Diabetes*, Wiley.

Mountjoy, M., Sundgot-Borgen, J.K., Burke, L.M., et al. (2018). IOC consensus statement on relative energy deficiency in sport (RED-S): 2018 update. *Br J Sports Med*, 52, pp. 687–697.

www.health4performance.co.uk—The British Association of Sport and Exercise Medicine (BASEM) resource on RED-S.

Elhakeem, A., Frysz, M., Tilling, K., Tobias, J.H., Lawlor, D.A. 2019. Association Between Age at Puberty and Bone Accrual From 10 to 25 Years of Age. *JAMA Netw Open*. 2(8), e198918. doi:10.1001/jamanetworkopen.2019.8918

Lowe, D.A., Baltgalvis, K.A and Greising, S.M. 2010. Mechanisms behind estrogen's beneficial effect on muscle strength in females. *Exerc Sport Sci Rev.* Apr; 38(2), pp. 61–67. doi: 10.1097/JES.0b013e3181d496bc. PMID: 20335737; PMCID: PMC2873087.L

Nicoll, J.X., Hatfield, D.L., Melanson, K.J and Nasin, C.S. 2018. Thyroid hormones and commonly cited symptoms of overtraining in collegiate female endurance runners. *Eur J Appl Physiol*. Jan; 118(1), pp. 65–73. doi: 10.1007/s00421-017-3723-9. Epub 2017 Nov 20. PMID: 29159669.

Riddell, M.C., Gallen, I.W., Smart, C.E., Taplin, C.E., Adolfsson, P., Lumb, A.N., Kowalski, A., Rabasa-Lhoret, R., McCrimmon, R.J., Hume, C., Annan, F., Fournier, P.A., Graham, C., Bode, B., Galassetti, P., Jones, T.W., Millán, I.S., Heise, T., Peters, A.L., Petz, A and Laffel, L.M. 2017. Exercise management in type 1 diabetes: a consensus statement. *Lancet Diabetes Endocrinol*. May; 5(5), pp. 377–390. doi: 10.1016/S2213-8587(17)30014-1. Epub 2017 Jan 24. Erratum in: Lancet Diabetes Endocrinol. 2017 May; 5(5):e3. PMID: 28126459.

Robitzsch, A., Schweda, A., Hetkamp, M., Niedergethmann, M., Dörrie, N., Herpertz, S., Hasenberg, T., Tagay, S., Teufel, M., Skoda E-M. 2020. The Impact of Psychological Resources on Body Mass Index in Obesity Surgery Candidates. *Frontiers in Psychiatry*, Vol 11.

Rheumatology 14

Anthony Hoban and Gui Tran

INTRODUCTION

Rheumatology as a speciality encompasses a variety of disorders that can affect any of the body's systems and can present at any age. Dysfunction typically arises from a systemic autoimmune or autoinflammatory pathology and it can be difficult to identify a precise diagnosis in the clinical setting. We often think of the rheumatoid arthritis hand as characteristic of this speciality but often the signs and symptoms are far more subtle. The role of the sport and exercise medicine clinician is to be able to identify signs and symptoms of potential rheumatological disorders and be cognisant of symptoms that may not be cited in the primary presenting complaint. A thorough systems review can help identify rheumatological disorders and one should keep an open mind toward systemic pathology when dealing with musculoskeletal presentations.

Some examples of systemic autoimmune diseases include rheumatoid arthritis, systemic lupus erythematosus, Sjögren's disease, scleroderma, polymyositis, and various vasculitides. However, there are in excess of 100 different types of autoimmune, autoinflammatory and musculoskeletal conditions. Over time, the rheumatologist has become versed in dealing with non-inflammatory disorders, chronic pain disorders (such as fibromyalgia) and may take a central role in advising on the management of non-autoimmune conditions such as osteoarthritis.

It can seem daunting when dealing with such a broad speciality and the potential for multisystem involvement. There can be significant overlap of abnormal laboratory values when arranging biochemical investigations. Changes found on imaging are not necessarily specific to any one diagnosis. The use of auto-antibody testing may narrow the differential diagnosis but will rarely pinpoint a diagnosis.

In practice, setting shared goals with the patient is key. Involving the patient, rheumatologist, general practitioner and SEM clinician in this process helps to ensure symptoms are monitored and therapeutic response maintained. Like any pathology and treatment programme, there will be successes and setbacks, but good planning will help predict these and adapt treatments to meet the patients' needs and expectations.

Rheumatology History

In assessing a potential rheumatological presentation there is often a musculoskeletal component to the examination. Pay attention to the pattern of joint involvement, the variation of symptoms with activity and rest, the duration of early morning stiffness, the patient's response to medications or the need to use these and the disruption of activities of daily living. Always ask about extra-articular symptoms if there is a question of a rheumatological condition.

RHEUMATOLOGY HISTORY

Patient age and demographics is important when considering the aetiology of a monoarthropathy. An acute infective cause or trauma is more likely than a chronic osteoarthritis in a child with a single joint pathology, whilst a symmetrical polyarthropathy is more likely to be rheumatoid arthritis than gout. Pattern recognition is important to guide your differential diagnosis and choice of investigations (Tables 14.1 and 14.2).

It is important to exclude an acute septic joint as this can have devastating effects if not promptly diagnosed and managed—typically in the inpatient orthopaedic setting.

DOI: 10.1201/9781003179979-14

RHEUMATOLOGY

Osteoarthritis (OA)

- Asymmetrical or symmetrical
- Worse with movement
- X-ray changes:
  L – Loss of joint space
  O – Osteophytes
  S – Subchondral sclerosis
  S – Subchondral cysts

- Shoulder
- Spine
- Hip
- Knee
- Ankle
- Distal interphalangeal (DIP)
- Carpometacarpal (CMC)

Psoriatic arthritis

- Psoriasis
- Morning stiffness, often better with movement
- Sacroiliitis, Dactylitis, Enthesitis
- Usually asymmetric
- 'Pencil-in-cup' deformity common on X-ray

- Shoulder
- Spine
- Sacroiliac joints
- Knee
- Distal Interphalangeal (DIP)

Rheumatoid arthritis (RA)

- Symmetrical
- Morning stiffness, often better with movement
- X-ray changes:
  L – Loss of joint space
  E – Erosions
  S – Soft tissue swelling
  S – Soft bones (Osteopenia)

- Shoulder
- Hip
- Knee
- Wrist
- Proximal Interphalangeal (PIP)
- Metacarpophalangeal (MCP)

Blood tests

- CRP/ESR – useful to help screen inflammatory vs. non-inflammatory pathology or to monitor treatment – low specificity
- Anti-cyclic citrullinated peptide antibodies (Anti-CCP) – The most specific and sensitive test in Rheumatoid arthritis, particularly in early disease ~80% RA patients
- Rheumatoid factor (RF) – Not specific for RA, higher levels suggest a worse prognosis ~80% RA patients
- Anti-nuclear antibodies (ANA) – Poor screening tool ~5-30% of the general population will have +ve ANA
- Anti-neutrophil cytoplasmic antibodies (ANCA) – Useful in confirming vasculitis
  - Granulomatosis with polyangiitis (GPA) +ve C-ANCA ~90%
  - Microscopic polyangiitis (MPA) +ve P-ANCA ~ 40-80%
  - Eosinophilic granulomatosis with polyangiitis (EGPA) +ve P-ANCA ~35-70%

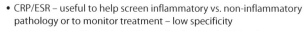
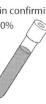
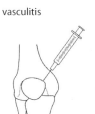
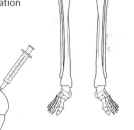

Joint fluid aspiration

	Colour	WBC count	Gram stain	Neutrophils	Crystals
Non-inflammatory	Straw-like	200–2000 cells/mm³	Negative	>25%	Negative
Inflammatory	Straw-like	2000–50,000 cells/mm³	Negative	>50%	Positive
Septic	Yellow/green purulent	>50,000 cells/mm³	Positive	>75%	Negative

- Monosodium urate (Gout) crystals $\rightarrow$ Needle shaped, negative birefringence
- Calcium pyrophosphate dihydrate deposition disease (CPPD/Pseudogout) $\rightarrow$ Rhomboid shaped, positive birefringence

Figure 14.1 Pictorial summary.

Table 14.1 Presentations of Joint Involvement

Articular symptoms	Extra-articular Symptoms
Joints	**Eyes**—Dry eyes/red eyes (ankylosing spondylitis)
Pain	**Mouth**—Xerostomia (Sjögren's)
Swelling	**Raynaud's Phenomenon**
Stiffness—Morning	**Rashes and Photosensitivity**
Loss of function	**Ulcers** (Behcet's)
Deformity	**Gastro** Ulcerative Colitis/Crohn's/reactive arthritis
Back Pain	**Urethritis** (reactive arthritis)
Loss of normal curvature	**Weight loss**
Reduced movement with flexion	**Night Sweats**
Muscle Pain	
Atrophy	

Table 14.2 Clinical Examination

Single joint	<5 joints	>5 joints	
		Symmetrical	**Asymmetrical**
Osteoarthritis	Psoriatic arthritis	Rheumatoid arthritis	Osteoarthritis
Trauma	Ankylosing spondylosis	Systemic infection (viral)	Reactive arthritis
Septic arthritis	Osteoarthritis		
Crystal arthropathy	Reactive arthritis		
(Gout/pseudogout)	Crystal arthropathy		

It is wise to consider limb examination from a rheumatological, orthopaedic, neurological and vascular perspective to form an accurate diagnosis. This, in addition to a review of extra-articular pathology, can be a burden on clinic time but consider it time well spent. The rheumatological system can be examined in a focused or full manner depending on your history with the patient and the nature of their presenting complaint. Always remember to **LOOK, FEEL and MOVE** the affected region and to compare the affected and non-affected side.

ADULT RHEUMATOLOGICAL CONDITIONS

Rheumatoid Arthritis (RA)

RA is a chronic disease characterised by inflammation of the lining, or synovium, of the joints. Females account for 75% of cases. It can lead to long-term joint damage, resulting in chronic pain, loss of function and disability. RA most often affects the small joints of the body symmetrically, aiding clinical diagnosis.

RA is a systemic auto-immune inflammatory disorder and patients may have extra articular symptoms:

- Loss of energy or appetite and associated weight loss
- Low fevers
- Dry eyes and mouth
- Rheumatoid nodules

DIAGNOSIS

This may be clinical and small joint arthritis can progress to characteristic deformity. Biochemistry and plain films showing soft tissue swelling, marginal erosions and juxta articular osteopenia, also aid diagnosis.

INVESTIGATIONS

- FBC may show anaemia and raised WCC
- CRP, ESR, complement and acute-phase reactants may be elevated
- Rheumatoid factor may be positive
- Anti-CCP may be positive

MANAGEMENT

Acute flares are managed with NSAIDs or corticosteroids. Remission should be maintained with DMARDs or biological agents in resistant disease. Patients should be directed to exercise interventions to maintain pain free range and proprioceptive control of affected joints.

Axial Spondyloarthropathies (Including Ankylosing Spondylitis)

A condition which primarily affects the spine and may lead to back stiffness and impaired mobility and function. The joints and ligaments of the back often become inflamed, beginning with episodic inflammation of the sacroiliac joints in late teens/early 20s. It has a characteristic presentation of prolonged morning low back pain (>1 hour) and stiffness, which improves on exercise. Extra-spinal features include peripheral joint involvement in about 25%, usually oligo-articular, large joints and asymmetric.

Six A's of ankylosing spondylitis (AS):

- Achilles enthesis
- Anterior uveitis
- Amyloidosis
- Aortitis and aortic insufficiency
- Apical fibrosis
- Aortic regurgitation

HLA-B27 is present in up to 90% and males are affected more than females (3:1).

'Rule of 2s'—AS occurs in: **2%** of the general population and **2%** of HLA-B27 positive people. **20%** of HLA-B27 positive people will have an affected family member.

EXAMINATION

- *Mobility:* reduced flexion in the lumbar spine.
- *Modified Schober's test:* distance between the midpoint of the posterior superior iliac spines and a point 10 cm vertically above when standing erect, following maximal forward flexion of the spine (normal >5 cm).
- Increased extension of the cervical spine.
- *Increased occiput to wall distance:* patient stands facing away from the wall with heels touching it. The occiput may not be able to touch the wall in ankylosing spondylitis.

- Reduced rotation at lumbar, thoracic and cervical spine and reduced expansion on chest wall movements.
- The Bath Ankylosing Spondylitis Disease Activity Index (BASDAI) is used to assess burden of active disease and response to treatment.

INVESTIGATIONS

- Inflammatory markers may be raised.
- Plain X-rays: loss of definition, then sclerosis, of the sacroiliac joints. Bilateral sacroiliac erosion on X-ray is the most suggestive feature of AS. Sclerosis of the intervertebral joints and intervertebral ligament insertions may be seen. Late changes include SIJ fusion, intervertebral discs, facet joints and syndesmophytes fuse causing 'Bamboo Spine.'
- MRI may detect earlier changes such as oedema at the SIJ and ligamentous insertions.

MANAGEMENT

Acute musculoskeletal complaints are managed with NSAIDs or corticosteroids. Patients may need biological therapies under the supervision of a Rheumatologist.

Psoriatic Arthritis (PsA)

PsA is a chronic disease, which often affects the joints at the end of the toes and fingers and can be accompanied by changes in the toenails and fingernails. The lumbar and sacroiliac joints may be involved. Patients do not need to have visible psoriasis to have psoriatic arthritis but the scalp should be examined thoroughly as plaques here may be missed. Onset is more common between 30–50 with equal incidence between genders.

INVESTIGATIONS

- Clinical examination and recognition of arthritic symptoms is sufficient to make a clinical diagnosis
- FBC may show anaemia and raised WCC
- CRP, ESR, complement and acute-phase reactants may be elevated
- X-rays of affected joints may show an erosive arthropathy

MANAGEMENT

Skin symptoms should be managed topically but active arthropathy often requires a DMARD to settle flares and prevent further joint damage. Resistant pathology requires consultant rheumatologist input for biological agents.

CLINICAL CONSIDERATIONS

PsA is associated with increased cardiovascular risk and mortality. Patients presenting with signs and symptoms should be screened for this and managed accordingly.

Reactive Arthritis

Reactive arthritis occurs in reaction to an infection by certain bacteria and presents as painful polyarthropathy. There is an association with HLA B27. Some patients will have inflammatory eye disease (e.g. uveitis), dysuria or a characteristic rash on the palms or soles of the feet (keratoderma blenorrhagicum).

DIAGNOSIS

Diagnosis is clinical in the presence of a known infective trigger. The most common bacterial causes are chlamydia trachomatis, campylobacter, salmonella, shigella and yersinia.

MANAGEMENT

Addressing the underlying pathogen is key and specialist input from the infectious diseases services may be needed. Treatment of the arthritis in the acute phase is typically with NSAIDs if renal function allows. Steroids may also be effective. Reactive Arthritis may become chronic and this may require treatment with DMARDs or with biologic agents in resistant disease.

CONNECTIVE TISSUE DISEASES

Bechet's Disease

Bechet's disease is an auto-inflammatory condition of unknown cause. It is characterised by oral and genital ulcer formation with uveitis. It is associated with arthritis/arthralgia, fever, malaise and non-erosive arthritis of the knees.

It is most prevalent in 20–30-year-olds and is associated with HLA-B51. Other risk factors are Mediterranean, Mid-eastern or East Asian ethnicity. One theory is that exposure to *Staphylococcus aureus* or to other pathogenic antigens may serve as a trigger for the development of the auto-inflammatory process.

This presents as a classic triad of painful oral and genital ulcers and uveitis.

These ulcers tend to heal over several weeks, although genital ulcers may scar. Uveitis may develop several years after the initial presentation of the disease and can progress to bilateral visual loss. Pathergy may be a feature.

Other symptoms may include:

- Erythema nodosum
- Acne-like spots on the limbs
- Late neurological symptoms of memory impairment and imbalance
- Mixed vessel vasculitis

INVESTIGATIONS

This is a clinical diagnosis but some results can help:

- HLA-B51
- FBC may show anaemia and raised WCC
- CRP, ESR, complement and acute-phase reactants may all be elevated during an acute attack
- Antiphospholipid antibodies are positive in 25%
- Pathergy test positive in up to 60%
- The role of imaging depends on the history and clinical examination but angiography may be required to identify aneurysms associated with vasculitis
- Sexually transmitted disease screening should be performed as differentials can include syphilis

MANAGEMENT

Management is aimed at controlling symptoms and inflammation in the affected systems. Corticosteroids (topical and oral) and colchicine are used as first-line agents in the treatment of oral and genital ulcers. Immunosuppressive agents should be used in select cases when initial measures are unsuccessful. Patients with eye symptoms should be referred to ophthalmology.

Underlying infections should be treated, with infectious disease specialist input as needed.

Polymyalgia Rheumatica (PMR)

PMR is a condition that causes aching, muscle stiffness and pain in the tendons, muscles, ligaments and tissues around the proximal muscle girdles, affecting the joints in the shoulders, hips, neck and lower back. It may occur with giant cell arteritis and this should be screened for during a consultation. Onset is typically in the 7th decade and women are more commonly affected than men.

DIAGNOSIS

This is based on the patient's history of upper girdle pain and prolonged early morning stiffness, which improves with exercise. CRP/ESR is typically raised and can be used as a marker of treatment response.

MANAGEMENT

Corticosteroids are the mainstay of treatment and these are usually prescribed at a lower dose (15–20 mg daily), which is then tapered to symptom response for prolonged periods—often for months. Daily exercise should be encouraged and can be supervised by a physiotherapist.

CLINICAL CONSIDERATIONS

Prescribers should be mindful of the risks associated with longer term steroid use and gastric protection should be considered (PPI prescription). PMR can be the first indication of giant cell arteritis, which is a disease of the arteries, and patients should be screened for this accordingly.

Myositis

Myositis is the name for a group of rare conditions that affect muscle function due to auto-immune dysfunction and inflammation. Symptoms are precipitated by exertion, causing pain and inflammation in the affected muscles. Other symptoms may include fatigue, weight loss and night sweats. There are several subtypes of myositis but the most common syndromes include:

Polymyositis

- Affecting the shoulders, hips and thighs most often.
- More common in women
- Onset 30–60 years old
- Where there is demonstrated muscle necrosis—a diagnosis of necrotizing myopathy can be considered. This is separate from polymyositis

Inclusion Body Myositis

- Distal muscle weakness
- Associated with dysphagia
- More common in men and those >50 years old

Dermatomyositis

- Similar to polymyositis but has a characteristic associated rash—heliotrope rash, Gottron's papules, shawl sign
- Heliotrope rash can be patchy red or purple in colour and is most commonly seen on the eyelids, cheeks and nose but can be seen on the back and chest.

INVESTIGATIONS

- A full history and examination are important to elicit symptoms of myositis. The characteristic heliotrope rash is noted clinically and does not warrant biopsy.
- FBC may show anaemia and raised WCC
- ALT may be raised
- CRP, ESR, complement and acute-phase reactants may be elevated
- Serum ANA may be raised and ENA studies may detect the anti-Jo-1 antibody
- EMG studies may show altered muscle contraction and electrical activity

- MRI may identify acute or chronic inflammatory change in the affected muscles
- Muscle biopsy can be used to identify necrosis and inflammation

MANAGEMENT

Aerobic exercise under supervision is key. Medical management consists of high dose steroids, which taper over weeks. DMARDs and biological agents may be used.

Scleroderma

Also known as systemic sclerosis, this is an autoimmune disorder that results in tightening of the skin, hence the name. Scleroderma is characterised by skin fibrosis. It can affect the skin, blood vessels, joints, respiratory and renal systems. Patients can present with localised or systemic symptoms and severity can vary.

Systemic sclerosis is the more severe form of Scleroderma, where there is multisystem involvement. There are two subtypes:

Limited Cutaneous Systemic Sclerosis (CREST Syndrome)

- C—Calcinosis
- R—Raynaud's phenomenon
- E—Esophagela dysmotility and reflux
- S—Sclerodactyly (skin thickening and tightness in the digits)
- T—Telangiectasias

Diffuse Cutaneous Systemic Scleroderma

This form of scleroderma more frequently involves internal organs, such as lungs, kidneys, or the gastrointestinal tract.

INVESTIGATIONS

- FBC may show anaemia and raised WCC
- U&Es to monitor renal function

- CRP, ESR, complement and acute-phase reactants may be elevated
- Serum ANA is often positive
- Anti-Scl-70 antibodies for systemic sclerosis, anti-centromere for localised scleroderma
- Serial BP measurements
- Baseline Pulmonary function tests (PFTs)

MANAGEMENT

Medications that treat other rheumatological disorders are often ineffective management options. Hypertension and scleroderma associated renal disease should be managed with ACE inhibitors. Raynaud's symptoms can be managed with calcium channel blockers, musculoskeletal symptoms with NSAIDs (as renal function allows), and reflux symptoms with PPIs or alginates.

Scleroderma associated lung disease (ILD, pulmonary hypertension) warrants review by a Respiratory specialist and treatment can involve PDE-5 inhibitors.

Sjogren's Syndrome

An autoimmune disease that causes dry eyes and a dry mouth. It may affect any part of the body and is more prevalent in females, occurring at any age. It is often associated with other autoimmune pathologies such as Systemic Lupus Erythematosus (SLE) or rheumatoid arthritis (RA) (secondary Sjogren's).

DIAGNOSIS

- Clinical examination
- Schirmer's test for lacrimation

INVESTIGATIONS

- ANA (Anti-SSA (ro), Anti-SSB (la) positive)
- Rheumatoid factor (RF)
- Biopsy of the affected glands can be performed

MANAGEMENT

Treatments involve symptom relief. Artificial tears and saliva can help reduce eye and oral irritation, PPIs can reduce gastric reflux and regular ophthalmic and dental review is advised.

Systemic Lupus Erythematosus (SLE)

SLE is a chronic autoimmune disease that affects joints, muscles and all organs. It most commonly affects females in their 20–40 s but 20% of sufferers develop the condition in the teens. SLE can be associated with general malaise, weight loss, fatigue and fever and its presentation can be difficult to readily diagnose in clinic. It often follows a relapsing and remitting course.

DIAGNOSIS

The American College of Rheumatology lists signs and symptoms to assess for:

- Rashes

  - Malar rash—butterfly-shaped rash over the cheeks
  - Discoid rash—red rash with raised round or oval patches
  - Rash on skin exposed to the sun
  - Mouth sores

- Arthritis
- Pleurisy and or pericarditis
- Renal involvement
- Neurologic problems—seizures, strokes or psychosis

INVESTIGATIONS

- FBC may show low neutrophils or lymphocytes
- U&Es to monitor renal function
- Complements can be low
- Serum ANA is often positive
- Anti-dsDNA and Anti-Sm are associated with Lupus
- Serial BP measurement
- Baseline PFTs

MANAGEMENT

There is no cure for SLE and regular patient review is important. Initially, tapered steroids are used to control symptoms acutely. DMARDs or biological agents are the mainstay of treatment to limit organ involvement and complications. For system specific symptoms, onward referral to the appropriate speciality is important where appropriate.

VASCULITIS

Large Vessel Vasculitis

The term large vessel vasculitis covers a series of disorders of the aorta and its major branches. These conditions result in granulomatous inflammation in the affected vessels. Inflammation is usually in the intimal layer of the vessel causing swelling, pain and subsequent reduction in distal perfusion.

Temporal Vasculitis—Giant Cell Arteritis

This commonly presents with pain and tenderness over the temples; it can be severe and bilateral. It may present with scalp tenderness, jaw pain, fever, fatigue, visual loss or double vision. There is a correlation with Polymyalgia Rheumatica in up to 20% of cases. Women are twice as likely to be affected, it is common in Northern Europeans and onset >50 years old.

INVESTIGATIONS

- Patients may have a raised CRP, ESR and plasma viscosity
- Diagnosis can involve temporal artery biopsy, although novel imaging modalities such as ultrasound, MR/CT angiography, or PET scans may be used

MANAGEMENT

Prompt recognition from the patient's history and clinical examination allow steroids to be commenced promptly to reduce serious complications of blindness or aneurysm formation (Aortic Aneurysm). Strokes are a rare complication. Relapse is common and prolonged tapered steroid courses are potentially needed.

Takayasu Vasculitis

A rare large vessel vasculitis that usually occurs between ages 15 and 50 years. 90% of patients are female. It affects the aorta and main branches causing inflammation and, in time, stenosis of the affected vessels.

PRESENTATION

- Headaches
- Presyncope or syncope
- Cardiovascular disease—chest pain, MI, Stroke

Diagnosis is typically by angiogram or CT/MR angiography. Diagnosis requires differentiation between atherosclerosis and vessel inflammation. This can be done on non-invasive angiography. Inflammatory markers such as ESR and CRP can be raised but this is not specific to vasculitis.

MANAGEMENT

Early steroid dosing is important to reduce inflammation and reduce complications. MDT input from the rheumatologist, cardiologist and vascular surgeon is important. There is a role for steroid sparing therapies such as DMARDs and biological agents. Low dose aspirin may be commenced to reduce thrombosis risk. Similarly, blood pressure control will reduce cardiovascular mortality.

Henoch—Schönlein Purpura (HSP)

HSP is defined as a vasculitis with immunoglobulin (Ig)A deposits in the small vessels of the body (Table 14.3). It can involve the skin, GI tract and renal glomeruli and is one of the most common vasculitis of childhood. It often presents between 3–10 years of age following an infective trigger.

DIAGNOSIS

The diagnosis should be considered in children with abdominal pain, arthritis or arthralgia. There is a characteristic purpuric rash of the lower limbs and renal involvement (proteinuria or haematuria on urinalysis). Red cell casts may be seen on microscopy.

INVESTIGATIONS

- IgA is typically elevated
- Elevated CRP and ESR
- Clotting is typically normal
- U&Es
- Urine dip

MANAGEMENT

This is symptom based as the condition resolves in time. Monitoring of renal function is important and arthralgia may be managed with tapering steroids to avoid renal insult from NSAID use. Steroids do not prevent renal involvement.

Osteoarthritis (OA)

OA is the most common type of arthritis. It is characterised by the breakdown of the joint's cartilage due to altered biomechanics, joint instability and trauma. Incidence increases with age and with certain occupations. Osteoarthritis can also be secondary to other rheumatological conditions.

Loss of cartilage causes increased bone wear and remodelling at the articular surfaces causing stiffness, pain and loss of range—ultimately leading to loss of function.

INVESTIGATIONS

Clinical history and examination will distinguish this from other arthropathies. Diagnosis can be aided by plain films, which show loss of joint space, subchondral cyst formation, osteophyte formation and

Table 14.3 Small and Medium Vessel Vasculitis		
Medium	**Small**	
Polyarteritis Nodosa (PAN) Kawasaki Disease	**ANCA +** Eosinophilic granulomatosis with polyangiitis Microscopic Polyangiitis Granulomatosis with Polyangiitis	**ANCA –** Henoch—Schönlein Purpura (HSP)

subchondral sclerosis. There is no role for biochemistry in diagnosis unless there is significant overlap with autoimmune rheumatological disorders.

MANAGEMENT

The mainstay of treatment is activity modification, weight management and strengthening of the muscles associated with the affected joints. Simple analgesia can help manage pain and allow activity and training. For those who are not managed with conservative treatment, referral to an orthopaedic surgeon for assessment of surgical intervention is warranted.

CLINICAL CONSIDERATIONS

Diagnosis of OA should be followed by early assessment by a physiotherapist where the treating doctor is not comfortable in prescribing exercise and lifestyle modification. For those diagnosed with well-established disease needing surgical intervention, pre-operative supervised exercise should be encouraged to expedite post-operative recovery.

CRYSTAL DISEASE

Gout

Intermittent and intensely painful swelling of joints (most often in the hallux) but can occur in any joint. This can be triggered by a diet high in purines, alcohol excess or dehydration. It is more common in those with renal impairment. Examination typically shows swollen painful monoarthropathy. Often, pain limits detailed joint examination in the acute setting.

Diagnosis

Finding the characteristic negatively birefringent crystals to polarised light in the fluid of joint aspirate is diagnostic. Clinically, a high serum urate and typical symptoms may allow diagnosis.

Investigations

- Inflammatory markers are typically raised in acute flares.

- Serum urate and renal function.
- Plain X-rays—more useful for larger joints. Pseudogout cases may show chondrocalcinosis in affected knees.

MANAGEMENT

Management should be tailored for each person, depending on kidney function, other health problems and personal preferences. Acute flares are usually managed with a short course of NSAIDs, colchicine or steroids. It is reasonable to start urate lowering medications during an acute flare once there is adequate prophylactic cover. Long term treatment can include allopurinol, febuxostat, probenecid or benzbromarone.

CLINICAL CONSIDERATIONS

Lifestyle changes such as controlling weight, limiting alcohol intake and limiting meals rich in purines can help control gout.

It is important to remember that patients with gout are more likely to suffer from cardiovascular disease and a full cardiovascular screen should be completed, assessing other cardiovascular risk factors e.g. cholesterol, smoking status, hypertension.

Calcium Pyrophosphate Deposition (CPPD)

Often called Pseudogout due to the overlap of symptoms, this condition occurs due to deposition of calcium pyrophosphate crystals in the joint cartilage. This triggers an inflammatory reaction and symptoms of joint pain and swelling.

Aetiology is unknown but the condition is associated with increasing age—3% of patients aged 60 years to 50% of those aged 90. Other associated disorders include:

- Haemochromatosis
- Hypercalcemia
- Hypomagnesemia
- Hyperparathyroidism
- Hypothyroidism

INVESTIGATIONS

- Diagnosis is made on clinical examination and joint aspiration (with CPP crystals on

microscopy). Crystals are positively birefringent to polarised light
- FBC may show anaemia and raised WCC
- CRP, ESR, complement may be elevated during an acute attack
- X-rays may show chondrocalcinosis

MANAGEMENT

Acute flares are typically managed with a short course of NSAIDs, colchicine or steroids. Management of any identified underlying cause is paramount as recurrence can occur.

BONE DISORDERS

Osteoporosis (OP)

Regular or frequent corticosteroid use is associated with early osteoporotic changes in bone density, amongst other side effects.

Patients on doses of >2.5 mg Prednisolone (or equivalent) for 3 months or more should have calcium and vitamin D supplementation daily. Patients with rheumatological conditions have an increased risk of osteoporosis due to the inflammatory nature of their disease.

Risk factors for steroid induced OP can be modifiable or non-modifiable (Table 14.4).

DIAGNOSIS

Ideally, this is a preventable condition so good prescribing and risk identification is key.

A DEXA scan will aid diagnosis and monitor treatment response.

MANAGEMENT

- Dietary supplementation of vitamin D and calcium
- Bisphosphonates (reduce bone turnover)
- Denosumab
- Romosozumab
- Teriparatide
- Hormone replacement therapy for post-menopausal women or testosterone treatment (where indicated) for men
- Selective oestrogen receptor modulators (SERMs)

CLINICAL CONSIDERATIONS

Regular review of patients who use steroids is important to limit steroid-related complications. Vitamin D levels can be easily checked in practice. Supplementation is important in both those on steroids and in general, over the winter months.

Calcium levels on biochemistry testing have little bearing on the progression of osteoporosis and combining calcium and vitamin D supplementation is safe in practice. Patients at risk should have DEXA screening.

Osteonecrosis

Osteonecrosis (ON) is death of bone cells leading to collapse of the bone structure. Typically, this is caused by a loss of blood supply to the affected bone (avascular necrosis) due to trauma, alcoholism, SLE or antiphospholipid syndrome. ON can also result from iatrogenic causes such as radiation therapy, bisphosphonate use and long-term steroid use.

DIAGNOSIS

- X-ray is first line
- MRI scan

Table 14.4 Risk Factors for Osteoporosis

Non-modifiable	Modifiable	Hormonal
White and Asian ethnicity	Physical inactivity	Hyperthyroidism
Parental history of hip fracture	Hypoandrogenism/hypoestrogenism	Hyperparathyroidism
	Anorexia or bulimia nervosa	Cushing's disease
	Tobacco or excess alcohol intake	
	Low dietary calcium and vitamin D	
	Medications—e.g. steroids/heparin/excess thyroxine/sex hormone antagonists	

- CT scans can allow 3D reconstruction of the affected bone prior to surgery

MANAGEMENT

ON is best prevented but analgesia is important in managing bone pain. Physiotherapy and orthopaedic input are important to manage pain and mobility. Bisphosphonates are used in some cases of pre-collapse avascular necrosis. Operative measures include core decompression, bone grafting and joint replacement. Evidence on these therapies is limited.

Paget's Disease of Bone

This is a chronic bone metabolism disorder, resulting in rapid isolated bone turnover at a rate disordered from normal remodelling. It can result in weaker sections of bone or disruption of normal articulation surfaces leading to arthritis. Patients are typically >40 years old and 30% of patients have a family history. Patients can present with a variety of symptoms ranging from loss of range, bone pain, fractures and hearing loss.

INVESTIGATIONS

- Serum biochemistry may show an elevated ESR. Serum alkaline phosphatase may be elevated where there is rapid bone turnover
- Imaging may show areas of increased bone density

MANAGEMENT

- Analgesia such and NSAIDs are useful in managing bone pain
- Bisphosphonates (can regulate bone turnover)
- Calcitonin (inhibits osteoclast function)
- Orthopaedic opinions should be sought where symptoms are not controlled or mobility is affected.

Hypermobility Syndrome

Hypermobility is when a joint can move beyond an expected range. Children may be more mobile than their adult counterparts but this does not equate to hypermobility unless the joint can exceed its predicted range. Hypermobility can predispose the affected area to pain and dysfunction due to altered biomechanics. Dislocation risk is higher.

Patients who are hypermobile should be screened for connective tissue disorders such as Ehlers-Danlos or Marfan's syndrome. These conditions are associated with systemic complications such as ocular and cardiac problems. Appropriate onward referral is important.

DIAGNOSIS

Beighton hypermobility assessment tool grades the severity of laxity experienced by the patient.

1. Passive dorsiflexion and hyperextension of the fifth MCP joint beyond 90°
2. Passive opposition of the thumb to the flexor aspect of the forearm
3. Passive hyperextension of the elbow beyond 10°
4. Passive hyperextension of the knee beyond 10°
5. Active forward flexion of the trunk with the knees fully extended so that the palms of the hands rest flat on the floor

A maximum score is 9, with the first four domains scored on the left and right.

MANAGEMENT

Supportive management of pain is important and supervised exercise within the limits of joint apprehension is the mainstay of musculoskeletal care.

Fibromyalgia

Fibromyalgia is a chronic pain disorder which is not caused by an autoimmune or inflammatory pathology. Often, it is classified as a complex neurological disorder characterised by widespread pain and sensitivity, or a central pain amplification disorder. These symptoms are typically migratory. Sleep disturbance and chronic fatigue are commonly associated.

Fibromyalgia is more common in women than men, typically noted in middle age. It is more common in patients with autoimmune disorders such as SLE, RA and AS. There is no specific genetic cause but physical and psychological stresses are thought to contribute.

INVESTIGATIONS AND DIAGNOSIS

This is a clinical diagnosis and there are no specific investigations needed. The American College of Rheumatology Symptom Severity Score and Widespread Pain Index may help.

MANAGEMENT

- Analgesia may be prescribed but focused exercise therapies are the mainstay of symptom control
- SSRIs and other antidepressants are shown to be of benefit and are licensed for use in fibromyalgia
- Medications that modulate nerve cell transmission of pain signals can be used with benefit
- Cognitive Behavioural therapy can help patients minimise their perception of symptom severity

CLINICAL CONSIDERATIONS

Fibromyalgia is a chronic disorder. There is a risk of polypharmacy as patients seek medications to manage their symptoms. Opioid medication has no role in managing pain in these cases. In practice, the role of the rheumatologist is limited and GP and psychologist input are important

PAEDIATRIC RHEUMATOLOGIC CONDITIONS

Juvenile Idiopathic Arthritis (JIA)

This is the most common form of arthritis in children. Common symptoms include pain, stiffness, swelling and loss of function in the joints. It can also be accompanied with fevers or rashes on various parts of the body. Whilst remission is possible, close monitoring of the child is important to maintain function and mobility and to manage extra-articular symptoms.

There are different classes of JIA including:

- Oligoarticular
- Polyarticular
- Psoriatic
- Enthesis related
- Systemic onset

DIAGNOSIS

History and clinical examination may detect a pattern of arthralgia similar to that of adult autoimmune arthritis. Extra-articular symptoms include eye irritation or abdominal pain. There can be an associated diffuse salmon coloured rash. Fever may be a feature—this needs to be distinguished from an infective arthropathy, particularly in an oligoarticular arthritis.

INVESTIGATIONS

- Clinical examination and recognition of arthritic symptoms is sufficient to make a clinical diagnosis
- FBC may show anaemia and raised WCC
- CRP, ESR, complement and acute-phase reactants may all be elevated
- Rheumatoid factor can often be negative
- ANA

MANAGEMENT

Referral to a paediatric rheumatologist with physiotherapy and occupational therapy input is important. The goal is to maintain function and to limit joint damage. Systemic steroid use may be necessary. Intra-articular steroids can be considered. DMARDs or biological agents may be used to manage symptoms and induce disease remission.

Juvenile Dermatomyositis

Similar to dermatomyositis of adulthood, although the characteristic associated heliotrope rash may be less frequently observed. A rash on the back, chest and upper limbs is more common. Investigations and treatments are similar for the adult variant.

OTHER

Bursitis

This is a condition that causes pain and tenderness in the location of bursae, which are small fluid-filled sacs that reduce the friction between bones and moving structures. Bursitis is not a standalone condition and is typically a result of either pathology, trauma or poor biomechanics.

INVESTIGATIONS

- Diagnosis is usually clinical
- Ultrasound imaging may be useful to confirm
- MRI may be of benefit to exclude associated regional pathology
- Aspiration may allow a fluid sample to be sent to the lab for analysis to exclude infective causes for diagnosis in conditions such as gout
- FBC may show anaemia and raised WCC
- CRP, ESR, complement and acute-phase reactants may be elevated during an acute episode

MANAGEMENT

- This may include rest or activity modification to offload the affected bursa
- Medication such as NSAIDs may alleviate pain and swelling
- Aspiration may alleviate symptoms rapidly and steroid injection into the bursa may be beneficial

Other Conditions

The rheumatology clinic may see and treat a variety of disorders including various localised soft tissue disorders (carpal tunnel syndrome), Ehlers-Danlos syndrome, hypermobility disorders and Lyme disease. Some of these conditions can be managed within primary care, physiotherapy, orthopaedics or infectious diseases, where appropriate. Furthermore, uncommon vasculitis may also be treated by the rheumatologist but due to the multi-systemic nature of these illnesses, there is typically shared care with specialities associated with the system of predominant dysfunction.

MULTIPLE CHOICE QUESTION (MCQ) QUESTIONS

1. A 52-year-old male with a tender and inflamed left first metatarsophalangeal joint attends your clinic. After completing a history and examination you diagnose gout. When giving dietary advice about gout, which of the following items is most appropriate to continue consuming?

    A. Alcohol
    B. Mussels
    C. Eggs
    D. Marmite
    E. Herring

2. You review a 62-year-old female in your musculoskeletal clinic. She has a history of haemochromatosis. She complains of a 3-week history of left knee pain, which has gradually worsened. On examination, her knee is swollen, warm and tender to touch. She is systemically well. What is the most likely diagnosis?

    A. Gout
    B. Pseudogout
    C. Septic arthritis
    D. Osteoarthritis
    E. Systemic sclerosis

3. A 32-year-old female skier complains of hand pain. The pains have affected both sides for 12 months, mainly in the small joints and the pain is often worse in mornings. She is struggling to hold her ski-poles. On examination, she has inflammation and tenderness over all of her metacarpophalangeal and proximal interphalangeal joints. Given the likely diagnosis, which of the following investigations is most specific?

    A. Rheumatoid factor
    B. Anti-CCP
    C. C-reactive protein
    D. Anti-neutrophil cytoplasmic antibodies
    E. Anti-histone antibodies

4. A 4-year-old boy has a history of spiking fevers. He has swelling present on multiple small finger joints in both hands, as well as a diffuse, pink rash and abdominal pain. There is no palpable lymphadenopathy. Blood tests are negative for autoantibodies; however, they reveal a mild anaemia and leukocytosis. What is the most likely diagnosis?

    A. Juvenile idiopathic arthritis
    B. Septic arthritis
    C. Kawasaki disease
    D. Rheumatic fever
    E. Scarlet fever

5. You are analysing some blood tests for a patient who presented to you with non-specific joint pain, fatigue and persisting cold-like symptoms. Which of the following vasculitidies is most strongly associated with C-ANCA (cytoplasmic antineutrophilic cytoplasmic antibody)?

   A. Kawasaki disease
   B. Granulomatosis with polyangiitis
   C. Microscopic polyangiitis
   D. Eosinophilic granulomatosis with polyangiitis
   E. Takayasu vasculitis

MULTIPLE CHOICE QUESTION (MCQ) ANSWERS

1. Answer C
   All of the items listed are high in purines apart from eggs (Answer C). Uric acid is a waste product from breaking down purines and so high amounts should be avoided in patients with gout.
2. Answer B
   Various endocrine and metabolic conditions can predispose to pseudogout including haemochromatosis, as mentioned in the stem. As she is systemically well, Answer C is unlikely. Gout (Answer A) can cause an inflammatory monoarthropathy but with the history of haemochromatosis, pseudogout is more likely. Rheumatic fever would usually present after a bacterial throat infection.
3. Answer B
   With PIP involvement, the most likely diagnosis is rheumatoid arthritis. Anti-CCP levels (Answer B) are the most specific test for rheumatoid arthritis, even though a number of the answers may be raised (A, C and D). Answer E may be raised in drug-induced Lupus.
4. Answer A
   This is juvenile idiopathic arthritis. Although fevers would be present in septic arthritis, it would be unlikely to affect multiple joints as in this case. Kawasaki disease is an important differential diagnosis, but often causes lymphadenopathy, conjunctivitis, skin peeling and a characteristic strawberry tongue. Rheumatic fever is usually preceded by a bacterial throat infection and Scarlet fever would usually involve a sore throat, strawberry tongue and lymphadenopathy.
5. Answer B
   C-ANCA is most strongly associated with granulomatosis with polyangiitis. This condition can cause renal, respiratory, nasopharyngeal and systemic symptoms.

Clinical Pharmacology 15

Luke McMenamin and Patrick Tung

Musculoskeletal pain, including its presentation and subsequent management, plays a huge role in athlete care. This ranges from acute pain to working alongside athletes in their management of long-term chronic pain. Pain management is often described as a 'multidisciplinary multimodal' treatment approach. This chapter reviews some of the commonly prescribed analgesic agents used in the world of sport.

PAIN

Pain by the International Association for the Study of Pain (IASP) as 'An unpleasant sensory and emotional experience associated with, or resembling that associated with, actual or potential tissue damage' (Raja et al., 2020).

Pain can be categorised by its timing:

- Acute pain is described as pain that is occurring for less than 12 weeks (<3 months).
- Chronic pain is pain that is occurring for greater than 12 weeks (>3 months).

CHRONIC PAIN IN SPORT

Unfortunately, many athletes develop chronic pain as a result of their actual or potential tissue damage. Many people will describe neuropathic pain, which is characteristically burning, (electrical) shocking, stabbing and gnawing in nature. Neuropathic pain is pain initiated or caused by a primary lesion or dysfunction in the peripheral or central nervous system.

The most common chronic pain manifestation from athletes is Chronic Regional Pain syndrome (CRPS). Complex regional pain syndrome is a post-traumatic disorder characterised by a non-dermatomal distributed, severe, continuous pain in the affected limb and is associated with sensory, motor, vasomotor, sudomotor, and trophic disturbances. Athletes with chronic pain should be identified early and referred to a pain specialist who can, with the multidisciplinary team, help the athlete manage their pain to hopefully regain their previous function.

DOPING

Doping can be used to improve the performance of an athlete. As mentioned in the 'Elite Sport' chapter, doping can be performed in a number of ways.

One category of 'performance enhancing drugs,' are 'narcotics' or painkillers used to mask pain and get the athlete back to training or competing, prior to them being physically or psychologically fit to return.

It is good practice to check that all analgesic agents are permissible with the World Anti-Doping Agency (WADA) prior to prescription or administration, and where appropriate, a Therapeutic Use Exemption (TUE) must be created and logged.

Doping Overview

S0 NON-APPROVED SUBSTANCES

These substances include pre-clinical drugs, usually under development.

- BPC-157 is a new, experimental compound with research underway for soft tissue healing. There are unproven claims it is performance enhancing.

DOI: 10.1201/9781003179979-15

CLINICAL PHARMACOLOGY AND THERAPEUTICS

Pain

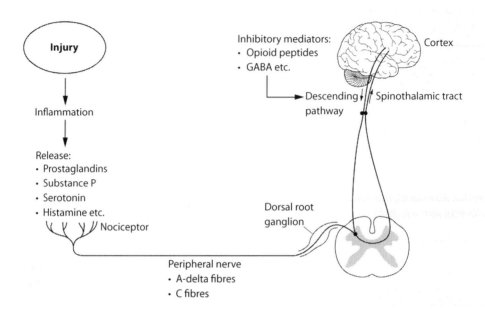

Non-steroidal anti-inflammatory drugs (NSAIDs)

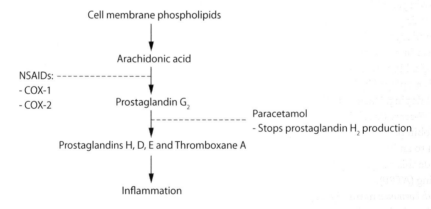

WADA prohibited list

S0 Non-approved substances
S1 Anabolic agents
S2 Peptide hormones, growth factors, related substances and mimetics
S3 Beta-2 agonists
S4 Hormone and metabolic modulators
S5 Diuretics and masking agents

Prohibited methods

M1 Manipulation of blood and blood components
M2 Chemical and physical manipulation
M3 Gene doping

In competition

S6 Stimulants
S7 Narcotics
S8 Cannabinoids
S9 Glucocorticoids

Figure 15.1 Pictorial overview.

S1 ANABOLIC AGENTS

Derivatives of testosterone, these drugs can increase lean muscle mass, reduce recovery time after exercise and increase aggressive, competitive edge. Side effects include breast enlargement and testicular atrophy in males, or increased facial hair and irregular menstruation in females. They can also cause liver dysfunction, hypercholesterolaemia and hypertension. Needle sharing carries the risk of blood-borne disease.

- Anabolic steroids: e.g. stanozolol, nandrolone, tibolone.
- Other anabolic agents: e.g. clenbuterol.

S2 PEPTIDE HORMONES, GROWTH FACTORS, RELATED SUBSTANCES AND MIMETICS

These hormones can have wide-ranging effects.

- *Erythropoietin:* is created by the kidneys in response to hypoxia and is licensed for treatment of certain conditions including kidney failure. It stimulates red blood cell production and subsequently increases haemoglobin levels, improving aerobic capacity. Side effects can be devastating, including thrombosis, encephalopathy and myocardial infarction. The UCI (Union Cycliste Internationale) introduced an Athlete Biological Passport (ABP) that is now more widely employed by WADA to tackle EPO and blood doping. Haemoglobin concentrations and an OFF-score (involving reticulocyte and haemoglobin percentages) are monitored and compared to an individually expected range. A result outside this range triggers an Atypical Passport Finding (ATPF).
- *Growth hormone:* naturally occurs from the anterior pituitary gland. It causes insulin-like growth factor (IGF-1) to be released from the liver, which encourages tissue growth and it is thought to have anabolic muscle effects. Risks include hypertension, diabetic complications and pancreatitis.
- *Human chorionic gonadotropin (HCG):* is also secreted by the pituitary gland. It is associated with pregnancy as well as certain cancers. HCG is thought to have a mild anabolic effect, as it increases the secretion of testosterone in males. It can cause renal failure, heart failure and hormonal imbalance.

S3 BETA-2 AGONISTS

These are common asthma treatments that cause bronchodilation. Evidence is mixed, but they may boost sprint and strength performance in athletes without asthma. Current maximum permitted inhaled amounts as per WADA (2023) include:

- *Salbutamol:* 1600 micrograms over 24 hours (in divided doses not to exceed 600 micrograms over 8 hours).
- *Formoterol:* 54 micrograms over 24 hours.
- *Salmeterol:* 200 micrograms over 24 hours.
- *Vilanterol:* 25 micrograms over 24 hours.

S4 HORMONE AND METABOLIC MODULATORS

Aromatase inhibitors, anti-oestrogens, meldonium, trimetazidine, insulins, AMPK activators and Activin receptor IIB activation preventers are prohibited.

- *Insulin:* lowers blood glucose and is produced by the pancreas. It is used as fuel in endurance athletes and to slow muscle tissue breakdown in power athletes. Overdose can cause hypoglycemia and death.

S5 DIURETICS AND MASKING AGENTS

These substances are used to mask doping and falsify test results. They include diuretics, which increase water and electrolyte excretion, probenecid acid and plasma expanders.

S6 STIMULANTS (IN COMPETITION)

Typically, stimulants increase sympathetic activity and are chemically similar to adrenaline. They decrease fatigue and increase mental or physical drive.

- Amphetamines: have historically been used for many years as a doping agent and can improve speed and power. They are highly addictive and risks include delirium, fluid loss, convulsions and myocardial infarction due to cardiovascular strain.
- Cocaine.

CLINICAL CONSIDERATIONS

Multiple over the counter decongestants contain ephedrine, which is a prohibited stimulant. Care should be taken when recommending treatments for athletes, and if used, a break of 48 hours should take place prior to competition.

S7 NARCOTICS (IN COMPETITION)

These generally act on the central nervous system and reduce pain perception. Opioid medications are highly addictive and overuse can cause respiratory depression.

S8 CANNABINOIDS (IN COMPETITION)

Naturally occurring, the main active component is tetrahydrocannabinol (THC). Cannabinoids increase dopamine centrally, which reduces brain excitability and causes relaxation and gratification. At high doses they can cause paranoia and anxiety. Long term use can cause psychiatric sequelae.

S9 GLUCOCORTICOIDS (IN COMPETITION)

Produced by the adrenal glands, these steroid hormones can reduce inflammation and trigger gluconeogenesis, as well as fat and protein breakdown. Side effects include osteoporosis, central obesity, increased diabetes risk and growth issues.

M1 MANIPULATION OF BLOOD AND BLOOD PRODUCTS

Tampering with blood products can increase haemoglobin and, subsequently, aerobic capacity. Blood borne viruses, as well as thrombotic events due to high haematocrit levels are risks.

- *Autologous doping:* this usually involves an athlete having some blood removed a number of weeks prior to competition. The body then regenerates lost red blood cells, and they are boosted with the transfusion of their old blood prior to, or in competition.
- *Homologous doping:* this involves an athlete being directly transfused from another person. Either blood or concentrated blood products can be used.

M2 CHEMICAL AND PHYSICAL MANIPULATION

- *Intravenous infusions:* more than 100 mL/12 hours is banned unless clinically required for hospital treatment.

M3 GENE AND CELL DOPING

Genetic material is introduced into an athlete, which may have far-reaching consequences such as influencing the growth of tissues or hormone production. Gene transfer and the modulation of existing genes is prohibited. Such alterations may not be reversible and cancers such as leukaemia are linked to genetic modification.

P1 B-BLOCKERS (IN PARTICULAR SPORTS)

These are banned in competition in automobile sport, darts, billiards, golf, underwater sports and skiing/snowboarding. They are banned at all times in archery and shooting, due to their effects of slowing heart rate and reducing tremors.

Medicines Storage in Sport

Sports physicians need to adopt strict governance rules when they are acquiring, storing, prescribing and dispensing medication. All medication stored for the use of sports teams must be ordered following local pharmacy guidelines. All medication must be logged in a drug book and accounted for before, during and after each training or competitive event. Use by dates must be adhered to and noted on the drug formulary.

All medication must be stored securely under lock and key at all times. Controlled drugs regulations classify controlled drugs into 5 schedules, with Schedule 1 being the most strictly regulated, and Schedule 5 being least strictly regulated. Controlled drugs should be stored in a locked cupboard that is secured to a wall and fixed with bolts that are not accessible from outside the cupboard. For competitive events that require transport of drugs (in particular, controlled drugs including weak opioids, such as codeine), they too must be securely locked in a separate drug box that only the physician caring for the team can access. Athletes must have all medication prescribed and logged. The indication of the medication, appropriateness, the athlete's past medical history and drug and allergy history should be considered. It is good practice to check all medication on the WADA formulary and follow the TUE process if clinically appropriate.

ANALGESIC AGENTS

Pain Management on the Field of Play

ENTONOX

Entonox is a gaseous 50:50 mix of nitrous oxide (N_2O) and oxygen (O_2). It comes in a blue and white cylinder.

It has a demand valve at the patient end allowing for self-administration. Nitrous Oxide is a strong analgesic agent. Contraindications to the use of Entonox include suspected facial or sinus fractures, head injuries, middle ear disease and pneumothorax. This is due to the risk of N$_2$O causing an expansion of air-filled cavities and subsequent deterioration of the clinical presentation. At a temperature of –6°C, Entonox separates into its constituents of liquid nitrogen and oxygen gas, making it unusable in these environments.

PENTHROX

Penthrox is the trade name of the anaesthetic agent Methoxyflurane. Methoxyflurane is an inhalational anaesthesia agent that displays both sedative and analgesic properties. It has been widely used in the

battlefield to provide immediate analgesia in the setting of significant trauma.

Contraindications to the use of Penthrox is that it must not be administered to patients who are at risk of malignant hyperthermia, as it may trigger an attack. In addition, it needs to be administered in well ventilated areas (such as pitchside) to prevent others from inhaling the anaesthetic agent. An activated charcoal chamber helps to ensure others don't get exposed to the drug.

Analgesic Agents Used in the Medical Room

Analgesic medication can be categorised into 'Simple,' 'Weak Opioid' and 'Strong Opioid;' widely adapted

Table 15.1 Common Analgesics

Medication	Mechanism of Action	Uses	Problems	Adult dose
Paracetamol	Inhibits the synthesis of prostaglandins	Generally very safe Good for mild pain but can be useful for most nociceptive pain	Not all patients are able to take oral liquids or tablets Can cause liver damage in overdose	Usually given PO but can be given PR PO or PR: 1G (two 500 mg tablets) QDS Maximum dose: 4G per 24 hours IV < 55 Kg = 15 mg/Kg
Aspirin	Irreversibly Inhibits COX1 & COX 2	Can be used with paracetamol Good for nociceptive pain	Side effects: Gastrointestinal problems, e.g. gastritis Kidney damage Fluid retention Increased risk of bleeding	PO: 600 mg (two 300 mg tablets) 4–6 hourly Maximum dose: 3.6 G per 24 hours
Diclofenac	Non-Selectively Inhibits COX1 & COX 2	As above for aspirin	As above for aspirin, but can be given IM or PR Caution in asthmatics	PO: 25–50 mg TDS PR: 100 mg OD IM: 75 mg BD Maximum dose: 150 mg per 24 hours
Ibuprofen	Non-Selectively Inhibits COX1 & COX 2	As above for aspirin	As above for aspirin Caution in asthmatics	PO: 400 mg TDS or QDS
Naproxen	Non-Selectively Inhibits COX1 & COX 2	As above for aspirin	As above for aspirin Caution in asthmatics	PO: 500 mg BD

Table 15.2 Weak Opioids

Medication	Mechanism of Action	Uses	Problems	Adult dose
Codeine	MOP receptor Agonist	Generally very safe Often added to paracetamol and/or NSAID for moderate pain	Not all patients are able to take oral liquids or tablets Similar side effects to other opioids: Constipation Respiratory depression in high dose Misunderstandings about addiction Different patients require different doses (variable dose requirement)	Usually given PO but sometimes given IM PO or IM: 30–60 mg 4-hourly
Tramadol	MOP receptor Agonist and weak inhibition of the reuptake of norepinephrine and serotonin.	Can be used with paracetamol and/or opioids for nociceptive pain Sometimes helpful for neuropathic pain Less respiratory depression and constipation than morphine	Not widely available Nausea and vomiting Confusion	PO or IV: 50–100 mg QDS

from the World Health Organisation's 'Analgesic Ladder,' which was first created for the management of cancer pain (Anekar and Cascella, 2022) see Tables 15.1–15.3. More recently, the role of 'Analgesic adjuncts' have come to the forefront. Recent research has proven these drugs help to potentiate classic analgesic agents or help modulate chronic pain pathways (Tables 15.4–15.5).

OTHER MEDICATIONS

- Fluoroquinolones (e.g. Ciprofloxacin), are commonly used antibiotics that act by inhibiting bacterial DNA gyrase. They have been associated with tendon rupture, so their use should be judicious, particularly in patients with musculoskeletal problems.
- Statin medication is used to lower cholesterol by slowing down LDL-cholesterol production in the liver. Their use has been associated with tendinopathy, muscle aches and rarely, rhabdomyolysis.

MULTIPLE CHOICE QUESTION (MCQ) QUESTIONS

1. You are the club doctor of a Rugby League team. At preseason, one of your players announces that he has started to take a painkiller that his friend has posted to him from Australia. You don't recognise the drug name. Which one of the following resources would you access to help determine if the drug complies with doping policy?

   A. The British National Formulary (BNF)
   B. The Drug Wise encyclopaedia
   C. The World Anti-Doping Agency (WADA) website
   D. The Rugby Football League (RFL) medical standards document
   E. The Global Drug Reference Online (Global DRO)

Table 15.3 Strong Opioids

Medication	Mechanism of Action	Uses	Problems	Adult dose
Morphine	MOP, DOP & KOP receptor Agonists	Very safe if used appropriately Often added to paracetamol and/or NSAID for moderate to severe pain Oral morphine very useful for cancer pain In general, should be avoided in chronic non-cancer pain Available as either fast release tablets or syrup, or slow release tablets	Similar problems to other opioids: Constipation Sedation and respiratory depression in high dose* Nausea and vomiting Myths about addiction Oral dose is not the same as the injected dose *Monitor respiratory rate and sedation, especially in elderly patients and patients receiving other sedating medications	Can be given PO, IV, IM or SC Different patients require different doses Oral dose is 2–3 times the injected dose PO (fast): 10–30 mg 4-hourly (e.g. for controlling cancer pain) PO (slow): BD dosing (may need high doses for cancer pain) IV: 2.5–10 mg (e.g. during or after surgery) IM or SC: 2.5–10 mg 4-hourly Use a lower dose (e.g. half-dose) in elderly patients
Oxycodone (Oxynorm, Oxycontin)	MOP, DOP & KOP receptor Agonists	As above for morphine Can be used for cancer pain Available as fast release (Oxynorm) or slow release (Oxycontin)	As above for morphine Not widely available	PO (fast): 5–10 mg 4-hourly PO (slow): 10 mg BD, increased as needed Use a lower dose (e.g. half-dose) in elderly patients

2. You are a club doctor for a football team. A new player with known asthma has arrived at the club. Unfortunately, during training he is tackled badly injuring his hamstring. At the pitchside he was given Entonox. In the dressing room he was given paracetamol and diclofenac by other players. He becomes more and more breathless over the next few minutes, complaining that his chest is 'tight.' There are no rashes, his heart rate is 97 bpm, and his blood pressure is 132/88 mmHg. There is widespread wheeze throughout his chest. What is the most likely diagnosis?

A. Anaphylaxis
B. Tension pneumothorax
C. Asthma attack
D. Fat embolism
E. Arrhythmia

3. You are providing medical cover for a mixed martial arts (MMA) tournament. A fighter has been knocked out and has sustained significant facial trauma around his eye and nose. He has also suffered a closed fracture of his tibia and fibula in the bout. He quickly regains consciousness and is now GCS 15. You notice the swelling around the eye and nose feels like 'bubble wrap' under the skin. He is in significant pain around his ankle and is asking for something. An ambulance is called but

Table 15.4 Other Analgesics and Adjuncts Used in Chronic Pain

Medication	Mechanism of Action	Uses	Problems	Adult dose
Amitriptyline	Increases norepinephrine and serotonin at presynaptic terminals	Useful in neuropathic pain. Also used to treat depression and improve sleep	Sedation Postural hypotension (low blood pressure) Anticholinergic side effects: Dry mouth Urinary retention Constipation	PO: Usually 25 mg at night 'Start low, go slow,' especially in elderly patients (e.g. start at 10 mg, increase every 2–3 days as tolerated)
Carbamazepine	Acts on the sodium channels to reduce the repetitive firing of action potentials	Anticonvulsant ('membrane stabiliser') Useful in neuropathic pain	Sedation Unsteadiness Confusion in high dose	PO: 100–200 mg BD, increased to 200–400 mg QDS as tolerated 'Start low, go slow,' especially in elderly patients
Clonidine	Alpha 2 receptor agonist which reduces norepinephrine release	May be useful if pain is difficult to treat	Not widely available Sedation Hypotension	IV: 15–30 mcg 15- minutely up to 1–2 mcg/kg PO: 2 mcg/kg
Gabapentin	Mimics the inhibitory neurotransmitter GABA	Anticonvulsant ('membrane stabiliser') Useful in neuropathic pain	Sedation	PO: 100 mg TDS, increased to 300–600 mg TDS as tolerated Maximum dose: 1800 mg per 24 hours
Ketamine	NMDA receptor antagonist	May be useful in severe pain (nociceptive or neuropathic) Also used as a general anaesthetic	Sedation (only need small dose for pain relief) Dreams, delirium, hallucinations	IV: 5–10 mg for severe acute pain SC infusion: 100 mg over 24 hours for 3 days, can be increased to 300 mg, then 500 mg per 24 hours
Sodium valproate	Blockade of voltage-gated sodium channels and increased brain levels GABA	Anticonvulsant ('membrane stabiliser') Useful in neuropathic pain	Gastrointestinal side effects, Sedation	PO: 200 mg 8–12 hourly

Table 15.5 Musculoskeletal Injections

Medication	Mechanism of Action	Uses	Problems	Adult dose
Corticosteroids (e.g. triamcinolone, methylprednisolone)	Blocks inflammatory mediators to reduce pain and inflammation	Useful in pain reduction, particularly in the short term. Often used in bursitis, osteoarthritis, spinal injections etc.	Infection risk Skin depigmentation Fat atrophy Short term exacerbation of symptoms Impairment of tendon healing Cartilage matrix degeneration	Intra-articular/ Intra-bursal: Methylprednisolone 10–80 mg, Triamcinolone 2.5–40 mg
High volume injections	Mechanical effects including neovessel stretching, denervation of sensory nerves	Used in tendinopathy	Infection risk Short term exacerbation of symptoms Further high-quality research required to confirm efficacy	Peritendinous injection: up to 40 mL normal saline. Local anaesthetic and steroid can be added
Hyaluronic acid	Replaces synovial fluid and modulates inflammatory response	Useful in pain reduction, particularly medium-long term in osteoarthritis	Infection risk Short term exacerbation of symptoms Allergy in rare cases	Intra-articular: Usually 2–4 mL
Prolotherapy (e.g. hyperosmolar dextrose)	Stimulates growth factor release and local inflammatory cascade	Used in treating musculoskeletal pain, including tendinopathy	Infection risk Mixed evidence regarding efficacy	Various concentrations and volumes are used depending on the location and injury type
Autologous blood injections	Introduction of blood, which contains growth factors	Used in treating musculoskeletal pain, including tendinopathy	Infection risk Mixed evidence regarding efficacy	Various volumes of blood injected depending on the location and injury type
Platelet-rich plasma (PRP)	Introduction of plasma, which contains growth factors	Used in treating musculoskeletal pain, including tendinopathy	Infection risk Mixed evidence regarding efficacy	Various concentrations and volumes are used depending on the location and injury type

it will be some time. You have cannulated and begun medication with IV paracetamol. The fighter is asking for more. Which of the following is the next best analgesic to prescribe and administer?

A. Entonox
B. Penthrox
C. PO Diclofenac
D. IV Morphine
E. PO Codeine

4. Which of the following irreversibly inhibits the COX pathway?

A. Aspirin
B. Ibuprofen
C. Diclofenac
D. Paracetamol
E. Naproxen

5. Which one of the following is NOT a controlled drug?

A. Ketamine
B. Gabapentin
C. Carbamazepine
D. Oxycodone
E. Pregabalin

MULTIPLE CHOICE QUESTION (MCQ) ANSWERS

1. Answer E
   The Global DRO resource allows health care professionals and players to search specific drugs (including brand names) and find out if they are banned in or out of competition for a large number of sports. Although Answer C will have some relevant information, it may not contain the drug you are looking for. The BNF (Answer A) may not include the Australian drug and will not give information about doping. Neither will Answer B or Answer D.

2. Answer C
   With a low velocity mechanism of injury to the lower legs, without long bone injury, a fat embolism (D) is ruled out. He is cardiovascularly stable; therefore, the possibility of a tension pneumothorax (B) is also slim. There are no

signs of shock or urticarial rash, so anaphylaxis (A) is unlikely. His heart rate is below 120 bpm, so an arrhythmia (E) is unlikely.
This is a known asthmatic who has recently ingested a NSAID, complaining of chest tightness with widespread wheeze. The safest action to take is to diagnose an asthma attack (C) and treat accordingly.

3. Answer D
   The fighter is displaying signs of subcutaneous emphysema communicating around his face, therefore excluding inhalational agents. Entonox (A) and penthrox (B) could cause an increased volume of gas to be trapped.
   He has suffered a significant trauma and head injury. As a result, he is at risk of losing consciousness or aspirating. Therefore, the oral route is risky, ruling out diclofenac (C) and codeine phosphate (E). The degree of trauma deserves robust, titrated strong opioids such as morphine (D) to manage his pain in incremental doses.

4. Answer A
   Aspirin irreversibly inhibits the COX pathway (A). All the other NSAIDs (B, C and E) inhibit the COX pathway but not irreversibly. Paracetamol (D) inhibits the actions of prostaglandins; however, future research is looking at a COX-3 pathway and the role of paracetamol.

5. Answer C
   From 2019, gabapentin (B) and pregabalin (E) are now controlled drugs alongside ketamine (A) and oxycodone (D). Carbamazepine (C) is not a controlled drug.

REFERENCES AND FURTHER READING

Anekar, A.A., Cascella, M. (2022 January). WHO analgesic ladder. [Updated 2021 May 18]. *StatPearls* [Internet]. Treasure Island, FL: StatPearls Publishing. Available at: www.ncbi.nlm.nih.gov/books/NBK554435/

Raja, S.N., Carr, D.B., Cohen, M., Finnerup, N.B., Flor, H., Gibson, S., Keefe, F.J., Mogil, J.S., Ringkamp, M., Sluka, K.A., Song, X.-J., Stevens, B., Sullivan, M.D., Tutelman, P.R., Ushida, T., Vader, K. (September 2020). The revised international association for the study of pain definition of pain: Concepts, challenges, and compromises. *PAIN*. 161(9), pp. 1976–1982. doi: 10.1097/j.pain.0000000000001939

Emergency Medicine **16**

Michael Cooke, Anita Vishnubala and Patrick O'Halloran

INTRODUCTION

'Prepare, or be prepared to fail,' is a mantra used by many sports professionals. This applies to clinicians working in both SEM and emergency care. Preparation is essential to every aspect of SEM: from team travel, developing an Emergency Action Plan (EAP), to the assessment and management of emergency situations as they arise.

Many situations involving emergency care require rapid assessment and simultaneous intervention to stabilise an athlete. There are numerous accredited courses for pitch side emergency care in sport within the UK and internationally, which focus on a minimum standard to work pitch side providing medical cover.

Clinical Considerations: Golden Rules

1. Practice your approach to an emergency situation regularly with your team. Pre-assign roles for a given emergency situation (e.g. cardiac arrest), and use simulation to familiarise the team with critical scenarios (e.g. extrication in cervical spine injury).
2. Get help early—under the pressure of dealing with an emergency, calling for help early is often forgotten. Consider where help might come from, and in what form, before it is needed—especially when travelling abroad. You could be the best emergency medicine physician but, working in isolation, you will never be as effective.

PRE-HOSPITAL CARE

Care of acutely unwell patients in the pre-hospital environment focuses on identifying life and limb threatening injuries for which we can improve outcomes and 'buy time' until the patient can reach definitive care. Many interventions might be simple, but can have a long-term impact. Focusing on a systematic approach to assessing and managing these patients is key, as evidenced by a similar theme running across international life support/trauma courses.

THE ACUTELY UNWELL PATIENT

The focus is on rapid systematic assessment with simultaneous resuscitation. It follows a standardised ABCDE approach with a few variations depending on environment, sport and situation. Have your emergency medical kit arranged in a structured way to support effective and efficient management, removing some of the non-technical aspects from an emergency situation.

Use of the 'SAMPLE' mnemonic to handover patients to other healthcare professionals will ensure pertinent information is transferred:

- Sex (+age)
- Allergies
- Medications
- Previous medical history
- Last meal
- Events preceding/mechanism of injury

DOI: 10.1201/9781003179979-16

EMERGENCY MEDICINE

The Acutely Unwell Patient

Handover information
S – Sex
A – Allergies
M – Medications
P – Past medical history
L – Last meal
E – Events leading to injury

Reversible causes of cardiac arrest

4 H's
• Hypoxia
• Hypovolaemia
• Hypothermia
• Hyper/Hypokalaemia

4 T's
• Thrombus
• Tension pneumothorax
• Toxins
• Tamponade (cardiac)

Life threatening chest injuries
A – Airway injury
T – Tension pneumothorax
O – Open pneumothorax
M – Massive haemothorax

F – Flail chest
C – Cardiac tamponade

Cardiopulmonary resuscitation (CPR)

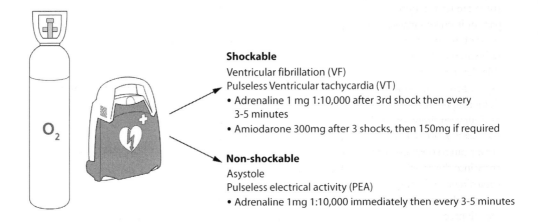

Shockable
Ventricular fibrillation (VF)
Pulseless Ventricular tachycardia (VT)
• Adrenaline 1 mg 1:10,000 after 3rd shock then every 3-5 minutes
• Amiodarone 300mg after 3 shocks, then 150mg if required

Non-shockable
Asystole
Pulseless electrical activity (PEA)
• Adrenaline 1mg 1:10,000 immediately then every 3-5 minutes

Concussion

• Traumatic brain injury
• Concussive symptoms following injury = remove from field of play
• SCAT-5 may be helpful

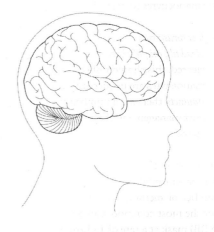

On field:
- Red flags
- Observable signs
- Memory assessment/Maddocks questions
- Examination (Glasgow Coma Scale and cervical spine assessment)

Off field:
- Athlete background
- Symptom evaluation
- Cognitive screening (orientation, immediate memory, concentration)
- Neurological screen and balance examination
- Delayed recall
- Decision

Figure 16.1 Chapter pictorial overview.

A list of pre-populated forms for this information is useful, where possible, so this can be accessed at short notice and other relevant information added at the time.

The initial approach follows the stepwise DR ABCDE assessment:

D—Danger—ensure safety for yourself and the medical team. Inadvertently increasing the number of casualties and reducing the number of medical personnel available is far from ideal.

R—Response—is the patient responsive or not? Caution is essential in scenarios involving an unwitnessed or traumatic mechanism, as cervical spine injury is possible. Verbally assessing for a response before controlling a patient's cervical spine can lead to unnecessary movement. If the patient is unresponsive, you should assess for signs of life for up to 10 seconds as per the Basic Life Support (BLS) guidelines covered, later in this chapter. If responsive, move to the next step.

A—Airway—alongside cervical spine control (at this stage, any catastrophic haemorrhage should be dealt with simultaneously). Take manual inline stabilisation (MILS) as you assess the airway. An airway can be clear, obstructed (silent with no air entry into the chest) or partially obstructed (noisy breathing). Look in the airway to assess for the cause of the obstruction, e.g. foreign body, blood/secretions, or the patient's tongue.

The most common cause of a partially obstructed airway in SEM is the athlete's own tongue and there are a few manoeuvres to deal with this:

- *Jaw thrust:* maintains MILS
- *Head tilt, chin lift:* if the cervical spine has not been cleared, this should only be performed if other manoeuvres are unsuccessful.
- *Adjuncts:* there are a number of adjuncts to support management of a patient's airway (discussed later).

Application of oxygen to acutely unwell patients in the pre-hospital environment is recommended. A number of methods of oxygen delivery are possible, but the most common would be via a non-rebreather (NRB) mask at a rate of 15 L/minute.

B—Breathing—having established an airway and administered oxygen, you need to assess for any breathing problems. In the first instance, having an adequate respiratory rate (RR) is important; less than 10 breaths per minute will need supporting with a bag valve mask (BVM) or equivalent. As well as assessing the RR, oxygen saturations can be obtained using a portable probe.

Assessment of the chest includes inspection, palpation, followed by percussion and auscultation (if able to, and the environment allows).

Inspection—look for bilateral chest movements, good rise and fall and adequate RR. Assess for any injuries suggested by bruising or abnormal chest movements. Distended neck veins and tracheal deviation are rare but important features to check for.

There are a number of life-threatening injuries in the chest, based on the mnemonic 'ATOM FC':

Airway injury—this can include laryngeal fracture.

Tension pneumothorax—decompression required via needle thoracocentesis in the fifth intercostal space, just anterior to the midaxillary line; or, failing that, the second intercostal space midclavicular line, just above the 3rd rib.

Open pneumothorax—bubbling chest wounds—cover any with a specialised dressing such as an Asherman seal or a simple dressing—making note this can become a tension pneumothorax if left occluded for a period of time—repeated assessment is required.

Massive haemothorax—suggested by chest injury with reduced air entry and dull percussion note, caused by blood in the underlying hemithorax (as opposed to a tension pneumothorax, which will have hyper-resonance to percussion). This requires expedited transfer to a trauma centre, with support of the patient's circulatory system as outlined in 'C.' Specific management requires a tube thoracostomy and is largely out of the scope of practice for most SEM clinicians.

Flail chest with pulmonary contusion—obvious chest wall injury with 'paradoxical' chest wall movement. These players need oxygenation, careful assessment for underlying chest injuries mentioned above and prompt transfer for definitive care. Analgesia is a simple, yet key, aspect in the management of this condition, and should be considered in the pre-hospital stage.

Cardiac tamponade—caused by blood accumulating inside the pericardium. As this increases, it has a tamponade effect on the heart, reducing cardiac output. This will present with muffled heart sounds, distended neck veins and hypotension. Such patients need support and transfer for drainage—a tamponade effect will likely develop over a period of time (rather than instantly), so be aware of the potential for this injury based on the mechanism and reassess regularly. Oxygen, circulatory support and rapid transfer to definitive care are the mainstays of pre-hospital pitch side management.

C—Circulatory Assessment

In the context of an injured athlete, the leading cause is haemorrhage (volume loss) until proven otherwise. Identifying the likely source forms part of the C assessment. It is important to consider other causes of circulatory issues—e.g. anaphylaxis and sepsis—leading to fluid shifts outside the intravascular space with circulatory compromise.

Regular palpation of the radial pulse—noting character, volume and rate—builds a picture of your patient's progress. Monitor evidence of deterioration (weaker pulse and increased HR despite termination of physical activity). An absent radial pulse should prompt assessment of a central pulse to exclude cardio-respiratory arrest. If a central pulse is present, absence of the radial pulse may be due to hypotension (symmetrical radial pulse absence) or vascular injury (asymmetrical). It is suggested that a systolic blood pressure below 80–90 mmHg would result in loss of a palpable radial pulse. While evidence for this is poor, it is agreed, in a pre-hospital environment, this is an indication for initiating fluid resuscitation. This is usually with cautious 250 mL fluid boluses of 0.9% saline. Supplementary measures of perfusion, as part of the C assessment, can be central capillary refill and skin changes (mottled and cold peripheries, suggesting hypoperfusion). These can be difficult to assess reliably in outdoor sporting environments.

Given compromise to C, the focus of the rest of the assessment looks to establish the source of potential blood loss. This is divided into 'the floor or 5 more':

- Looking at the **floor** for signs of external bleeding from wounds.
- **Chest:** which you have already assessed in 'B.'
- **Abdomen** and **retroperitoneum**—evidence of injury, or pain on palpation, suggests potential bleeding from underlying structures.
- **Pelvis:** asymmetrical leg lengths with pelvic pain should prompt suspicion. Do not mechanically assess this with palpation or passive movement if injury is suspected—this might disrupt any clotting process—'the first clot is the best clot.' If no obvious injury is apparent, then it is accepted that gentle palpation of the pelvis—once only—to assess for injury can be undertaken. Concern for pelvic injury should prompt internal rotation of the lower legs and application of a pelvic binder (or improvised device fashioned using a sheet or similar to provide support). This attempts to close the 'open book,' reducing the volume of the pelvis (to tamponade haemorrhage), and keep the injury stabilised until definitive care.
- **Long bones:** inspection and palpation of the long bones for deformity is important—fractures can lead to significant blood loss. Identification of a suspected long bone fracture should prompt a neurovascular assessment and splinting, both to reduce blood loss and to help with pain, pending definitive management. There are a variety of methods for splinting fractures, with a number of devices on the market.

D—Disability

This section includes an assessment of the patient's conscious level using the Glasgow Coma Scale (GCS). This scores three domains—motor response (1–6), verbal response (1–5) and eye opening (1–4), with a maximum score of 15 and a minimum score of 3. Initially, at pitch side, it is acceptable to use the less comprehensive AVPU scale (Alert, responsiveness to Voice, Painful stimuli or Unresponsive). It is generally accepted in the pre-hospital environment, that a score of P is equivalent to a GCS of 8. This is important: a patient's ability to maintain their own airway is impaired at a GCS of 8 or below. Continuous assessment of the airway (or use of an adjunct) is required.

In addition, assess pupillary response—noting size, symmetry and reaction to light. An assessment for gross neurology of the four limbs can be carried out.

E—Exposure/Everything Else

This should include assessment for other injuries—e.g. fracture/dislocations of the extremities, keeping the patient warm and obtaining further information like capillary blood glucose.

Regular reassessment, recognising changes in clinical condition or parameters, are imperative to promptly manage deterioration, whilst awaiting definitive care.

Basic Airway Management

Having already discussed the initial assessment of an airway, there are a number of skills and adjuncts to be aware of. In the scope of SEM, these remain relatively simple measures, which—when employed effectively—enable most airways to be managed adequately.

Manoeuvres: Jaw thrust and head tilt, chin lift as mentioned previously.

Adjuncts—portable suction device, naso- or oro-pharyngeal airway (NPA/OPA), supraglottic airway devices e.g. I-gel, endotracheal tube (ETT).

Oxygen Delivery—NRB mask with flow rate 15 L/Minute, Nebuliser at 6 L/Minute, BVM to deliver assisted or mechanical ventilations at 15 L/Minute.

Emergency—needle cricothyroidotomy: surgical airway via anterior neck access.

Cardiorespiratory Arrest (CRA)

CRA is a scenario you hope to never encounter. Prior preparation is essential if it does occur. Basic life support refers to the initial steps in the management of someone in cardiorespiratory arrest. They are only basic by the nature of requiring no specialist kit; otherwise, they are critical aspects to maximise likelihood of return of spontaneous circulation (ROSC). Identification of CRA is the first stage; early recognition allows commencement of effective CPR

as soon as possible. Approaching a patient with the DR ABCDE approach will allow rapid identification of CRA in its initial stages, when the patient is unresponsive and has no definite signs of life. These steps, in combination with early defibrillation, are recognised as key factors in maximising the chances of ROSC.

In the event of drowning and in paediatric patients, there should be five rescue breaths before CPR is commenced. For paediatric patients, the ratio of compressions to breaths is 15:2 (as opposed to 30:2 in adults).

Advanced life support considers BLS skills with more advanced training. This maintains a focus on performing BLS well and pausing to reassess every 2 minutes. The ALS algorithm looks to determine if the patient is in either a 'shockable' or 'non-shockable' rhythm, with two separate arms of management. There may be the concurrent administration of drugs (e.g. adrenaline), if available, during ALS. Alongside resuscitation efforts, the team leader will consider potentially reversible causes for CRA, which are remembered as the four H's and 4T's:

- Hypoxia, Hypovolemia, Hypothermia, Hyper/hypokalaemia
- Tension pneumothorax, Toxins, Thrombus, Tamponade

Adrenaline—given intravenously at a dose of 1 mg (10 mL of 1:10000 concentration). It is administered immediately on identification of a non-shockable rhythm and after the 3rd shock on the shockable algorithm. Once administered on either algorithm, the patient should continue to receive the same dose every 3–5 minutes, whilst they remain in CRA and with ongoing CPR.

Amiodarone (300 mg) can be given for 'shock resistant' rhythms whilst following the shockable algorithm and is administered after the third attempt at defibrillation. A further dose of 150 mg can be given after a further two shocks (after the fifth shock), if the patient continues in a shockable rhythm.

For ongoing CPR attempts, consider upgrading the airway. More advanced airways, like the I-gel, allow provision of continuous CPR alongside delivery of 10–12 breaths per minute for the duration of each 2-minute cycle, minimising interruptions to chest compressions.

Adult basic life support in community settings

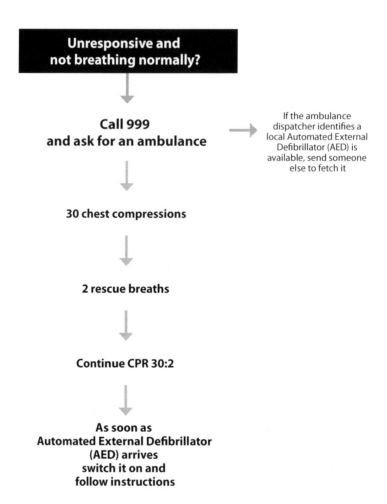

Unresponsive and not breathing normally?

↓

Call 999 and ask for an ambulance → If the ambulance dispatcher identifies a local Automated External Defibrillator (AED) is available, send someone else to fetch it

↓

30 chest compressions

↓

2 rescue breaths

↓

Continue CPR 30:2

↓

As soon as Automated External Defibrillator (AED) arrives switch it on and follow instructions

Figure 16.2 BLS algorithm. (Perkins et al., 2021.)

The key points for CRA are to defibrillate early and minimise interruptions to good BLS, maintaining adequate perfusion (Figure 16.2).

SUDDEN DEATH IN SPORT

Sudden death in sport receives attention via media coverage of high-profile elite events. It is always a concern for any doctor working in SEM.

Different sports and nations have their own approaches to screening. Most high-level athletes will undergo discussion of cardiac risk factors and previous screening history during a 'medical.'

Causes can be divided into *traumatic* and *atraumatic*. *Traumatic* conditions may be supported whilst awaiting definitive care. These include, but are not limited to: tension pneumothorax, massive haemothorax and cardiac tamponade.

Atraumatic causes refer (usually) to cardiac conditions, and are more common in over 35's due to underlying ischaemic heart disease. Other cardiac causes can sometimes be identified through screening. These are discussed in more detail in the cardiology chapter.

- *Hypertrophic obstructive cardiomyopathy (HOCM):* the most common cardiac cause in younger athletes.
- *Long QT:* QT segment prolonged at >0.44 seconds, predisposing to ventricular arrhythmia during exercise or stress. Pharmacological management can be considered.
- *Wolff-Parkinson-White:* characteristic delta wave on ECG with a short PR interval <0.12 seconds; accessory myocardial electrical pathways can lead to ventricular arrhythmia.
- *Coronary artery anatomical variations* can lead to compression of the coronary arterial ostia during exercise, causing syncope and possible sudden death. Identification may involve echocardiogram or coronary angiography.

MANAGEMENT OF FRACTURE DISLOCATIONS

With significant load involved in sport, fracture dislocations are possible. Definitive management occurs in the emergency department or operating theatre. General principles apply to managing these injuries in the pre-hospital environment. First, you should consider the type of injury and its mechanism. Injuries do not always occur in isolation, and understanding common associated complications and injury patterns can help identify other injuries. For example, clavicle fractures are associated with pneumothorax in a small proportion. Sometimes, significant fracture dislocations can distract professionals from the initial stepwise approach to assessment of the patient, and other problems can be overlooked.

Once you have assessed for other life-threatening injuries, you can address the fracture dislocation itself. An initial neurovascular check can inform the next management steps. Any movement or change in position should prompt a repeat neurovascular assessment. This involves checking perfusion, peripheral pulses and sensory and motor function.

If a patient is neurovascularly intact, you must evaluate their analgesia requirements. Splinting may be enough, and patients will often present in a position of relative comfort. Deciding whether to attempt a reduction pre-hospital will depend on a few variables. If a neurovascular check identifies compromise, restoring the limb to its anatomical position could salvage a threatened limb. Reducing a neurovascularly intact, closed injury depends on your level of experience and the athlete (e.g. some athletes have recurrent dislocations).

Take caution: medicolegal issues can ensue if X-rays following attempted reduction show associated fractures (without proof of their existence pre-reduction). Splinting and transfer for full assessment (with access to imaging) should occur if there is any uncertainty.

The most common fracture dislocations include:

- Shoulder dislocations (predominantly anterior).
- *Ankle fractures:* some require minimal manipulation due to minor talar shift and these can wait for the ED. However, significant talar shift can lead to neurovascular compromise and require urgent reduction.
- *Tibia/fibula fractures:* perform assessment of neurovascular status before splinting to an anatomical position.
- *Femoral fractures:* shortening or thigh deformity may occur in mid-shaft fractures. External rotation with shortening can indicate a neck of femur fracture. Large volume blood loss with haemodynamic compromise can occur—these require urgent splinting.

SPINAL INJURIES AND SAFE RETRIEVAL

Spinal injuries often cause significant morbidity and mortality. Initial assessment of any injured patient assumes spinal injury, until proven otherwise, for this reason. A significant proportion of spinal injuries will have associated head injury. Most spinal injuries occur to the cervical spine, with the rest evenly distributed throughout thoracic, lumbar and sacral levels.

Spinal injury should prompt concerns for other organ system effects and be assessed for using the ABCDE approach. For example, respiratory failure from high cord injury with subsequent hypoventilation, and a reduced ability to perceive pain, can mask other significant injuries, such as abdomino-pelvic trauma.

Following initial insult to the spine, subsequent care focuses on minimising movement. Neurological symptoms may occur some time later, due to cord ischemia or oedema, and can progress—careful reassessment and good documentation for trends of neurological deficit are important. In the context of pre-hospital care, emphasis is on initial assessment and monitoring, along with careful handling, to reduce risk of further damage. Specific extrication techniques are discussed during sport specific pre-hospital courses.

Spinal shock and neurogenic shock are often confused and are important to understand:

Neurogenic shock occurs with high spinal cord injury at or above the T6 level, which disrupts the sympathetic chain. The main two effects are:

o Hypotension, caused by venous pooling from loss of vasomotor tone and reduced peripheral vascular resistance.

o An inability to mount a tachycardic response to hypovolemia, or even bradycardia from unopposed parasympathetic activity to the heart. It is important to exclude haemorrhage in the context of an injured athlete, without presuming abnormal haemodynamics are secondary to spinal injury alone.

Spinal shock describes the initial loss of reflexes and muscle tone with spinal cord injury. This progresses to spasticity over time.

ENT EMERGENCIES

With ENT injury, there should be assessment for facial trauma and head injuries.

Epistaxis and Nasal Bone Fracture

These can occur in isolation, with the potential formation of a septal haematoma. Breakdown and perforation of the septum can occur, if not recognised and managed appropriately.

Epistaxis itself can lead to large volumes of blood loss and airway compromise if not controlled. Most commonly, bleeding comes from the anterior septum at 'Little's area.' Simple first aid measures, using direct pressure to 'pinch' the nose, will control most anterior bleeds. Patients with hypertension, or those on anticoagulation, must be cautiously managed; they have the potential for significant blood loss.

If simple direct pressure is ineffective, there is a stepwise approach to stop haemorrhage. Initially, a nose clip can replace fingers to apply pressure more evenly and consistently. Nasal tampon type devices range from simple tampons to those requiring balloon inflation once in situ. Referral to ENT is required; once any pack has been placed, it should not be removed until ENT review, unless the bleeding is ongoing. The final step, if feasible, is to place two Foley catheters, one in each nostril, and inflate the balloons in the posterior nasopharynx in an attempt to control haemorrhage. This technique is reserved for significant bleeding and often indicates a posterior source.

Quinsy can require urgent care and must be a differential for sore throat or tonsillitis. A retropharyngeal abscess can cause airway compromise and sepsis, requiring admission with intravenous antibiotics and drainage under the care of ENT.

OPHTHALMOLOGICAL EMERGENCIES

Eye examination following trauma should be completed immediately and include visual acuity for both eyes (if a Snellen chart is unavailable, a distance from a readable text should be recorded), eye movements, visual field assessment, light assessment and ophthalmoscopy.

A simple torch can evaluate anterior structures. A difference in the depth of the anterior chamber may suggest a leaking injury (e.g. corneal laceration). An irregular pupil may indicate injury to the iris, ciliary body, or vitreous prolapse. Corneal abrasion can be detected under blue light assessment after fluorescein staining.

Visual field assessment can assess injury to posterior structures. Direct and consensual response to light should be checked and, if there is significant damage to the optic nerve, a relative afferent pupillary defect will be observed.

An ophthalmoscope can be used to assess the red reflex. An abnormal reflex may indicate injury to the lens, cornea, vitreous haemorrhage or retinal detachment. Fundoscopy may suggest vitreous haemorrhage, detachment or retinal tear. Gonioscopy is a specialist test using a lens and slit lamp to assess the eye's drainage angle (anterior chamber angle) and can show signs of glaucoma.

Hyphema is an accumulation of blood in the anterior chamber, usually after blunt trauma. Uncomplicated hyphemas can be managed conservatively (head elevation, protection, avoiding contact sport). Topical corticosteroids may be used to reduce inflammation. When intraocular pressure is elevated, topical aqueous suppressants such as beta-blockers or alpha-agonists may be used, with surgery reserved for cases where pressures are not controlled.

Orbital floor fractures usually occur due to trauma. Examination may reveal enophthalmos, numbness in the ipsilateral trigeminal (maxillary) nerve distribution, restricted ipsilateral up-gaze (less often down-gaze), ptosis and swelling. CT scan is diagnostic. Surgery is delayed in most adult cases to allow oedema to resolve; however, paediatric cases with signs of muscle entrapment or vagal stimulation require urgent surgical intervention.

SKIN CLOSURE AND SUTURING PITCH SIDE INJURIES

When to Close

The nature of sport and the equipment involved make wound management a core skill of SEM clinicians. The first decision involves when to close the wound. In many sports, a temporary dressing is sufficient to cover the wound and provide pressure whilst play continues. A more thorough assessment, with definitive wound management, can occur after activity completion. This is not always possible; if there is ongoing bleeding or the location of the wound is not amenable to dressings, definitive management may be needed at the time of injury. This can put time pressure on the clinician.

How to Close

Options include steristrips for more superficial skin tears, wound glue for some injuries, and sutures. More advanced dressings are available, which are applied over the wound and oppose the edges under tension. Before closing, there are important general considerations:

1. Regardless of closure method, a neurovascular check must be carried out and underlying structures assessed for damage.
2. Clean the wound thoroughly, with any necessary debridement prior to closure.
3. Check the patient's tetanus status and consider a booster.
4. Does the wound require prophylactic antibiotic cover? Any bite would warrant this. Assess blood-borne virus risk.
5. Following wound closure, give clear advice regarding follow up and management for the athlete: e.g. signs of infection, caring for a glued wound.

Sutures

There are a wide range of suture techniques. Standard interrupted sutures and mattress sutures will manage most wounds (Figure 16.3). A mattress suture can be used vertically for deep wounds, and, in a horizontal

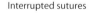
Interrupted sutures
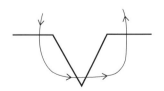

Mattress sutures (vertical)
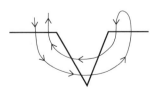

Figure 16.3 Sutures.

orientation, can be useful for avoiding tension across the suture. This also reduces the risk of sutures pulling through or breaking. A plan for suture removal should be made and communicated. This should consider time for wound healing based on location and sporting competition. For example, a player who may need suture removal in 7 days, but has a fixture to play, might keep them until after the game, to reduce the chance of the wound reopening.

ENVIRONMENTAL FACTORS IN COLLAPSE OR SUDDEN DEATH

Exercise associated collapse is common. Most cases are benign with full and rapid recovery after cooling, hydration and rest. This does not warrant further investigation or onward referral. However, patients who do not recover quickly, or with concerning features (e.g. seizures), need investigation into underlying causes (hyponatremia, hypoglycaemia, heat-related illness).

Exercise associated hyponatremia (EAH) is a condition occurring in athletes predominantly in endurance sports. The mechanism is excessive water intake versus fluid losses during prolonged activity. Fluid shifts manifest as peripheral oedema and central oedema—with altered mental state (cerebral) or shortness of breath (pulmonary). Endurance athletes with confusion, seizures or unconsciousness could be secondary to EAH. Point of care testing (POCT) capabilities should be available at endurance events. The treatment of choice is intravenous hypertonic saline (e.g. 3% saline) to correct sodium levels (where significant or symptomatic e.g. <135 mmol/L). Rapid correction of sodium is inadvisable due to the risk of central pontine myelinolysis (CPM). However, there are no known case reports of CPM in athletes with hyponatremia. Confused patients must be treated promptly; observation with oral replacement is inadequate. Furthermore, normal saline administration can exacerbate the situation. It is important to understand that patients can develop EAH up to 24 hours after exercise.

Activity in extreme temperatures is common within certain sports e.g. marathon de Sables or mountaineering. While an acute change in temperature might be obvious—e.g. jumping into icy water and resultant shivering—be aware of gradual changes to weather conditions on exposed routes, where effects may be subtle.

Hypothermia—Core Temperature <35°C

Below 35°C, vasoconstriction acts to preserve core temperature. Accurate temperature reading will require a core thermometer (e.g. rectal probe), which must be factored in the inventory for events where hypothermia is a risk.

Severe low body temperature can cause arrhythmias such as ventricular fibrillation. Any large movements (such as log rolling) or procedures (like catheterisation) increase the risk of cardiac dysrhythmia and, where possible, should be avoided until the patient is warmed. Hypothermia can be subdivided into mild (33–35°C), moderate (31–33°C) and severe (<31°C). Treatment ranges from passive rewarming e.g. removing wet clothes and insulating, to active rewarming such as administering warmed fluids, hot packs to torso and hot tubs. Peripheries should not be warmed; this would counteract vasoconstriction aimed at maintaining core temperature. In addition, hot tubs provide hydrostatic pressure, supporting haemodynamics. Extrication of patients from cold water should be done whilst maintaining a horizontal position to avoid cardiovascular collapse and CRA. Hypothermic patients in CRA must be actively warmed—they are said to be 'not dead until they are warm and dead.' There are several case reports of good neurological recovery following significant periods of prolonged resuscitation in hypothermic patients.

Hyperthermia—Core Temperature ≥40°C

Exertional heat illness (EHI) often presents with athlete collapse and can range from self-limiting Exertional Heat Exhaustion (EHE) to life-threatening Exertional Heat Stroke (EHS). As well as an elevated core temperature ≥40°C, EHI will manifest with organ dysfunction. Central nervous system involvement, such as delirium or seizures, will be present in EHS. These patients can be relatively asymptomatic up to temperatures just below 40°C, before rapid deterioration. Treatment consists of rapid cooling—most effectively achieved with ice water baths or cold water immersion. Ice packs to the groin and axillae are helpful before there is access to more substantial methods. For sporting events, the American College of Sports Medicine guidelines

(Roberts et al., 2021) outline safe levels of exercise, based on the wet bulb globe temperature (WBGT). This considers a number of environmental aspects: recorded ambient temperature, humidity, wind speed, sun angle and cloud cover (solar radiation).

CONCUSSION

Sport related concussion is a form of Mild Traumatic Brain Injury. It is commonly encountered in the pre-hospital environment, particularly in contact and collision sports. It may result from either direct impact to the head or impact to the body with rapid acceleration and deceleration of the head.

In 10% of cases, this presents with loss of consciousness. However, more frequently, the presentation is subtle or, especially given the distances involved, the patient may have partially recovered before a first responder arrives.

Symptoms of headache and dizziness are most commonly reported, but issues such as language barriers, or players intentionally or unintentionally under-reporting, can make this unreliable. Reliance only on the Maddocks Questions (which venue are we at? which half is it? etc.) is also discouraged.

Despite intensive research, there remains no single objective test which is diagnostic of concussion, so practitioners must rely on their judgement combined with a multi-modal clinical evaluation of the athlete. This may be supported by evidence from video replay, reports from other players regarding behaviour and reports from coaches regarding performance.

When managing concussion, firstly it is important to be vigilant for the injury. Particularly in the case of facial wounds, there is often time pressure on the medic to return the player promptly. However, it is important to consider that the trauma required to produce such injuries may also result in concussion.

Secondly, a cautiously low threshold for removing a player from play, if concussion is suspected, is important. Continuing sport after concussion is associated with: a reduction in performance; a dose-response relationship with a longer recovery time post injury and, particularly in adolescents, cases of 'Second Impact Syndrome.' This is a rare and somewhat contentious condition in which sustaining further head trauma shortly after the index event results in catastrophic cerebral oedema and, usually, death.

Thirdly, since the signs and symptoms of concussion can take time to develop, the diagnosis should remain under consideration for at least 48 hours after the inciting head impact has occurred.

Therefore, if a concussion is suspected, athletes should be removed from play immediately and not return to play again until evaluation by a healthcare professional. This evaluation does not make use of brain imaging and instead will usually rely on neurological examination, tests of cognitive function and self-reported symptoms.

All athletes suffering a concussion should follow a period of absolute rest, followed by a graduated return to play protocol. The purpose of this is to expose athletes to progressively increasing cognitive and physical load to ensure a safe return to sport. The degree to which the completion of this return indicates recovery of the brain is hotly debated.

Different sporting codes have produced their own guidelines for the identification and management of concussion, usually supported by the four-yearly Concussion In Sport Group Consensus meetings.

MULTIPLE CHOICE QUESTION (MCQ) QUESTIONS

1. You are working as a medical officer at the London Marathon and encounter a number of competitors with heat-related illness. Which one of the following principles contributes the least to heat loss in runners?

    A. Evaporation via respiration
    B. Evaporation via skin losses
    C. Convection
    D. Conduction
    E. Radiation

2. You are preparing your medical equipment prior to covering a Netball match. Approximately how long will a full, standard oxygen cylinder provide oxygen for, at 15 L/minute?

    A. 10 minutes
    B. 20 minutes

C. 30 minutes

D. 40 minutes

E. 60 minutes

3. You are first on the scene to a boxer who has been knocked unconscious in a bout. He has suffered a blow to the face, and a pool of blood lies between him and the ringside. Which one of the following would be the most appropriate first step?

   A. Remove his gum shield

   B. Apply a head tilt, chin lift

   C. Place a towel over the blood that is present on the ring canvas

   D. Apply a jaw thrust

   E. Feel for a carotid pulse

4. An endurance runner attends the medical tent with confusion and drowsiness. His friend tells you he hasn't stopped drinking water all day. On assessment, his heart rate is 128 bpm, blood pressure is 100/65 mmHg and core temperature is 37.9 °C. Point of care blood testing reveals a Sodium of 128 mEq/L, Potassium 4.2 mmol/L and blood sugar 4.4 mmol/L. What treatment should you initiate?

   A. 250 mL intravenous NaCl 0.9%

   B. 100 mL intravenous NaCl 3%

   C. 250 mL intravenous Glucose 5%

   D. Cold water immersion

   E. 500 mL Compound Sodium Lactate

5. A nearby spectator collapses so you begin assisting with cardiopulmonary resuscitation. The paramedic on scene is working through reversible causes. Which one of the following is NOT considered one of the 'Four H's'?

   A. Hypoxia

   B. Hypovolaemia

   C. Hypo/Hyperkalaemia

   D. Hyperglycaemia

   E. Hypothermia

MULTIPLE CHOICE QUESTION (MCQ) ANSWERS

1. Answer D

   Evaporation is the primary heat loss mechanism in runners. Convection (E), is the transfer of heat between the air around the runner's body surface and air with a differing temperature, and is thought to play a role in heat loss. Conduction is the transfer of heat between two surfaces in direct contact, with differing temperatures. This would be a more significant factor of heat loss in swimmers.

2. Answer B

   A full, standard oxygen cylinder should supply around 20 minutes of high flow oxygen.

3. Answer C

   As part of DR ABC, assessing danger should be the first action. Blood is potentially hazardous and you should make the necessary steps of protecting yourself before you assist your patient.

4. Answer B

   This is exercise associated hyponatremia. The treatment of choice is intravenous hypertonic saline in a pre-hospital setting.

5. Answer D

   Hyperglycaemia is not recognised as one of the 'Four H's.'

REFERENCES AND FURTHER READING

Perkins, G.D., Colquhoun, M., Deakin, C.D., Smith, C., et al. (2021). Adult basic life support guidelines. *2021 Resuscitation Guidelines*.

Roberts, William O; Armstrong, Lawrence E; Sawka, Michael N; Yeargin, Susan W; Heled, Yuval; O'Connor, Francis G. 2021. ACSM Expert Consensus Statement on Exertional Heat Illness: Recognition, Management, and Return to Activity. *Current Sports Medicine Reports* 20(9):p 470–484, DOI:10.1249/JSR.0000000000000878

Primary Care **17**

Emma Jane Lunan and Andrew Duncan Murray

MANAGEMENT OF COMMON PRIMARY CARE PROBLEMS

The management of primary care problems is an integral component of sport and exercise medicine. It helps maintain athlete health, avoids time away from sport, shortens recovery time and reduces long term sequelae. A wide range of clinical issues are encountered within primary care, and it should be remembered that athletes suffer from the same conditions as the general population. Many athletes require ongoing support and treatment for chronic medical conditions and a broad knowledge of these, with an awareness of when to refer to specialist services for input, is essential.

INFECTIOUS DISEASES

Infectious diseases are extremely common and cause significant morbidity in both the general and athletic populations, often affecting ability to train and compete. Respiratory conditions occur most frequently, however, all body systems can be affected. Certain factors can increase an athlete's risk of infection: close contact with others, over-training, inadequate recovery, stress, travel, trauma and poor nutrition. Consideration must be given to diagnosis and treatment, but also to infection prevention, limiting spread, and return to play following illness.

Upper Respiratory Tract Infections (URTIs)

These are predominantly self-limiting infections of the upper airways, usually resolving within 7–10 days. Symptoms include nasal discharge, low grade fever, cough, sore throat and these spread via respiratory droplets and aerosols. URTIs are common, with adults having an average of 3 common colds per annum. The pathogens are viral in 95% of cases: rhinovirus, adenovirus, coronavirus. COVID-19 will typically cause URTI symptoms, including cough, temperature and change in taste or smell, but some variants are associated with more significant complications such as pneumonia and thrombotic sequelae. Athletes are also at higher risk of sudden cardiac death whilst training or competing following some variants of COVID-19 infection.

Pharyngitis (Sore Throat)

Aside from viral URTI, there are other causes of sore throat. Acute tonsillitis is particularly common and may be viral or bacterial; with *Group A Streptococcus* the usual bacteria. Malaise, fever, lymphadenopathy, absence of cough and enlarged tonsils with pus may help indicate bacterial infection. Penicillin V is the antibiotic of choice, with amoxicillin best avoided if glandular fever is a differential, because a rash can occur. Rarely, tonsillitis can lead to rheumatic fever, renal failure, sepsis or quinsy (a collection of pus in the peri-tonsillar space).

Infectious Mononucleosis or Glandular Fever (Caused by *Epstein-Barr* Virus)

This occurs more frequently in adolescents and exudate in the pharynx with cervical lymphadenopathy is common. Splenomegaly is a key feature and should be assessed. Splenic rupture is reported in up to 0.5% of cases and usually occurs in the first 3 weeks, although

DOI: 10.1201/9781003179979-17

PRIMARY CARE

Infectious diseases

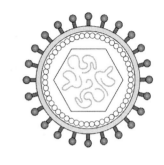

'Neck check'
- If above neck symptoms e.g. nasal congestion, sore throat
- 10 minutes of moderate exertion
- If OK, permitted to continue
- Myalgia, systemic symptoms or temperature ≥38°C = Don't exercise

Common Organisms
- Upper respiratory tract infection – Rhinovirus, Adenovirus, Coronavirus
- Bacterial tonsillitis – Group A streptococcus
- Glandular fever – Epstein-Barr virus
- Urinary tract infection – E. Coli, Klebsiella pneumoniae, Proteus mirabilis, Staphylococcus saprophyticus
- Gastroenteritis – Adenovirus, Norovirus, Rotavirus, Campylobacter, Salmonella, Shigella
- Sexually transmitted diseases – Chlamydia trachomatis, Neisseria gonorrhoea
- Skin infection – Staphylococcus aureus, Streptococcus pyogenes
- Otitis media – Haemophilus influenzae, Streptococcus pneumoniae
- Otitis externa – Pseudomonas aeruginosa, Staphylococcus aureus

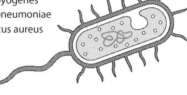

Vaccination

United Kingdom National Health Service schedule
- Babies <1
  8 weeks – 6-in-1 (Diphtheria, Hepatitis B, Haemophilus influenzae, Polio, Tetanus, Pertussis), Rotavirus, Meningitis B
  12 weeks – 6-in-1, Pneumococcal (PCV), Rotavirus
  16 weeks – 6-in-1, Meningitis B

- Children (1- 15)
  1 year – Haemophilus influenzae B (Hib)/Meningitis C, Measles, Mumps and Rubella (MMR), Pneumococcal (PCV), Meningitis B
  2-10 years – Influenza (annual)
  3 years 4 months– MMR, 4-in-1 (Diphtheria, Tetanus, Polio, Pertussis)
  12-13 years – Human Papilloma virus (HPV)
  14 years – 3-in-1 (Tetanus, Diphtheria, Polio), Meningococcal (MenACWY)

- Adults
  50 years and annually thereafter- Influenza
  65 years – Pneumococcal (PPV)
  70 years – Shingles

- Pregnancy
  Flu season – influenza
  16 weeks- Pertussis

- Covid-19 vaccinations

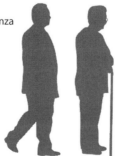
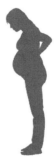
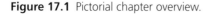

Figure 17.1 Pictorial chapter overview.

it has been reported at up to 8 weeks. Full blood count and heterophile antibody (monospot) tests can confirm the diagnosis. Advice should be given about avoiding sharing utensils and kissing. Occasionally, glandular fever may result in chronic fatigue syndrome, which can have a significant impact on quality of life. Contact sport should be avoided until the athlete has physically recovered and the spleen is not palpable. Splenomegaly is typically fully resolved at 4–6 weeks.

Urinary Tract Infection (UTIs)

Lower UTIs of the bladder, termed cystitis, present frequently to primary care. Females are more commonly affected than males, primarily due to a shorter urethra. Symptoms of uncomplicated, lower UTI include urinary frequency, dysuria, urgency, haematuria and suprapubic tenderness. If an upper UTI or pyelonephritis is suspected, patients may have a high temperature, loin pain, rigors, and vomiting. Uncomplicated UTIs in females do not usually hamper athletic training. Risk factors include dehydration, previous UTI, sexual intercourse and alcohol. UTIs are secondary to common gastrointestinal bacteria such as gram-negative *Escherichia coli*. Uncomplicated UTIs in young, healthy females can be diagnosed and treated based on symptoms alone. Urinary dipstick can aid diagnosis—if positive for nitrite, leukocyte or red blood cells, UTI is highly likely. A mid-stream urine sample can be sent for culture if the diagnosis is unclear or in recurrent cases. Simple UTI is treated empirically according to local guidelines; trimethoprim is a common choice. Upper UTIs require a longer duration of treatment with alternative antibiotics such as co-amoxiclav.

CLINICAL CONSIDERATIONS

In sexually active young females with urinary symptoms, remember to consider chlamydia trachomatis infection and pregnancy. Enquiring about vaginal discharge/irritation may be helpful.

Gastroenteritis

Gastroenteritis is frequently a highly contagious infection, causing a diarrhoeal and vomiting illness.

The majority of cases are caused by viral infections such as *norovirus, adenovirus* and *rotavirus*. However, bacterial infection can occur secondary to pathogens such as *Campylobacter* and *Salmonella* and may cause more invasive disease. Symptoms of gastroenteritis include vomiting, diarrhoea, abdominal cramps and fever, which are usually self-limiting. It spreads easily within team sports and when travelling; transmission occurs through contaminated food or drink, contaminated water source, or direct contact, and often occurs in food service places. Prevention is key when working with athletes, particularly when travelling.

CLINICAL CONSIDERATIONS

Ensuring food is cooked thoroughly, avoiding shellfish, maintaining scrupulous hand washing, and drinking bottled water, may be helpful. Athletes should avoid sharing bottles and immediately isolating individuals with symptoms is important to reduce spread. Treatment is supportive and aims to maintain hydration status with oral fluids. Electrolytes or oral rehydration salts may be required.

Sexually Transmitted Infections (STIs)

Every day, over 1 million STIs are acquired across the globe, with the majority in young adults. Over 30 different viral, bacterial and parasitic agents can be transmitted through sexual contact. *Chlamydia trachomatis* infection is the most common bacterial pathogen in the UK, followed in prevalence by *Neisseria gonorrhoea*. Symptoms in men include dysuria, frequency and penile discharge. Females may present with vaginal discharge, bleeding, urinary symptoms and pelvic pain; however, a significant 70% of infected females and 50% of males are asymptomatic. Diagnosis and treatment are essential, as pelvic inflammatory disease caused by STIs can lead to tubal infertility and ectopic pregnancy. If an athlete tests positive for chlamydia, treat with oral antibiotics, and refer to genitourinary medicine clinic for partner notification and contact tracing. As well as genital symptoms, infections can lead to reactive arthritis, uveitis and enthesopathies, which can impair sporting performance, leading to long term morbidity.

Blood Borne Infectious Diseases

Worldwide, blood borne infectious diseases are prevalent and cause a significant proportion of global disease burden. There is a very small, but theoretical risk, of contracting blood borne infections during sports participation. Transfer is potentially increased during close contact and collision sports where open and bleeding wounds may occur and, although risk is minimal, appropriate preventative procedures should be in place. Timely treatment of wounds and blood injuries should be undertaken as well as disposal of contaminated materials. Transmission is primarily the same in athletes as the general population. Focus should be on education regarding reducing risky behaviours such as unprotected sexual intercourse, multiple sexual partners and sharing of needles between athletes (blood doping, steroids, vitamin infusions).

Human Immunodeficiency Virus (HIV)

HIV is an RNA virus transmitted via unprotected sexual intercourse, sharing of infected needles (injecting equipment), and infected blood products, or via mother to baby transmission. Untreated, it can lead to acquired immune deficiency syndrome (AIDS), the late stage of HIV, which is the cause of significant immune deficiency and a variety of opportunistic infections. Antiretroviral medications, which prevent viral replication, are used to treat the virus. HIV testing is mandatory in sports such as boxing, as per the International Boxing Federation.

Hepatitis

Hepatitis is inflammation of the liver secondary to infection (viruses ABCDE), drugs, alcohol, or autoimmune conditions. Viral hepatitis is common worldwide. Acute infection can cause symptoms including myalgia, malaise, high temperature, vomiting, fatigue, abdominal pain and jaundice. Chronic infection with hepatitis B and C can lead to further complications, like cirrhosis or hepatocellular carcinoma. Athletes living in, or travelling regularly to areas with, a higher incidence of hepatitis B (endemic infection) are at increased risk. Vaccination against hepatitis B

is 95% effective and is the most important method of prevention.

CLINICAL CONSIDERATIONS

If an athlete is having repeated infections, this may be an indication of overtraining and a thorough history should be taken, including the volume and intensity of exercise.

EFFECT OF ILLNESS ON ACTIVITY CAPACITY

Exercise and Immunity

Numerous theories have been proposed to describe the relationship between exercise and immunity. Evidence suggests that individuals who partake in regular moderate physical activity have a reduced risk of infection compared to being sedentary. This may be secondary to increased endorphins, interleukins and T-cell lymphocytes. The link between exercise and immunity is complex and athletes who participate in regular high intensity training or endurance exercise can be more susceptible to infection in the days afterwards. Strenuous exercise has been shown to cause neutrophilia, lymphopenia and increased pro-inflammatory cytokines which may increase gut permeability.

Effects on Activity Capacity

Several factors contribute to impairment of athletic capacity during and following an acute illness. Symptoms such as lack of sleep, cough and congestion may hamper training, fever can impair body temperature regulation and increased fluid losses may occur. Inadequate nutrition may also occur during an acute illness causing an energy deficit. The psychological wellbeing of an athlete may be affected; they may be concerned about missing training and competitions. Deconditioning of athletes occurs within 4 weeks of cessation of training, although VO_2 max can drop much faster. It is essential that despite these factors, athletes and coaches are educated on the risks of returning to training prematurely, as this may lead to further illness, injury and be detrimental in the longer term. Ensuring that an athlete is managed appropriately during illness and during the graduated return to sport is fundamental.

CLINICAL CONSIDERATIONS

It is possible that even mild infections may reduce exercise capacity and athletic performance, however studies have not consistently demonstrated substantive differences. It is generally accepted that if an athlete has a mild URTI, they should be able to train. The 'neck check' is often used: if an athlete reports above neck symptoms, such as nasal congestion, sore throat, mild cough, then they should be able to try 10 minutes of moderate exertion and, if ok, continue. Any below neck or systemic symptoms would prevent an athlete from training: myalgia, severe cough, high temperature (>38°C). Intense exercise during an infectious illness has been shown to increase the risk of myocarditis and heat exertional illness.

Chronic Illness

Chronic illness can affect any system: diabetes, asthma, coeliac disease, inflammatory bowel disease are a few common examples. The mainstay of treatment is aimed at symptom management, prevention and treatment of acute relapse and maintenance of optimum physical health. Careful monitoring of pharmacotherapy and liaison with secondary care may be required. Athletes exist in a careful homeostatic balance between training load, recovery and competition. Sleep, nutrition and stress levels need to be continually assessed and modified in order to optimise training and competition.

DERMATOLOGY

Dermatological issues present frequently in primary care with one in four patients attending their GP each year. As well as common acute presentations, skin disorders are often chronic, requiring education, self-care and monitoring. Often, athletes' unique environmental and physical conditions increase the risk of various dermatological issues due to close contacts.

Eczema

Atopic dermatitis, or eczema, is the most common inflammatory skin condition with a lifetime prevalence of over 15%. The condition is frequently seen in children, often with a history of atopy—asthma, hay fever, eczema and a positive family history. Atopic dermatitis in children classically presents as an itchy, erythematous, flexural rash, however in adults it may take a number of forms. Several factors, including sweating, heat and chlorine, can exacerbate symptoms. Athletes need to be educated regarding maintaining hydration, topical emollient therapy and avoiding allergens. Treatment may also require topical corticosteroid therapy. TUEs are not required for topical corticosteroids.

Psoriasis

Psoriasis is an immune mediated disease causing a chronic, inflammatory skin condition with multiple associated health conditions. It is classified into types including: plaque, guttate, palmoplantar, nail and erythrodermic psoriasis, but usually presents with symmetrical erythematous, scaly plaques on the extensor surfaces and scalp. Guttate psoriasis often follows a streptococcal infection of the throat and causes a characteristic rash of multiple small red scaly plaques over the torso and limbs. Athletes may notice a flare of symptoms when under stress or if taking certain medications e.g. antimalarials, B-blockers and NSAIDs. Psoriatic arthritis occurs in up to 30%, which can be extremely disabling. Treatment depends on severity but includes topical therapy, phototherapy, disease-modifying medications and biologic preparations, many of which reduce immunity, therefore increasing susceptibility to infection.

SKIN INFECTIONS

Bacterial

Numerous sport-related bacterial infections occur and are commonly secondary to *Staphylococcus aureus* and *Streptococcus pyogenes*. They may be contagious, particularly in close contact sport conditions e.g. wrestling. Folliculitis is an infection of the hair follicles causing a typical rash with multiple small papules and pustules. It often occurs after shaving or waxing, causing irritation and inflammation of the follicles. This is usually treated with topical or oral antibiotics. Impetigo is characterised by an erythematous rash with typical golden crusted lesions, often in the perioral region and can be treated with topical Fucidin, or oral Flucloxacillin if more extensive.

Viral

Herpes gladiatorum (otherwise known as herpes rugbiorum or scrumpox) is a highly infectious condition, which spreads easily through direct skin contact, common in rugby scrums and between wrestlers. Clinically, it causes a painful, vesicular rash often on the face or neck and is secondary, most frequently, to *herpes simplex one (HSV-1)*. Primary infection may cause myalgia, fever and lymphadenopathy. Episodes usually last 7–10 days and treatment is with antiviral medications, e.g. acyclovir. The infection remains dormant in the dorsal root ganglion of the nervous system and can reactivate, particularly when stressed, tired and in sunshine. Some individuals suffer from recurrent infection, which may be treated using prophylactic antivirals.

Molluscum Contagiosum

This is a benign condition secondary to a *pox virus* causing clusters of small, clear papules with a central punctum. The rash is often asymptomatic, although can be itchy. Athletes in close contact are susceptible to spread. The lesions self-resolve, though this may take more than 12 months. Cryotherapy can be used.

Verrucae

Palmar and plantar warts, caused by *human papillomavirus*, are common in swimmers due to direct skin spread. When skin and changing room floors are wet, this acts as a viral reservoir. Verrucae are small, painful lesions with central tiny black dots (thrombosed capillaries). Athletes are advised to use personal footwear to avoid spread. Topical salicylic acid, filing and cryotherapy are used.

Fungal

Dermatophytosis is an extremely common condition, caused by dermatophytes or fungi that invade and live in dead keratin. The common species are *Trichophytons*, *Microsporum* and *Epidermophyton*. Various body parts can be affected and clinical classification depends on site.

CLINICAL CONSIDERATIONS

Fungal transmission is due to shedding of spores from infected skin and is encouraged by damp, warm environments, and close contact with sharing of fomites in towels, clothing and bedding.

Tinea Corporis or ringworm causes a typical annular or 'ring like' red lesion with a raised scaly edge. Asymmetric or solitary initially, multiple lesions may develop over time. Diagnosis is by inspection of the skin surface including scalp and nails. If the diagnosis is uncertain, skin scrapings can be obtained and viewed under microscopy for hyphae and spores. Dermatoscopy can be helpful. Differential diagnoses include eczema, psoriasis, pityriasis and seborrheic dermatitis. Treatment is ensuring skin is clean and dry. Topical antifungal agents, e.g. terbinafine, can be used.

Tinea Pedis, otherwise known as athlete's foot, is the most common dermatophyte condition, with young males frequently affected. Transfer to groin causes Tinea Cruris. It often starts as an asymmetrical, unilateral, itchy, scaly rash often between the fourth and fifth toes. It can cause scale on the sole and sides of the foot. Vesiculobullous tinea pedis can occur, with small blisters on the inner aspect of the foot. Treatment includes careful drying of feet to avoid spread, wearing sandals, avoiding wet shoes and using topical antifungal cream or powder.

Onychomycosis is a fungal nail infection caused by yeasts, dermatophytes and moulds. Incidence increases with age. Issues are mainly cosmetic due to nail discolouration and loss. Athletes are commonly affected. It is diagnosed with clippings and microscopy, prior to treatment. Topical agents or oral antifungal agents may be used. Laser treatment may be effective.

Swimmer's Itch—Cercarial Dermatitis

An itchy rash in open water swimmers, it is more likely to occur in freshwater than the sea. It is caused by an allergic reaction secondary to parasites that burrow under the skin. The normal hosts are waterfowl and some mammals. Overall, the condition is short lived. Treatment with antihistamines may help.

Blisters

Blisters are common. Painful, fluid filled skin lesions develop secondary to prolonged friction, contact and pressure (between surfaces). Shearing forces leads to separation of the epidermal cell layers causing a subepidermal bulla. They cause pain, may impair concentration in athletes and can cause secondary infection. They most frequently occur on the extremities. Predisposing factors include prolonged exercise and sweating. Prevention is key: Footwear should be well fitted; double layers may help and moisture absorbent socks, or a barrier such as Vaseline, can be used. The majority of blisters can be left alone, but padding can help discomfort. Avoid de-roofing, which will increase the risk of infection and potentially cause more pain due to exposed nerve fibres. Hydrocolloid dressings are helpful. If large, the blister can be drained after thorough cleaning, with appropriate dressing afterwards.

OPHTHALMOLOGY

Eye problems can cause significant and preventable disability. Acute traumatic issues are most likely to be encountered whilst working pitch side, however an awareness of non-traumatic conditions is also important.

Conjunctivitis

A highly contagious but usually self-limiting condition, most frequently seen in children. Irritation and inflammation of the conjunctiva can be viral, bacterial and allergic in origin, with one or both eyes affected. Patients complain of pain, grittiness, redness (pink eye), itch, swelling and discharge. Vision is not usually affected. Close contact between athletes can increase spread, so care should be taken. Viral (often *adeno-virus*) conjunctivitis often occurs with concurrent common cold symptoms, spreads easily and resolves

without treatment within 3–5 days. Bacterial conjunctivitis (*streptococcus*) is also extremely infectious and often causes a thick purulent discharge. Both can be treated by careful wiping, avoiding make up and hand hygiene. Topical antibiotics (chloramphenicol), can be used for bacterial cases. Suspect allergic conjunctivitis in those with a history of atopy or if complaining of severe itch. It is often secondary to pollen, grass and animal dander. Treatment is allergen avoidance. Topical sodium cromoglicate drops and oral antihistamines may be beneficial.

Blepharitis

Inflammation of the eyelids, usually bilateral, causes itching, swelling, irritation, and lid crusting. It can be acute or chronic, and can be associated with other conditions such as seborrheic dermatitis, atopy, contact dermatitis or bacterial infection with *Staphylococcus aureus*. Eye hygiene and consistent cleaning is the treatment. Warm compress 10-minutes daily with 30-second eyelid massage is advised. Using a small amount of baby shampoo to clean often helps and, if not improving, topical antibiotics may be required.

Stye

Small, tender, red swellings on the eyelid edges, which are usually secondary to bacterial infection, and may occur with blepharitis. These are treated with warm compresses and analgesia. Topical antibiotics can be used, although have little penetrance.

Corneal Abrasion

A tear or defect of the corneal epithelial surface can be caused by a scratch to the eye in contact sports or from a foreign body. Pain, watering, and foreign-body sensation are reported. Diagnosis can be undertaken after instilling fluorescein drops using cobalt blue light via ophthalmoscope. It is important to evert the lid when examining to exclude foreign bodies. Treatment depends on size, position and pain. If uncertain, an Emergency Department review with a slit lamp can confirm. Small, superficial abrasions heal quickly in 3–5 days. Topical antibiotics and regular lubricant drops can prevent recurrent corneal abrasion syndrome.

EAR, NOSE AND THROAT (ENT)

ENT conditions account for around 25% of adult GP consultations, and even more in children. The close relationship between ear, nose and throat with the respiratory system means such conditions can impact on exercise and physical activity.

Acute Otitis Media

Inflammation in the middle ear, usually as a result of infection, causes acute otitis media (AOM). This can present with pain, fever, hearing loss and discharge. It is more common in children but can occur in adults. The eustachian tube is more horizontal and shorter in children, meaning infection can track more easily from the pharynx. Typical organisms include various viruses and bacteria including, *Haemophilus Influenzae* and *Streptococcus pneumoniae*. As infection progresses, the middle ear fills with pus, causing pressure on the eardrum. This pain is relieved if there is tympanic membrane perforation, and discharge becomes apparent. If patients are systemically unwell, antibiotics may be indicated. Those with discharge, bilateral infection or an age of less than 2 years are more likely to benefit from antibiotics; typically, illnesses are self-limiting and usually resolve within 3 days, but may last a week. Rarely, AOM can cause mastoiditis or spread to the facial nerve or brain.

Otitis Externa

Infections of the external auditory canal (otitis externa) are common, more so in children. Typical symptoms include pain, itching, hearing loss and discharge. Swimming is an important risk factor, as is trauma to the canal skin, such as with inappropriate cleaning. The most common responsible organisms include *Pseudomonas aeruginosa* or *Staphylococcus aureus*. Treatments include antibiotic ear drops, with acetic acid, aminoglycosides and quinolones being acceptable choices. Fungal infections (Otomycosis) are possible. Persistent or significant cases may need referral for micro suction.

Otitis Media with Effusion (Glue Ear)

If fluid is present in the middle ear with no signs of inflammation, this is classed as otitis media with effusion. It is the most common cause of hearing loss in children and is thought to be triggered by an initial otitis media infection and perpetuated by eustachian tube dysfunction. The condition usually resolves spontaneously over months. In persistent cases, or when education is affected by hearing loss, hearing aids may be used temporarily until improvement, or grommets (small tubes) inserted to equalise pressure.

Perforated Eardrum

The tympanic membrane may be perforated by trauma, such as a blow in contact sports, or following infection. In AOM rupture, the membrane usually heals; however, occasionally, chronic suppurative otitis media occurs. Perforation may cause no symptoms, but sudden hearing loss is common. A perforated eardrum is also more predisposed to discharge, particularly after swimming. Often, conservative management by avoiding water exposure is all that is needed. In some cases, topical antibiotics may be useful. Ciprofloxacin may be preferred to aminoglycosides due to ototoxicity risk. If there are issues with recurrent infections or problems with frequent water exposure, such as in swimmers, a myringoplasty may be required by an ENT specialist.

Epistaxis

Significant epistaxis must be taken seriously as it can be fatal. Kiesselbach's plexus or Little's area is a vascular network that is prone to bleeding anteriorly. It comprises the anterior ethmoidal artery, posterior ethmoidal artery, sphenopalatine artery, greater palatine artery and septal branch of the superior labial artery. Its location is exposed to the drying effect of inspiration and finger trauma. Management comprises resuscitation and stopping bleeding. Nasal packing, cauterisation or other intervention may be required. When evaluating a nosebleed, it is important to assess for fracture and examine the posterior pharynx for signs of a posterior bleed. These features may be enough to exclude an athlete from returning to the field of play.

GASTROENTEROLOGY

Many gastrointestinal (GI) disorders are diagnosed and treated within primary care. Careful evaluation and assessment of GI symptoms is essential to determine whether exercise is the cause of symptoms or whether there is an underlying issue. A large proportion of athletes report GI disturbances during exercise with symptoms increasing with duration and intensity. Numerous physiological changes contribute, such as diversion of blood flow from the GI tract to muscles and skin, increased motion of internal organs and increased gut permeability.

Gastro Oesophageal Reflux Disease (GORD)

GORD may follow relaxation of the lower oesophageal sphincter, allowing reflux of gastric contents back into the oesophagus. Acidity causes inflammation of the oesophageal mucosa and symptoms include heartburn, water brash, epigastric or retrosternal pain, halitosis and dental erosion. Risk factors are commonly related to lifestyle such as stress, smoking and obesity. GORD is also common amongst athletes, with exercise that increases intra-abdominal pressure e.g. weight lifting, high intensity workouts or with endurance exercise. Athletes with GORD should adopt strategies such as avoiding eating 1–2 hours before exercise, limiting triggering foods, eating slowly and not lying flat. H2 antagonists and Proton Pump Inhibitors can be used to treat GORD.

Irritable Bowel Syndrome (IBS)

A common, chronic disorder of the lower gastrointestinal tract with no clear structural or pathological cause. Symptoms fluctuate and include abdominal cramps and pain, especially with defaecation or after eating, change in bowel habit, bloating and mucus per rectum. The prevalence of IBS is around 5–20%. Young adult females are most likely to have the condition and research suggests endurance athletes may be disproportionately affected. Diagnosis is based on history and examination, considering diet, stressors, exercise, symptoms and excluding red flags. Initial treatment includes education, lifestyle advice such as modifying dietary triggers and stress reduction techniques. Pharmacotherapy can be used as second line treatment for pain or specific symptoms.

Coeliac Disease

Coeliac disease is a common multisystem disorder causing gluten sensitive enteropathy. In genetically susceptible children and adults, the immune system reacts to gluten ingestion, causing gut inflammation and malabsorption. Gastrointestinal symptoms are frequent, such as abdominal pain, bloating, constipation, diarrhoea and nausea. Mouth ulcers, weight loss, anaemia and fatigue also feature. In the UK, the prevalence is 1 in 100, with around 30% of cases undiagnosed. Diagnostic tests need to be undertaken whilst continuing with a gluten-containing diet. Autoantibody tests are 90% sensitive and 95% specific. The gold standard test is a small bowel biopsy demonstrating villous atrophy and crypt hyperplasia. Management is with a lifelong gluten-free diet, excluding wheat, rye, and barley. Diagnosis is important to avoid malabsorptive issues, vitamin deficiencies (vitamin D, calcium, folate) and consequent osteoporosis, poor training, fatigue and stress fractures.

Inflammatory Bowel Disease (IBD)

Crohn's disease (CD) and Ulcerative colitis (UC) are the two main inflammatory bowel diseases causing chronic inflammation of the bowel. CD can affect the entire GI tract (mouth to anus) and UC affects the large intestine and always the rectum. Symptoms include abdominal pain, bloody diarrhoea and weight loss. Crohn's disease can also present with obstructive symptoms: strictures, constipation and perforation. Extra-intestinal manifestations can affect all systems and are related to disease activity. IBD is often diagnosed in young adults, usually with a family history and genetic predisposition. Diagnosis is with intestinal biopsy confirming typical pathological characteristics. Acute disease episodes often require treatment with oral corticosteroids, which needs to be carefully considered in an athlete subject to doping control, including the need for TUE. Other pharmacotherapy includes disease-modifying drugs and biologic preparations, which often require careful monitoring, including regular blood tests.

Travellers' Diarrhoea

Increase in stool frequency to three or more daily whilst travelling abroad, also associated with one other feature such as nausea, vomiting, abdominal pain and fever. The majority of cases are benign and self-limiting. 80–90% are due to bacteria, with Enterotoxigenic E-coli (ETEC) being the most common pathogen worldwide. Primary prevention prior to travel, and secondary prevention once cases are discovered in the travelling group are important. Treatment is supportive, ensuring adequate hydration. Standby antibiotics are useful.

CLINICAL CONSIDERATIONS

Increasing evidence reports protective benefits of probiotic use to improve gut health. *Lactobacilli* is thought to colonise the GI tract quickly after ingestion and may be helpful in travellers' diarrhoea and other conditions. Probiotics are thought to promote a healthy immune response, decreasing infection and potentially increasing energy availability and performance.

RENAL AND URINARY TRACT

Patients present frequently with urological complaints. Additionally, exercise induces changes in renal physiology. The kidneys receive 20% of cardiac output and are composed of metabolically active cells that are sensitive to hypoxia. The kidneys and urinary tract are also susceptible to trauma, despite their anatomical protection from the lower ribs and flank muscles.

Renal Colic

The incidence of urolithiasis or kidney stone disease is increasing worldwide. Patients present with sudden onset spasms of severe colicky pain, often loin to groin and associated with nausea and vomiting. Risk factors include dehydration, genetic factors, previous renal stones and medications. Diagnosis is usually clinical. There may be microscopic haematuria on urinary dipstick. The majority of stones are radiopaque and CT KUB is the imaging modality of choice. Initial treatment is analgesia, ensuring normal urinary function and treatment of concurrent infection. Small stones may pass themselves but further treatment includes shock wave lithotripsy, percutaneous stone removal or ureteroscopy.

Haematuria

Haematuria, or blood in the urine, can be visible or non-visible and picked up on urine dipstick. Various pathologies are responsible, including infection, stones, trauma, malignancy and inflammatory conditions. In sport, haematuria can occur spontaneously or secondary to trauma. The lower poles of the kidneys are more susceptible, due to their position, and injuries are often mild (contusion) and graded according to severity. Haematuria is the most common clinical symptom following trauma. Most cases are benign, with the majority of athletes suffering contusion. Treatment is usually conservative, with observation until resolution of haematuria. Imaging is not usually required. If an athlete develops increasing loin pain, reduced urinary output or hypotension they require immediate referral to secondary care. Contact should be avoided for a minimum of 6 weeks after renal trauma.

Exercise-induced haematuria ('runner's bladder') is a benign condition more likely after endurance events with high intensity and poor hydration. Usually, athletes are asymptomatic and resolution occurs within 24–72 hours post-event with rest and hydration. Persistent cases require investigation.

Non-Steroidal Anti-Inflammatory Drugs (NSAIDs)

The risk of renal impairment with exercise can be exacerbated by NSAID use as they cause renal vasoconstriction, reduced urine output and salt and water retention. This risk is increased with prolonged, high intensity exercise, high heat, humidity, and dehydration. It is therefore key that athletes are aware of these risks.

VACCINATION

Vaccinations are the most important way of protecting ourselves against infectious disease and the World Health Organisation (WHO) states that vaccine hesitancy is a significant threat to global health.

The UK offers a routine immunisation schedule starting in infancy. All immunisations are voluntary and should be undertaken with informed consent. The Department of Health Green Book, available online, provides all up-to-date information regarding vaccinations and the schedule. This covers a number of diseases including: COVID-19, diphtheria, haemophilus influenzae type b (Hib), hepatitis B, human papillomavirus (certain serotypes), influenza, measles, meningococcal disease (certain serogroups), mumps, pertussis (whooping cough), pneumococcal disease (certain serotypes), polio, rotavirus, rubella, shingles and tetanus. Athletes and patients with underlying conditions may require additional vaccination such as post-splenectomy. If travelling abroad, vaccinations may be required depending on the destination (Yellow fever, typhoid, hepatitis A). www.travelhealth.pro provides useful advice for travel vaccinations. Athletes may require proof of vaccination via the International Certificate of Vaccination or Prophylaxis (ICVP).

Hepatitis A

A common and highly contagious, self-limiting infection. It is spread by the faecal-oral route, therefore easily passed between athletes travelling in groups and present in close quarters. It occurs worldwide, most commonly in countries with poor hygiene. Hepatitis A vaccination is recommended prior to travel. Two doses confer long term protection. The vaccination can be given in combined preparations with Yellow Fever and Typhoid.

Tetanus

A rare but life threatening condition, secondary to the bacteria *Clostridium tetani*. Infection is due to environmental spores in soil and manure contaminating wounds or burns. It affects the central nervous system. Immunisation is key in prevention. Primary immunisation consists of three doses of inactivated tetanus toxoid vaccine, most commonly at 2, 3 and 4 months of age in the UK. Two reinforcing booster doses are given usually at three years after the primary course (age 5 years), then another dose at 10 years after the booster (age 15 years). Following this, if an individual sustains a tetanus prone wound, additional vaccine and/or immunoglobulin doses may be required.

MULTIPLE CHOICE QUESTION (MCQ) QUESTIONS

1. An 18-year-old male rower presents with a 3-day history of dysuria and urinary frequency. On examination, his temperature is 37°C. Abdomen is soft and non-tender. Based on this history, what is the most likely causative organism?

   A. *Escherichia coli*
   B. *Chlamydia trachomatis*
   C. *Gonorrhoea*
   D. *Proteus mirabilis*
   E. *Herpes simplex*

2. A 21-year-old male fencer presents with a recent onset widespread macular rash covering his trunk and arms. It is mildly itchy. He denies any recent illness and has no past medical history. The most likely diagnosis in this case would be:

   A. Pityriasis versicolour
   B. Tinea corporis
   C. Eczema
   D. Pityriasis rosea
   E. Guttate psoriasis

3. A 17-year-old academy rugby player complains of a sore throat, raised glands in her neck and a temperature. You order some blood tests and a monospot test is positive. You review her 2 weeks later and she is symptom free and keen to return to play. You assess the player and find that her temperature is 36.5°C, heart rate is 68 bpm, her throat appears normal and her abdomen is soft and non-tender. You discuss returning to play. Which of the following is the most appropriate advice?

   A. Splenic rupture is no longer a risk in return to play now that she is feeling better.
   B. If you organise an ultrasound today you can exclude splenomegaly and then allow the player to return to play.
   C. The player is not at risk of splenic rupture if she avoids contact sport.

D. Because your examination findings are normal, splenomegaly is excluded.

E. The player should wait a further 4 weeks and avoid non-contact training sessions such as weightlifting.

4. A 28-year-old male track athlete complains of upper respiratory tract symptoms. For which of the following symptoms would you exclude the athlete from exercise?

A. Nasal congestion
B. Myalgia
C. Temperature 37.4°C
D. Sore throat
E. Cough

5. A 25-year-old female footballer has been investigated for ongoing tiredness and has had a number of bloods checked. Her results reveal: Haemoglobin 115 g/l (low), Serum ferritin 20 ug/L (low), Folate 3.2 ng/mL (low), Vitamin B12 175 pg/mL (low), CRP <5 mg/l (normal), ESR 4 mm/hr (normal). What is the most likely cause of her symptoms?

A. Ulcerative colitis
B. Crohn's disease
C. Relative energy deficiency syndrome (RED-S)
D. Menorrhagia
E. Coeliac disease

MULTIPLE CHOICE QUESTION (MCQ) ANSWERS

1. Answer B
Chlamydia trachomatis infection is responsible for around 50% of non-gonococcal urethritis (NGU) cases in young adult males with symptoms typically presenting around 1–3 weeks after contracting the STI. *Herpes simplex* virus may present with NGU and *E. coli* and *Proteus* frequently cause UTIs. Gonorrhoea is the second most common bacterial STI in the UK after *Chlamydia*. Men often report urethritis as well as penile discharge and inflammation of the foreskin.

2. Answer A
All of the conditions listed can cause a widespread itchy rash; determining which is the cause can be difficult. Eczema (C) is unlikely to present suddenly as a widespread rash in an athlete with no past medical history. The fact that he has been well with no clear preceding illness makes guttate psoriasis (E) and pityriasis rosea (D) less likely. The fencing suit is occlusive, which can increase the chance of fungal infections. Pityriasis Versicolour is the likely cause, with tinea corporis often causing less widespread and gradual onset rash.

3. Answer E
The diagnosis here is infectious mononucleosis. Splenic rupture can remain a risk up to 8 weeks following illness so Answer A is incorrect. Although an ultrasound scan may be useful to assess for splenomegaly, without a baseline scan this limits its utility, and ultrasound does not help determine risk of rupture (B). Splenic rupture may occur spontaneously, so Answer C is incorrect, and physical examination is not sensitive for excluding splenomegaly (D). A total of 6 weeks return to play may seem cautious but is the most appropriate answer. Weight lifting can also increase intra-abdominal pressure, increasing rupture risk, so should be avoided.

4. Answer B
The majority of options here are upper respiratory tract symptoms that may cause an athlete some problems with engaging in exercise. Myalgia (B), however, is a symptom that suggests systemic involvement and so should exclude an athlete from exercise outright.

5. Answer E
Coeliac disease is most likely to cause multiple deficiencies due to malabsorption, so mild iron deficiency anaemia as well as a combination of vitamin B12 and folate deficiency can occur. Menorrhagia (D) can cause an iron deficiency anaemia. Ulcerative colitis (A) and Crohn's (B) affecting the terminal ileum can cause iron/vitamin B12 and folate deficiencies, however, inflammatory markers such as ESR and CRP are often raised. RED-S is less likely to show multiple abnormalities of blood profile.

Physical Activity 18

Ashley Ridout, Hamish Reid, Justin Varney, Andy Pringle,
Camilla Nykjaer, Katie Marino and Dane Vishnubala

*If physical activity were a drug, we would refer to it as a miracle
cure, due to the great many illnesses it can prevent and help treat.*
UK Chief Medical Officers, 2019.

INTRODUCTION

Increasing physical activity (PA) levels, reducing sedentary behaviour and improving muscle strength and
balance are critical for improving health outcomes
and preventing morbidity and mortality. Despite the
strong evidence for benefit, activity levels continue to
decrease in the UK and globally. The World Health
Organisation (WHO, 2010) have reported inactivity as
the fourth leading risk factor for global mortality (after
hypertension, tobacco use and high blood glucose).
Physical inactivity is responsible for 1 in 6 deaths in the
UK and costs an estimated £7.4 billion/year. A quarter
of adults worldwide are not meeting physical activity
recommendations and in some countries (especially
high-income countries) this is much higher.

What Is Physical Activity?

While each of us will have an understanding of what
physical activity is, it is useful to have shared standardised definitions so we have a common language
for discussion. The definitions in Table 18.1 are drawn
from the WHO guidelines on Physical Activity and
Sedentary Behaviour (2020):

Table 18.1 Physical Activity Definitions

Term	WHO Definition
Physical Activity	Any bodily movement produced by skeletal muscles that requires energy expenditure.
Physical Inactivity	Less than 150 minutes of moderate-intensity activity per week, or equivalent.
Exercise	A subcategory of PA that is planned, structured, repetitive and purposeful – in the sense that the improvement or maintenance of one or more components of physical fitness is the objective.
Muscle-strengthening activity	PA and exercises that increase skeletal muscle strength, power, endurance and mass – strength training, resistance training or muscular strength and endurance exercise
Balance Training	Static and dynamic exercises that are designed to improve an individual's ability to withstand challenges from postural sway or destabilising stimuli caused by self-motion, the environment, or other objects.
Metabolic Equivalent (MET)	A physiological measure expressing the intensity of physical activities. One MET is the energy equivalent expended by an individual while seated at rest.

(Continued)

DOI: 10.1201/9781003179979-18

Table 18.1 (Continued)	
Term	**WHO Definition**
Light-intensity PA	1.5-3 METs – slow walking
Moderate-intensity PA	3-5.9 METs – walking, cycling, shopping
Vigorous-intensity PA	≥6 METs – running, dancing, swimming
Sedentary Behaviour	Any waking behaviour characterised by an energy expenditure of 1.5 METs or lower whilst sitting, reclining, or lying: – desk-based office work, driving a car, watching television (these can also apply to those unable to stand, such as wheelchair users)

PHYSICAL ACTIVITY RECOMMENDATIONS

The UK Chief Medical Officers (CMOs) have issued PA guidance, summarised below in Table 18.2 (Department of Health, 2019). While the recommendations specify targets, some activity is always better than none. This applies across all ages, and, even if people are not able to reach the recommended targets, any increase in aerobic and muscle-strengthening activity is beneficial and should be encouraged.

Table 18.2 Physical Activity Recommendations	
Children and Young People (0-18 years)	
Infants <1y	Should be physically active several times a day, in a variety of ways including interactive floor-based activity/crawling • If not yet mobile include >30 minutes of tummy time whilst awake, as well as reaching, grasping, pushing and pulling themselves independently, or rolling over
Toddlers 1-2y	≥180 minutes/day in a variety of physical activities at any intensity, including active and outdoor play, spread throughout the day
Pre-schoolers 3-4y	≥180 minutes/day in a variety of physical activities at any intensity, including active and outdoor play • To include >60 minutes of moderate-vigorous intensity PA
Children and Young People	An average of ≥60 minutes/day of moderate-vigorous intensity PA/week • This can include all activities such as physical education, active travel, after-school activities, play and sports • A variety of types and intensities of PA across the week to develop movement skills, muscular fitness, and bone strength is ideal • Minimise sedentary time and, when physically possible, break up periods of not moving with at least light PA
Disabled Children and Young People	20 minutes of PA/day • Do challenging but manageable strength and balance activities 3 times/week
Adults (19-64 years)	≥150 minutes of moderate intensity or 75 minutes of vigorous intensity activity per week, or shorter durations of very vigorous activity (or a combination) • Aim to be physically active every day (any activity is better than none) • Do activities to maintain strength in the major muscle groups on ≥2 days/week • This could include activities such as carrying heavy shopping, heavy gardening or resistance exercise • Minimise sedentary time, when possible, interrupt long periods of inactivity with at least light PA

Table 18.2 (Continued)	
Other groups	
Older Adults (>65 years)	≥150 minutes of moderate intensity aerobic activity, building up gradually from current levels • Participate in daily PA to gain health benefits, wellbeing and social functioning • Those who are already active can achieve these benefits from 75 minutes of vigorous intensity activity, or a combination. • Undertake activities aimed at improving or maintaining muscle strength, balance and flexibility on at least 2 days/week • Break up prolonged sedentary periods with light activity when physically possible, or by standing instead of sitting
Disabled Adults	Aim for ≥150 minutes of moderate intensity activity/week • Strength and balance activities on at least 2 days per week • Reduce sedentary time
Pregnancy	Aim for ≥150 minutes of moderate intensity PA per week • Muscle strengthening activities twice/week • If not active, start gradually
Post-Partum (Birth-12 months)	Aim for ≥150 minutes of moderate intensity PA per week • Start pelvic floor exercises as soon as possible and continue daily • Build back up to muscle strengthening activities twice/week.

Behaviour Change

Addressing behaviour change is fundamental to successful PA intervention. It is vital that messages around PA are delivered in a person-centred way, addressing individual perspective, understanding, previous experience, hopes and concerns. Choice of language is important in successfully engaging people, since those who are not regularly active may negatively perceive words such as 'exercise'. Words like this are commonly associated with negative past experiences or inappropriate expectations and represent an avoidable barrier to engagement. People living with medical conditions may experience social stigma around PA participation and have additional perceptions or fears about becoming active, such as exacerbating pre-existing medical conditions. Fears in this group commonly incorporate symptom exacerbation, such as pain or shortness of breath. When this occurs, it is helpful to address these fears, reassure and empower patients, focussing on how activity can actually help these symptoms.

CLINICAL CONSIDERATIONS

When discussing PA, initial assessment should involve determining if the person is receptive to

increasing activity levels. An individualised intervention should be developed, ideally based on their interests – an understanding of current activity levels can inform initial recommendations and help identify these interests. For those who are not active, creating a good rapport and simply introducing the topic of PA may promote more successful discussion later. Resolving their reasons for lack of engagement, while evoking reasons for change, can be powerful towards encouraging readiness and self-efficacy. If there are previous levels of regular activity, finding out why these have reduced can form the basis of quantifying readiness and confidence to change. Goal setting and understanding of individual motivators and barriers encourages autonomy.

After the initial discussion, follow-ups can be planned to assess ongoing levels of activity, discuss relapses (which should be expected) and periodic review depending on individual progress. Anticipating and planning how to overcome relapses can help prevent longer-term lapses in the PA journey.

Physical Activity Levels and Benefits

The benefits of increasing and maintaining PA levels are significant at all ages (Table 18.3). As well as benefits

PHYSICAL ACTIVITY

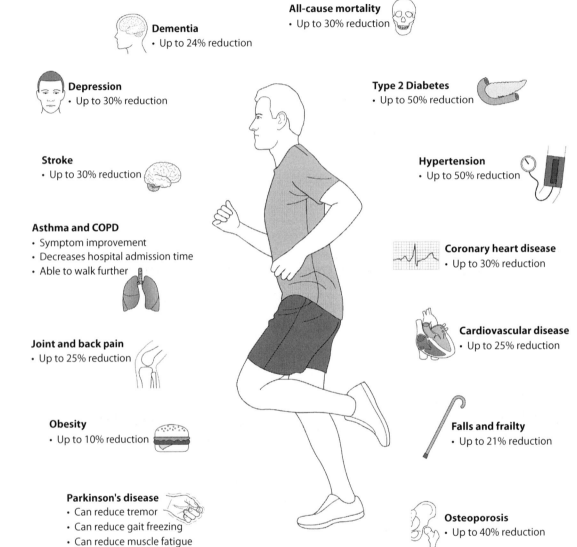

All-cause mortality
• Up to 30% reduction

Dementia
• Up to 24% reduction

Depression
• Up to 30% reduction

Type 2 Diabetes
• Up to 50% reduction

Stroke
• Up to 30% reduction

Hypertension
• Up to 50% reduction

Asthma and COPD
• Symptom improvement
• Decreases hospital admission time
• Able to walk further

Coronary heart disease
• Up to 30% reduction

Cardiovascular disease
• Up to 25% reduction

Joint and back pain
• Up to 25% reduction

Obesity
• Up to 10% reduction

Falls and frailty
• Up to 21% reduction

Parkinson's disease
• Can reduce tremor
• Can reduce gait freezing
• Can reduce muscle fatigue

Osteoporosis
• Up to 40% reduction

Pregnancy and Postnatal
• Improves blood pressure control
• Improves cardiovascular fitness
• Improves pelvic floor muscles
• Reduces risk of gestational diabetes
• Improves mood
• Helps control weight gain

Cancer (Breast, colon and others)
• Up to 25% reduction

Figure 18.1 Pictorial chapter overview.

Table 18.3 Benefits of physical activity

Physical Health Benefits	• Reduced premature mortality, all-cause mortality and cardiovascular disease mortality
	• Dose-response relationship – mortality drops with increased aerobic capacity
	• Improved cardiorespiratory fitness and function
	  ○ Increased central and peripheral oxygen uptake; improved vascular endothelial function; decreased minute ventilation, myocardial oxygen consumption, heart rate and blood pressure at a given intensity; increased capillary density in skeletal muscle and increased exercise threshold
	• Improved cardiovascular risk profile
	  ○ Decreased systolic and diastolic hypertension, reduced resting heart rate, decreased total peripheral resistance (increased muscle capillarisation), increased serum HDL cholesterol and reduced triglycerides, reduced total body and intra-abdominal fat, improved glucose tolerance and decreased inflammation
	• Reduced risk and better control of long-term medical conditions
	  ○ including cardiovascular disease, hypertension, stroke, diabetes, metabolic syndrome, osteoporosis and cancer
	• Improved bone health
	  ○ Can prevent, slow or reverse the effects of osteopaenia/osteoporosis and associated fracture
	• Improved body composition
	  ○ NB physical activity in isolation rarely results in weight loss without dietary intervention
	• Improved motor function, strength and balance
	  ○ Decreased MSK pain, improved physical function and reduced work absence
	  ○ Prevention of functional limitations, reduced risk of falls, frailty and associated injury. Maintenance of independence for older adults

Mental Health Benefits	• Prevention and treatment of anxiety and depression • Improved symptoms, quality of life and cognition in schizophrenia • Improved wellbeing, self-esteem and self-efficacy • Improved sleep • Reduced fatigue and increased energy • Improved cognitive function and prevention of neurodegenerative disease

for physical and mental health, there are social, economic and environmental benefits for both individuals and communities. PA can help to reduce social isolation and tackle health inequalities. Multimorbidity is very common and the number of people in the UK with four or more long-term conditions is predicted to double by 2032 (Kingston et al., 2018). Inactivity increases with age and in those with long-term conditions (including chronic health conditions, disability, mental health and sensory impairments). According to the 2020-21 Active Lives survey, only 45% of disabled people or those with a long-term condition reported ≥ 150 minutes of PA per week (Sport England, 2022a). Both regular aerobic and muscle-strengthening activity (muscle strength, endurance and power) is widely recommended for adults with long-term medical conditions and safely promotes physical health, mental health and general wellbeing.

PRESCRIBING PHYSICAL ACTIVITY

Healthcare professionals have been identified as central to the promotion of PA in the CMO guidelines. They are well placed to address PA and provide trusted advice, even to the most sedentary individuals with long-term medical conditions (Kime et al., 2020). Inactive and sedentary individuals have the most to gain from increasing their PA, as demonstrated by the dose-response curve (Figure 18.2).

Increased sedentary time is associated with higher all-cause and cardiovascular mortality, cardiovascular and type 2 diabetes disease incidence, and there is an association between increased risk of endometrial, colon and lung cancer, cancer mortality and obesity.

Prescribing PA can enable a more structured approach to starting, increasing and maintaining activity levels. Despite the known benefits, healthcare professionals can be reluctant to advise PA because of fears it might exacerbate existing conditions, cause unwanted side-effects or lead to adverse events; however, evidence suggests this is very rare and the benefits of being active far outweigh the risks in almost all scenarios (Vishnubala et al., 2022). People should, of course, be advised to seek medical attention if their symptoms deteriorate or they develop new symptoms of concern.

Initial assessment should include current and past medical history, including any symptoms of cardiovascular, respiratory or metabolic disease, drug history and allergies, family history (such as sudden or unexplained death, cardiovascular risk factors or significant features) and lifestyle factors (smoking, alcohol, and recreational drugs). Any special circumstances (such as pregnancy) and red flags should be identified. There are validated questionnaires, such as the PAR-Q+, which can be used as part of the risk stratification process (Warburton et al., 2011). The American College of Sports Medicine (ACSM)

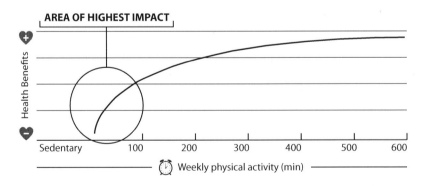

Figure 18.2 Dose-response curve of physical activity and health benefits.

Source: Taken from UK Chief Medical Officers' Physical activity guidelines.

Table 18.4 Absolute and Relative Contraindications to Symptom-Limited Maximal Exercise Testing (Reibe et al., 2018)

Absolute Contraindications
Myocardial infarction within 2 days
Ongoing unstable angina
Uncontrolled cardiac arrhythmia with haemodynamic compromise
Active endocarditis
Symptomatic severe aortic stenosis
Decompensated heart failure
Acute pulmonary embolism, pulmonary infarction, or deep venous thrombosis
Acute myocarditis or pericarditis
Suspected or known dissecting aneurysm
Physical disability that precludes safe and adequate testing

Relative Contraindications
Known obstructed left main coronary artery stenosis
Moderate to severe aortic stenosis with uncertain relationship to symptoms
Tachyarrhythmias with uncontrolled ventricular rates
Acquired or advanced complete heart block
Recent stroke or transient ischaemic attack
Mental impairment with limited ability to cooperate
Resting hypertension with systolic >200 mmHg or diastolic >110 mmHg
Uncorrected medical conditions, such as significant anaemia, important electrolyte imbalance and hyperthyroidism

recommends the use of such questionnaires when initiating or progressing aerobic exercise prescription, with any active signs or symptoms of cardiovascular, renal or metabolic disease requiring medical clearance (Reibe et al., 2018).

There is no evidence regarding contraindications for PA, but there are some established contraindications that preclude exercise testing (Table 18.4).

There is a slightly increased risk of adverse cardiac events with increasing age and activity levels, especially during and shortly after vigorous activity in the most sedentary, or in those with undiagnosed cardiovascular disease. The reported absolute risk remains very low (1 sudden cardiac death in every 1.5 million episodes of vigorous activity in men and 1 in every 36.5 million hours of moderate to vigorous intensity activity in women), especially if activity levels are increased gradually from each individual baseline and unaccustomed vigorous activity is avoided. Risk decreases as cardiovascular fitness improves.

Measuring Physical Activity

PA can take many forms and includes routine daily activities. This can include active travel (walking/cycling), housework, gardening, sport and fitness activities, family activity and work activities, as well as structured exercise. Community groups and group activities may provide a social aspect to increasing PA and convey additional wellbeing or safety benefits. The exercise vital sign (EVS) is a validated tool that can be used to quantify current weekly levels of PA activity, by multiplying active minutes per day by the number of active days per week (Coleman et al., 2012). It consists of two questions:

1. On average, how many days per week do you engage in moderate intensity or greater PA (like a brisk walk) lasting at least 10 minutes?
2. On those days, how many minutes do you engage in activity at this level?
   An additional question for muscle strengthening activity can be included:
   "How many days per week do you perform muscle strengthening exercises such as bodyweight exercises or resistance training?"

The FITT (Frequency, Intensity, Time, Type) Principle

The FITT framework can be used to provide a structure for individualised PA recommendation, depending on baseline level of activity, functional status, comorbidities, and individual goals.

> **Frequency**—how many times per week?
> **Intensity**—how vigorous is the activity?
> **Time**—how long should the activity be done for?
> **Type**—what type of activity should be done?

Intensity level can be used to gauge and recommend PA in a practical way. The 'talk-test' represents the increasing breathlessness with increasing intensity of PA and can be an effective method for discussion with patients (Table 18.5).

PHYSICAL ACTIVITY IN SPECIAL GROUPS

Under 5's, Children and Young People

UK CMO PHYSICAL ACTIVITY GUIDELINES—UNDER 5'S, CHILDREN AND YOUNG PEOPLE (0–18)

Infants <1y

- Should be physically active several times a day, in a variety of ways including interactive floor-based activity/crawling.
- If not yet mobile, include >30 minutes of tummy time whilst awake, as well as reaching, grasping, pushing and pulling themselves independently, or rolling over.

Toddlers (1–2y)

- >180 minutes per day in a variety of physical activities at any intensity, including active and outdoor play, spread throughout the day.

Pre-schoolers (3–4y)

- >180 minutes per day in a variety of physical activities at any intensity, including active and outdoor play; this should include >60 minutes of moderate to vigorous intensity PA.

Children and Young People (5–18y)

- An average of >60 minutes per day of moderate to vigorous intensity PA per week.
  - This can include all activities such as physical education, active travel, after-school activities, play and sports.

Table 18.5 Measures of Physical Activity Intensity

	Moderate Intensity Walking/Cycling/Shopping	Vigorous Intensity Running/Dancing/Swimming
'Talk Test'	Able to talk, but not sing	Not able to say more than a few words or speak in full sentences
Borg Scale—a self-reported scale of perceived exertion from 6 (no exertion) to 20 (maximal exertion)	12–14	>14
Metabolic Equivalent (METs)	3–5.9 METs	≥6 METs

○ A variety of types and intensities of PA across the week to develop movement skills, muscular fitness, and bone strength.

○ Minimise sedentary time, when physically possible, break up long periods of not moving with at least light PA.

The benefits of PA in children and adolescents encompass physical health conditions, psychological and social wellbeing (Table 18.6). Sport England report that only 47.2% of children and young people in England self-reported an average of at least 60 minutes of activity per day in the academic year 2021/22 and it is estimated that up to 81% of adolescents globally do not do enough PA to derive health benefits (Sport England 2022b). Establishing age and ability-appropriate PA and other healthy behaviours in childhood significantly increases the likelihood of continuing healthy behaviours throughout life. Increased activity levels are also beneficial for children and adolescents living with long-term conditions or obesity.

Any amount of PA is beneficial compared to none, even if not meeting the age-specific recommendations. Activity can be incorporated into daily life (in recreation, at school (where interventions demonstrate significant improvement in diastolic BP and fasting insulin), physical education, transportation or helping with household jobs). Sedentary behaviour (screen time, sitting) is associated with poorer physical fitness and cardiometabolic health, worse health outcomes and sleep disruption in children and adolescents. Increased sedentary time is associated with poorer mental health and behaviour. Some sedentary behaviours (such as reading, homework, crafts, puzzles and music) are beneficial for cognitive development and so should be encouraged in addition to activity.

When children and adolescents increase their activity levels, risk of adverse events are very low, and the benefits of increasing PA and reducing sedentary time outweigh the risks. Potential risk can be reduced by building up gently, following recommended guidance and seeking medical attention if any new symptoms develop. Current evidence does not clarify the effect of activity duration, exercise modality, ratio of rest or volume of activity on aerobic fitness, therefore vigorous activity should be encouraged to optimise cardiovascular fitness (Füssenich et al., 2016).

Some sports have age-specific directives in place to prevent injury. The England and Wales Cricket

Table 18.6 Benefits of Physical Activity in Children and Adolescents	
Physical Fitness	• Increased vigorous-intensity activity is associated with improved cardiovascular fitness. • Increased muscle-strengthening exercise is associated with improved muscular fitness.
Metabolic Health	• Improved serum lipid profile and glucose, decreased insulin resistance.
Bone Health	• Improved bone mineral density and bone structure with weight-bearing/impact activity. • Almost 90% of peak bone mass is achieved by 18y – optimising this in adolescence is protective against osteoporosis and associated morbidity into adulthood.
Cognitive Outcomes	• Improved cognitive function and academic outcomes. • Improved memory and executive function.
Mental Health	• Reduced depression, possibly as effective as psychological and medication therapy.
Improved Body Composition	• Improved body composition (especially with structured interventions of longer duration with an aerobic component). • Reduced visceral and intra-hepatic fat (improved liver enzymes) with supervised aerobic or combined interventions. • Maintenance of healthy weight.

Board (ECB) has guidance for fast bowling including number of overs bowled, technique and equipment. The Football Association (FA) specify that no heading is allowed during training in primary school children, with a graduated approach in the U12-U16 age groups. This involves between 5 (up to U13) to 10 headers (up to U18) in one training session per week. Heading drills should be reduced for U18s, to account for heading during matches. Footballs should be inflated to the lowest authorised pressure. Defensive body checking in ice hockey is introduced later in adolescence.

WOMEN

Physical Activity in Pregnancy

UK CMO PHYSICAL ACTIVITY GUIDELINES—PREGNANCY

- Aim for ≥ 150 minutes of moderate intensity activity/week
- Muscle strengthening activities twice a week

Pregnancy is a 'teachable moment,' when women may be more motivated to make behavioural changes around lifestyle, including PA (Phelan et al., 2010). Multiple healthcare contacts provide opportunities for positive reinforcement. Despite the known benefits

of PA in pregnancy for both maternal and newborn health, women may lack confidence in becoming more physically active due to fear of pregnancy complications and social stigma. Few women meet PA guidelines during pregnancy, and this declines with increasing gestation. Healthcare professionals report a lack of knowledge and confidence for giving PA advice, resulting in inaccurate or conflicting information (Lowe et al., 2022). The benefits of being active during pregnancy outweigh the risks (once specific contraindications are excluded—see Table 18.7).

Pregnant women are advised to aim for the same amount of PA as the general population, but this will vary depending on the stage of pregnancy, and pre-pregnancy activity levels. Women who were active before pregnancy can continue as tolerated. Inactive women should start slowly and increase according to tolerance—cardiovascular fitness can be increased during pregnancy. Strengthening activities are important. The WHO also recommends gentle stretching (WHO, 2020). Women should be advised to consult a medical professional if they develop any new or concerning symptoms, including persistent or excessive shortness of breath, chest pain, regular painful uterine contractions, vaginal bleeding, loss of fluid from the vagina (suggesting membrane rupture) or dizziness/presyncope that does not resolve with rest.

Table 18.7 Absolute and Relative Contraindications to Physical Activity in Pregnancy (adapted from Meah et al., 2020)

Absolute Contraindications	Relative Contraindications
Severe respiratory disease (COPD, restrictive lung disease, cystic fibrosis)	Mild respiratory disease, congenital or acquired heart disease
Severe heart disease (acquired or congenital) with exercise intolerance, or uncontrolled arrhythmia	Well controlled Type 1 Diabetes
Uncontrolled Type 1 Diabetes	Mild pre-eclampsia
Placental abruption	Preterm premature rupture of membranes (PPROMs)
Vasa praevia	Placenta praevia after 28/40 weeks
Severe pre-eclampsia	Symptomatic, severe eating disorder
Cervical insufficiency	Multiple nutrient deficiencies and/or chronic undernutrition
Intrauterine growth restriction (IUGR)	Untreated thyroid disease
Active preterm labour	Moderate/heavy smoking (> 20 cigarettes/day) in the presence of comorbidities

Specific Considerations in Pregnancy

- Avoid excessive heat and humidity (e.g. hot yoga), and vigorous activity in these conditions, especially during the first trimester.
- Avoid exercising at high altitude (> 2500 m) if not usually living above that level.
- Avoid scuba diving.
- Avoid contact activities, or those with a high risk of falling or trauma.
- Ensure adequate hydration and nutrition, as demands are increased by both the pregnancy and increased PA levels.
- Be aware of musculoskeletal symptoms that may occur (neck/back pain, pelvic pain, carpal tunnel syndrome, diastasis recti). Avoid activities that may exacerbate pain, such as pelvic girdle pain.
  - Appropriate PA will help in management of these conditions (e.g. back pain).
- Increased hormone-related ligamentous laxity may increase the risk of injury, therefore thorough warm up and cool down should be recommended.
- Lying supine during exercise after 20 weeks gestation may cause decreased venous return due to compression from the gravid uterus. This can lead to hypotension and should be considered when providing exercise advice in pregnancy.

Contraindications to Physical Activity During Pregnancy

Guidelines for absolute contraindications can be variable and have often been based on expert opinion. More recently, evidence for specific conditions associated with harm from PA have been investigated in more detail, highlighted as absolute contraindications in Table 18.7 (Meah et al., 2020). Pregnant women with pre-existing health conditions or complications of pregnancy are very likely to be under specialist obstetric care and therefore should seek advice from their obstetrician. For absolute contraindications, activities of daily living can be continued but moderate or vigorous physical activity should be discouraged. For relative contraindications, it is a risk benefit conversation to be had between the pregnant woman and her healthcare provider. PA can be adapted and reduced in intensity, duration or volume.

Benefits of Physical Activity in Pregnancy

The benefits for PA in the general adult population can be extrapolated to pregnant women, including improved cardiovascular fitness and muscle strength, management of cardiovascular risk factors, primary and secondary prevention of long-term medical conditions and mental health benefits (Table 18.8). There is no evidence for increased risk of miscarriage, stillbirth, complications of delivery or effects on birth weight. There is moderate certainty evidence for reduced risk of preterm birth in women undertaking vigorous-intensity PA. There is no difference in caesarean section in overweight or obese pregnant women in PA intervention groups compared to standard antenatal care (Oteng-Ntim et al., 2012).

Physical Activity Postpartum

UK CMO PHYSICAL ACTIVITY GUIDELINES—POSTPARTUM (BIRTH-12 MONTHS)

- Aim for $\geq$ 150 minutes of moderate intensity activity/week.
- Start daily pelvic floor exercises as soon as possible.
- Build back up to muscle strengthening activities twice a week.

Specific Postpartum Considerations

- Women should build activity levels up gradually, according to tolerance.
- Complications during the pregnancy or delivery, as well as mode of delivery, should be considered.
- Consider musculoskeletal symptoms present during the pregnancy, such as pelvic girdle pain, and whether diastasis recti is present. Women may benefit from healthcare professional guidance in the return to activity, including women's health physiotherapy.
- Ensure good hydration, especially if breastfeeding.
- Wear a supportive bra for comfort.

Table 18.8 Benefits of Physical Activity in Pregnancy	
Cardiovascular Fitness	• Regular aerobic activity is associated with maintenance or improvement of cardiovascular fitness. • Increased aerobic capacity is associated with improved maternal health after delivery, reduced labour and delivery complications and faster maternal recovery. • Better self-reported fitness levels are associated with less body pain, low back and sciatic pain and reduced disability from pain.
Prevention and Treatment of Gestational Diabetes (GDM)	• First degree prevention: decreased risk of GDM (high certainty evidence – Davenport et al., 2018) in women of normal weight and overweight/obese women. • Management of GDM: improved glycaemic control and insulin sensitivity.
Reduced Excessive Gestational Weight Gain	• Reduced overall and excessive gestational weight gain (high certainty evidence – McDonald et al., 2016) in women of normal weight and overweight/obese. • Higher maternal BMI between pregnancies is associated with significantly higher maternal and fetal/neonatal complications in subsequent pregnancies.
Blood Pressure Control	• Regular aerobic activity is associated with decreased risk of hypertensive disorders including pre-eclampsia.
Improved Mental Health and Wellbeing	• Activity during pregnancy can reduce symptoms of depression both during and after pregnancy. • Improved sleep

Benefits of Postpartum Activity

As with pregnancy, the benefits for PA in the general adult population can be extrapolated to postpartum women (Table 18.9). There is no evidence for harm with increasing PA levels after pregnancy and childbirth, or for a negative effect on breastfeeding.

Older Adults

• Participate in daily PA to gain health benefits, wellbeing and social functioning.
• Aim to accumulate ≥ 150 minutes of moderate intensity aerobic activity, building up gradually from current levels. Those who are already active can achieve these benefits from 75 minutes of vigorous intensity activity, or a combination of the two.

• Undertake activities aimed at improving or maintaining muscle strength, balance and flexibility on at least 2 days per week.
• Break up prolonged sedentary periods with light activity when physically possible, or with standing.
  ○ Older adults with high levels of physical fitness may benefit from very vigorous physical activities performed in short bursts, interspersed with rest or lower intensity activity breaks (High Intensity Interval Training or HITT).

Levels of PA decrease with age. Only 39% of people over 75 were meeting the activity recommendations in the most recent Active Lives survey (Sport England, 2022a). Associated frailty has a significant impact on functional status, ability to carry out activities of daily living, risk of falling and quality of life. The benefits of PA extend beyond physical health, and activity is a very important component of healthy ageing. This includes opportunities for social interactions, preventing isolation, and empowers people to manage their health. Low levels of PA in middle age are a

Table 18.9 Benefits of Physical Activity in the Postpartum Period (Birth-12 months)	
Cardiovascular Fitness	• Regular aerobic activity is associated with maintenance or improvement of cardiovascular fitness. • Increased aerobic capacity is associated with improved maternal health after delivery.
Improved Mental Health	• Reduced postpartum depression, especially in those who had symptoms of depression before starting PA. • Improved emotional wellbeing. • Improved sleep.
Improved Body Composition	• Decreased postpartum weight gain. • Sooner return to pre-pregnancy weight.

predictor for frailty, and people who are more physically active in middle age have reduced frailty and long-term health conditions.

Capacity to increase activity levels depends on functional status, symptoms of long-term conditions and previous activity levels, as well as psychological motivations and barriers. Older adults, especially those who were previously sedentary, should start slowly, build up gradually and ensure adequate recovery time. The messaging of the 2019 CMO PA guidelines reflects inclusivity that 'some PA is good, more is better'. Even for the most sedentary, lighter-intensity activity (sit-stand exercise, short walks and stair climbing, as appropriate) and reduced sedentary time convey health benefits.

Specific Considerations in Older Adults

- Identifying the PA levels, needs, preferences and experiences of older people.
- Individuals may be highly sedentary or frail, with ≥ 1 long-term medical condition and associated symptoms; therefore, activity should be increased gradually, according to tolerance.
- The physical consequences of ageing may increase risk of injury, including sarcopenia (a marker of frailty defined as 'progressive and general loss of muscle mass and muscle function, defined by either low muscle strength or low physical performance'), lower bone mineral density, degeneration of connective tissues and skin quality.
- Reduced balance and coordination can be associated with increased risk of falling and injury.

- Supervised activity may be required for those who require support, education, or who have cognitive impairment.
- Physiological changes in older age include reduced maximum heart rate and cardiac output, higher blood pressure, lower maximal aerobic capacity (therefore older people will be exercising at a relatively higher intensity), higher residual lung volume, lower vital capacity, increased work of breathing and decreased lung perfusion quality.
- Reduced glucose tolerance.
- Longer recovery time.

Benefits of Physical Activity in Older Adults

As well as extrapolating the benefits of PA for all adults to the older population, there are some additional benefits, with high certainty evidence for combined PA including balance, strength, gait and functional training (Table 18.10).

Disabled Adults

UK CMO PHYSICAL ACTIVITY GUIDELINES—DISABLED ADULTS

- Aim for ≥ 150 minutes of moderate intensity activity/week.
- Do strength and balance activities at least 2 days/week.
- Reduce sedentary time.

Table 18.10 Benefits of Physical Activity in Older Adults

Improved Physical Function	• Improved cardiovascular fitness is independently associated with reduced morbidity and mortality. • Improved strength, balance and flexibility. • Functional improvements mitigate against age-related deterioration in the general population. • Reduced progression of disability affecting activities of daily living. • Increased independence.
Improved Muscle Strength	• Muscle strength decreases with age and is a major limiting factor for independence – strength and balance activities are very important in maintaining physical function.
Decreased Risk of Falls	• Combined strength and balance programmes are associated with reduced risk of falls/falls-related injuries, increased confidence, and increased levels of moderate-intensity activity.
Improved Bone Health	• Improved lumbar spine and femoral neck bone mineral density. • Prevention of osteoporosis.
Cognitive Benefits	• Reduced cognitive impairment and dementia.
Improved Mental Health	• Improved wellbeing. • Reduced social isolation. • Reduced depression.

Table 18.11 Specific Considerations and Benefits of Physical Activity in Disability Groups

Spinal Cord Injury	
Specific Considerations	• Functional ability will depend on the level of the spinal cord lesion and whether it is complete or incomplete. • Increased risk of associated conditions that may increase injury risk (pressure ulcers, low BMD/osteopenia/osteoporosis, urinary tract infection, pain (shoulder pain, chronic pain), spasticity and joint contractures). • There is an increased risk of depression and cardiovascular risk factors (obesity, T2DM, cardiovascular disease), which may influence physical activity advice. • Autonomic dysreflexia (in people with spinal lesion at T6 or above)—the autonomic response to a painful or irritating stimulus below the level of the cord lesion, and is a medical emergency that can cause rapid severe hypertension with significant morbidity and mortality if untreated. • Joint contractures may develop due to muscle spasticity, wheelchair use and muscle strength imbalance.
Specific Benefits	• Improved walking, muscular strength and upper extremity function. • Improved health-related quality of life. • Improved vascular function in paralysed limbs. • Reduced shoulder pain.

Multiple Sclerosis	
Specific Considerations	• Fatigue is common, but improves with overall fitness levels; exercise tolerance may also be reduced. • Maximal aerobic capacity, heart rate and blood pressure response to activity may be reduced. • Lower muscle strength and power. • Issues with hydration (people may limit fluid intake in order to manage urinary symptoms). • Short-term memory loss or cognitive impairment. • Risk of hyperthermia. • Potential side effects of medications.
Specific Benefits	• Improved physical function, muscle strength and endurance, balance, walking speed and endurance, mobility and cardiorespiratory fitness. • Reduced fatigue. • Improved cognitive function. • Improved health-related quality of life.
Parkinson's Disease	
Specific Considerations	• Potential effects of medications, especially after dose changes. • Cognitive impairment. • Falls prevention and balance training are important.
Specific Benefits	• Improved motor function, mobility, endurance, reduced gait freezing and walking speed. • Improved cognitive function with moderate/vigorous-intensity activity. • Improved quality of life.

Adults living with a disability are much more likely to be inactive than adults living without disability (Sport England, 2022a). Furthermore, rates of inactivity increase with the number of disabilities. Only 45% were meeting activity recommendations in the most recent Active Lives survey (Sport England, 2022a). The benefits of PA for the general adult population can be extrapolated to those living with both physical and cognitive impairments (Table 18.11). Aerobic, strength, balance and stretching activities are all beneficial. There is no evidence to suggest increased risk for increasing PA levels in disabled adults, if started slowly (depending on baseline), progressed according to tolerance (increasing frequency, duration and then intensity), and specific abilities and comorbidities are considered.

CONCLUSION

Despite the well documented and hugely broad-reaching benefits of increasing PA levels, the global population is becoming more inactive. It is vital that this is addressed, for both individual and societal benefit. Health care professionals are well placed to promote PA. In almost all cases, the benefits of increasing activity levels outweigh the risks, at all ages, in pregnancy and postpartum, and in those living with long-term medical conditions and disability.

MULTIPLE CHOICE QUESTION (MCQ) QUESTIONS

1. You are counselling one of your patients about the benefits of physical activity. You explain that there is evidence to suggest exercise can prevent cancer. Which cancers have the strongest evidence of primary prevention with exercise?

   A. Prostate and cervical cancer
   B. Colon and breast cancer
   C. Colon cancer and leukaemia
   D. Oesophageal cancer and sarcoma
   E. Thyroid and endometrial cancer

2. A 34-year-old patient attends your clinic. She is 10 weeks pregnant and previously enjoyed running 5 kilometres on a weekly basis. Which statement is the best advice to give to this patient with regard to physical activity?

    A. If she continues to exercise on a regular basis in the third trimester, she is more likely to need a caesarean section at birth.
    B. If she continues with regular physical activity of a vigorous intensity, there is a reduced risk of preterm birth.
    C. She should reduce the amount of exercise she is doing for the remainder of the 1st trimester as there is an increased risk of miscarriage in this time period.
    D. Physical activity has an association with improving high blood pressure, so she should continue, even though there is no evidence that it helps hypertension in preeclampsia.
    E. All forms of physical activity should be encouraged throughout pregnancy including sit ups and scuba diving.

3. Which of the following best describe the UK Chief medical officer's physical activity guidelines for disabled adults?

    A. ≥ 150 minutes of moderate intensity activity per week with strength and balance exercises on at least 2 days per week.
    B. ≥ 30 minutes of moderate intensity activity each day with strength and balance exercises on at least 2 days per week.
    C. ≥ 150 minutes of moderate intensity activity per week with strength and balance exercises on at least 1 day per week.
    D. ≥ 150 minutes of low-moderate intensity activity per week with strength exercises on at least 1 day per week.
    E. ≥ 90 minutes of vigorous intensity activity per week with strength exercises on at least 1 day per week.

4. You are providing a structure for a physical activity prescription for one of your patients. You decide to use the FITT framework. What does the acronym FITT stand for?

    A. Frequency, Impact, Time, Total
    B. Function, Intensity, Task, Total
    C. Function, Impact, Task, Type
    D. Frequency, Intensity, Time, Type
    E. Follow-up, Interval, Time, Total

5. You attend a cardiac service in a tertiary hospital to help provide exercise testing for its patients. Which one of the following is considered an absolute contraindication to exercise testing?

    A. Myocardial infarction 4 weeks ago
    B. Blood pressure 200/100 mmHg
    C. Angina controlled with Ranolazine 375 mg twice daily, Bisoprolol 5 mg once daily and Isosorbide mononitrate 50 mg twice daily
    D. 5.4 cm Abdominal aortic aneurysm
    E. Acute pericarditis

MULTIPLE CHOICE QUESTION (MCQ) ANSWERS

1. Answer B
    Although evidence is emerging that physical activity is associated with reducing the risk of many cancers, the highest quality evidence is with breast and colon cancer.
2. Answer B
    Keeping physically active in pregnancy has many benefits, including reducing the risk of preeclampsia (D is incorrect) and preterm birth (B). After 16 weeks, prolonged periods of time spent supine should be avoided due to the risk of obstructing vena cava blood flow. There is also no protection against decompression sickness for an unborn baby so scuba diving should be avoided (E is incorrect).
3. Answer A
    Although disabled adults are more likely to be inactive than non-disabled adults, the recommendations remain the same.
4. Answer D
    FITT is an acronym that stands for Frequency, Intensity, Time and Type.
5. Answer E
    According to the American College of Sports Medicine (ACSM), acute pericarditis is considered an absolute contraindication to exercise testing. A myocardial infarction within the last 2 days, unstable angina and a suspected dissecting aneurysm are other absolute contraindications. Severe hypertension is considered a relative contraindication.

REFERENCES AND FURTHER READING

Coleman, K.J., Ngor, E., Reynolds, K, et al. Initial validation of an exercise "vital sign" in electronic medical records. *Med Sci Sports Exerc.* 2012;44:2071–2076.

Davenport, M.H., et al. 2018. Prenatal exercise for the prevention of gestational diabetes mellitus and hypertensive disorders of pregnancy: a systematic review and meta-analysis. *Br J Sports Med.* 52(21). 1367–1375.

Department of Health (2019) A report from the Chief Medical Officers in the UK on the amount and type of physical activity people should be doing to improve their health. Available from: https://www.gov.uk/government/publications/physical-activity-guidelines-uk-chief-medical-officers-report

Füssenich, L.M., Boddy, L.M., Green, D.J., Graves, L.E.F., Foweather, L., Dagger, R.M., McWhannell, N., Henaghan, J., Ridgers, N.D., Stratton, G and Hopkins, N.D. 2016. Physical activity guidelines and cardiovascular risk in children: a cross sectional analysis to determine whether 60 minutes is enough. *BMC Public Health.* 2016 Jan 22;16:67. doi: 10.1186/s12889-016-2708-7. PMID: 26801090; PMCID: PMC4724140.

Kime, N., Pringle, A., Zwolinsky, S. et al. 2020. How prepared are healthcare professionals for delivering physical activity guidance to those with diabetes? A formative evaluation. *BMC Health Serv Res* 20, 8. https://doi.org/10.1186/s12913-019-4852-0

Kingston, A., Robinson, L., Booth, H., Knapp, M and Jagger, C. 2018. for the MODEM project, Projections of multimorbidity in the older population in England to 2035: estimates from the Population Ageing and Care Simulation (PACSim) model, Age and Ageing, Volume 47, Issue 3, 374–380, https://doi.org/10.1093/ageing/afx201

Lowe, A., Myers, A., Quirk, H., Blackshaw, J., Palanee, S and Copeland R. 2022. Physical activity promotion by GPs: a cross-sectional survey in England. *BJGP Open 2022*; 6 (3): BJGPO.2021.0227. DOI: 10.3399/BJGPO.2021.0227

McDonald, S.M., et al. 2016. Does dose matter in reducing gestational weight gain in exercise interventions? A systematic review of literature *J Sci Med Sport.* Apr;19(4)323–35.

Meah, V.L., Davies, G.A., Davenport, M.H. 2020. Why can't I exercise during pregnancy? Time to revisit medical "absolute" and "relative" contraindications: Systematic review of evidence of harm and a call to action. *Br J Sports Med*, 54, pp. 1395–1404. doi: 10.1136/bjsports-2020-102042

Oteng-Ntim, E., Varma, R., Croker, H. et al. 2012. Lifestyle interventions for overweight and obese pregnant women to improve pregnancy outcome: systematic review and meta-analysis. *BMC Med* 10, 47.

Phelan, S. 2010. Pregnancy: a "teachable moment" for weight control and obesity prevention. *Am J Obstet Gynecol*, 202, 135.e1–8.

Reibe, D., Ehrman, J., Liguori, G., Magal, M. 2018. *ACSM Guidelines for Exercise Testing and Prescription.* 10th ed. Philadelphia: Wolters Kluwer. Available at: www.academia.edu/36843773/ACSM_Guidelines_for_Exercise_Testing_and_Prescription_10th

Sport England. (2022a). Active Lives Adult November 2020–21 Report, pp. 1–43. Available at: https://sportengland-production-files.s3.eu-west-2.amazonaws.com/s3fs-public/2022-04/Active%20Lives%20Adult%20Survey%20November%202020-21%20Report.pdf?VersionId=nPU_v3jFjwG8o_xnv62FcKOdEiVmRWCb

Sport England. (2022b). Active lives: Children and Young People Survey Academic Year 2021/22 Report, pp. 1–51. Available at: https://sportengland-production-files.s3.eu-west-2.amazonaws.com/s3fs-public/2022-12/Active%20Lives%20Children%20and%20Young%20People%20Survey%20Academic%20Year%202021-22%20Report.pdf?VersionId=R5_hmJHw5M4yKFsewm2vGDMRGHWW7q3E

Vishnubala, D., Iqbal, A., Marino, K., Whatmough, S., Barker, R., Salman, D., Bazira, P., Finn, G., Pringle, A and Nykjaer, C. 2022. UK Doctors Delivering Physical Activity Advice: What Are the Challenges and Possible Solutions? A Qualitative Study. *Int. J. Environ. Res. Public Health.* 19, 12030.

Warburton, D.E.R., Jamnik, V.K., Bredin, S.S.D and Gledhill, N. 2011. PAR-Q+ Research Collaboration The Physical Activity Readiness Questionnaire (PAR-Q+) and electronic Physical Activity Readiness Medical Examination (ePARmed-X+) Health Fitness J Can. 4(2):3–23

The Physical Activity Readiness Questionnaire for Everyone is available at: https://eparmedx.com/

WHO Guidelines on Physical Activity and Sedentary Behaviour. Geneva. (2020). Available at: www.who.int/activities/developing-new-guidelines-on-physical-activity-and-sedentary-behaviour-for-youth-adults-and-sub-populations

World Health Organization. 2010. *Global Recommendations on Physical Activity for Health.* doi: 10.1080/11026480410034349

Population and Public Health **19**

*Linda Evans, Hamish Reid, Justin Varney, Andy Pringle,
David Eastwood and Dane Vishnubala*

WHAT ARE PUBLIC HEALTH AND PUBLIC HEALTH ORGANISATIONS?

Public health refers to the organised measures of promoting health and preventing disease amongst populations. It can be defined as three activities (Figure 19.2):

- *Health protection:* preserving the health of the population.
- *Health improvement:* enhancing health at the individual and population level.
- *Health services delivery:* ensuring consistently high-quality health resources, which are evidence-formed and value-based.

This chapter covers definitions and scope of public health, with a specific focus on physical activity. The above definitions can be applied to physical activity: ensuring the safety of the air and environment to allow outdoor activity could be considered a protective measure; introducing physical activity interventions at hospital discharge could be an improvement measure and employing a skilled workforce to advise and guide the population to be more active could be a health services delivery initiative.

Within the UK, there are two main government agencies which are responsible for public health: the UK Health Security Agency (UKHSA) and Office for Health Improvement and Disparities (OHID). UKHSA is responsible for protecting every member of every community from the impact of infectious diseases, chemical, biological, radiological and nuclear incidents and other health threats. OHID focuses on preventing ill health in the regions and communities where there are the most significant needs.

UK SCREENING PROGRAMMES TO PROMOTE HEALTH

Screening programmes are encompassed by the health protection aspect of public health. National Health Service (NHS) screening programmes invite individuals to be tested for a range of specific diseases (UK Government, 2023). As well as testing for disease, patients will be provided with information and referral for treatment, if required. This differs from health promotion, which involves advice or guidance to reduce risk of disease.

OHID is currently responsible for three national cancer screening programmes (breast, bowel and cervical), six antenatal and newborn programmes (foetal anomaly, infectious diseases in pregnancy, sickle cell anaemia and thalassaemia, newborn and infant physical examination, newborn blood spot and newborn hearing) and two adult programmes (abdominal aortic aneurysm and diabetic eye). These screening programmes provide relatively simple and low-invasive procedures with clear benefits of early detection. Healthcare providers benefit from early detection, with more efficient provision of care.

All Our Health is a government resource by OHID, which provides a framework to guide healthcare professionals in preventing illness, protecting health and promoting wellbeing. The NHS Health Check is one way that All Our Health can be applied (UK Government, 2023). The NHS Health Check offers advice to help prevent the onset of cardiovascular disease for eligible people (those not currently on a cardiovascular disease register or being treated as at-risk, aged between 40 and 74). It comprises an extended primary care appointment with a healthcare assistant

DOI: 10.1201/9781003179979-19

POPULATION AND PUBLIC HEALTH

International society for physical activity and health (ISPAH)

Eight Investments

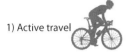

1) Active travel

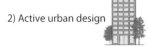

2) Active urban design

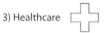

3) Healthcare

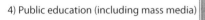

4) Public education (including mass media)

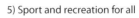

5) Sport and recreation for all

6) Workplaces

7) Community-wide programmes

8) Whole-of-school programmes

Barriers

- Inadequate knowledge about physical activity and the benefits
- Misconceptions exercise can make health conditions worse
- Fear of injury
- Living environments have little space
- Limited access to clubs or equipment
- Inadequate public transport
- Time constraints
- Lifestyle means a reliance on own vehicles
- Health inequalities

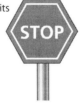

Physical activity consultation
The 5A guidelines are useful: Ask about (or Assess), Advise about, Agree upon, Assist, and Arrange follow up

1) Ask – "Is it OK if we spend a moment talking about something that patients in your position find helpful?"
2) Clear message about health benefits – "Walking briskly for 30 minutes each day can improve your depressive symptoms."
3) Encourage reflection – "What do you make of that?" "Are there any other reasons you would decide to become more active?"
4) Establish engagement – "So, what do you want to do?"
5) If in agreement, plan and set goals
6) Signpost – local clubs, public health bodies, online resources etc.
7) Arrange follow up

Figure 19.1 Pictorial overview.

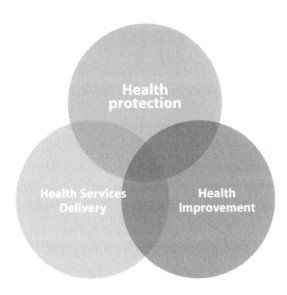

Figure 19.2 Public Health Domains

or nurse with a discussion about lifestyle, family history, a blood pressure check, measure of height and weight and a blood test. Based on the findings, personalised advice is given on how to lower an individual's risk of heart disease, stroke, diabetes and kidney disease. The NHS Health Check provides an opportunity for healthcare professionals to discuss physical activity with patients.

WHAT IS POPULATION HEALTH?

Population health sits within the health improvement aspect of public health. Population health is the model of improving health outcomes within a defined population and has important implications for physical activity. It aims to reduce health inequalities and address the wider determinants of health by working in collaboration with communities, governments and healthcare providers. Population health recognises that these wider health determinants are associated with lifestyle, behaviours, social circumstances and environmental exposure. It extends beyond providing medical care, to improving the wellbeing of everyone within the population. This has implications for physical activity.

A population is, at its most simple, a group of people. Populations may be defined geographically, by identity, medical condition or disease risk factors. Individuals may belong to more than one population.

Increasingly, healthcare is focused on optimising patient care and outcomes at the population level. Collaboration can improve efficiency and reduce costs. Chronic conditions tend to be well suited to management at a population level because of the associations with lifestyle, behaviour and both social and environmental circumstances.

In the UK, demand on the National Health Service (NHS) continues to grow due to the increasing number of people needing NHS care and the intensity of support they require. In 2019, the NHS set out the Long-Term Plan. This places significant emphasis on the prevention of avoidable illness and population health as a strategy to improve overall healthcare. It takes a proactive approach to improving health by targeting cohorts of people rather than individuals. The Long-Term Plan aims to deliver interventions within the interaction of a patient and healthcare professional, such as health promotion, community engagement and risk factor modification. In this way, these patient contacts can be used as positive opportunities to help people to improve their health.

Table 19.1 The individual and population benefits of improving population health

Individual benefits	Population benefits
Reduced risk of long-term conditions	Supporting social inclusion
Better management of existing conditions	Reduced health inequalities
Maintaining physical and mental function	Reduced congestion
Maintain a healthy weight	Safer roads

Table 19.1 provides examples of the physical, mental and social benefits of improving individual and population health. Physical activity has important implications for how these benefits are derived.

By reframing society's perceptions of physical activity, more people can benefit from the improved physical and mental wellbeing, reduced stress, new motor skills, wider social networks and improved self-confidence that are associated with being physically active.

EPIDEMIOLOGY AND PHYSICAL ACTIVITY LEVELS

Physical inactivity has been recognised by the World Health Organisation as the fourth leading risk factor for mortality behind hypertension, smoking and high blood glucose. Physical inactivity is responsible for 6% of deaths globally. Physical inactivity is associated with a 30% increased risk of ischaemic heart disease, a 27% increased risk of type 2 diabetes and cancers, such as of the breast and colon.

The World Health Organisation (WHO) estimates that, globally, 81% of adolescents and 25% of adults do not do enough physical activity and up to 5 million deaths per year could be avoided if the global population was more active. People who do not meet physical activity requirements are at a 20–30% increased risk of death (WHO, 2022).

GLOBAL PHYSICAL ACTIVITY

Across the world, there are multiple organisations working to improve physical activity levels, such as WHO, ACSM and Exercise is Medicine. Another, is the International Society for Physical Activity and Health (ISPAH), which is the leading global society of researchers and practitioners focused on promoting physical activity across the lifetime. The Toronto Charter for Physical Activity: A Global Call for Action (ISPAH, 2022), was produced in 2010 to create sustainable opportunities to promote global physical activity. The charter was developed by 55 countries and launched out of the City of Toronto in 2010. It is an influential guiding document that "is a call for action and an advocacy tool to create sustainable opportunities for physically active lifestyles for all."

The Charter provided a framework for action across four key areas:

1. Implementing national policy and action plan
2. Introducing policies to support physical activity
3. Reorienting services and funding to prioritise physical activity
4. Developing partnerships for action

Within the charter, governments, professional associations, the private and voluntary sector, communities and academic institutions were all identified as stakeholders in improving access to physical activity.

Building on this work over the last decade, ISPAH, working with partners with international and national agencies to promote global health, have identified the eight most effective investments for increasing population physical activity:

1. Active travel/transport
2. Active urban design
3. Healthcare
4. Public education (including mass media)
5. Sport and recreation for all
6. Workplaces
7. Community-wide programmes
8. Whole-of-school programmes

In order to reverse the downward trend in physical activity, the government, local councils, schools, communities, voluntary and private sectors and professional bodies need to commit to a combination of these strategies aimed at populations as a whole.

World Health Organisation

The World Health Organisation (WHO) introduced the global recommendations for physical activity for health in 2010. This aimed to prevent noncommunicable diseases through physical activity at the population level.

Physical inactivity has negative impacts on health systems, the environment, economic development, community wellbeing and quality of life.

More recently, the 'WHO Global Action Plan on Physical Activity 2018–2030: more active people for a healthier world (GAPPA)', provides effective policies to increase physical activity (WHO, 2018). GAPPA recognises that progress to increase physical activity has been slow due to lack of awareness and investment. As countries develop economically, activity levels fall due to changing patterns of transport, urbanisation and reliance on technology. Often, the populations who could have the greatest benefit from being more physically active are those which have least access to being physically active. GAPPA recognises there are multiple opportunities and benefits to being more physically active and that digital innovations can promote physical activity across all age groups.

GAPPA's mission is to ensure all people have access to safe and enabling environments and to diverse opportunities to be physically active in their daily lives. In this way, physical activity can contribute to social, cultural and economic development globally, whilst improving individual and community health.

GAPPA aims to reduce the global prevalence of physical inactivity in adults and adolescents by 15% by 2030 through the creation of: a) active societies; b) active environments, by creating spaces within communities with equal access for people, and c) active systems, to implement physical activity and reduce sedentary behaviour.

Sedentary lifestyles have been increasing as a result of environmental changes. The urban design and infrastructure are key factors. Redesigning cities to promote active travel with provision of safe crossings, footpaths and cycle infrastructure, as well as open spaces and parks – to create safe environments for physical activity – can empower people to live healthier lives.

Improving school and workplaces – with the introduction of purposeful and incidental physical activity, along with spaces that promote active breaks – provides vital opportunities to increase activity. By incorporating physical activity into buildings' design, workspaces and schools can influence the opportunities and choice of users to change physical activity and sedentary behaviours, such as by taking the stairs or ramps rather than the lifts, using standing workstations or encouraging walking meetings.

A range of barriers, such as perceived lack of time, can also be overcome by thoughtful design and employer emphasis. Successful strategies include providing safe storage facilities for bicycles and showering facilities, to make active travel easier for employees.

Communities designed with mixed land use – involving the co-location of residential developments alongside shops, recreational facilities and schools – are paramount to reducing the reliance on car transport.

Changes to our work and leisure activity over the years has influenced society to be more sedentary. The Chief Medical Officer's Physical Activity Guidelines, discussed in the Physical Activity chapter, describe the minimum recommendations for health (Department of Health, 2019). However, it is widely accepted that there is a dose-response curve – any activity is deemed better than none. This reflects the importance of physical activity messaging that is both inclusive and which captures people who are working towards the optimal CMO physical activity guidelines. The CMO guidelines emphasise that every minute of physical activity matters; this should be reinforced, especially to the least active members of society. Whilst a global guideline for sedentary behaviour does not yet exist, the consensus is that it should be limited. This is recognised in the UK Chief Medical Officer's updated 2020 Physical Activity guideline.

International Olympic Committee

The International Olympic Committee (IOC) recognised the public health implications of physical inactivity at the 2009 Congress in Copenhagen. As a result, an expert group was formed in 2011, with the purpose of critically evaluating scientific evidence, identifying potential solutions and providing recommendations towards young people's physical activity levels.

The IOC has since collaborated with international federations, national Olympic committees, WHO, international physical activity networks, governments, non-government organisations, healthcare systems and the education sector to improve child and adolescent involvement in physical activity.

One example of how the IOC has collaborated with the Active Well-being Initiative, is the Global Active City programme (Active Well-being Initiative, 2018). This programme aims to recognise the implementation of the Global Active City management system; it has been successful in significantly improving the health of cities' inhabitants and increasing participation in physical activity. The Active Well-being Initiative includes standards, supporting tools and training modules to enable cities to enhance the well-being of their population.

Liverpool was the first IOC Active City in 2005 (Active Well-being, 2017). At the time, fewer than one in five occupants of the city exercised for 30 minutes three times per week. As part of the Active City programme, the profile of active living was increased – with mass media campaigns – and healthcare professionals were trained in the benefits of physical activity. There was improved coordination of existing services and, in consultation with local communities, collaborative groups highlighted new services that would provide the most benefit.

Whilst it is recognised that cities will have individual structure and culture, growing urbanisation and increasing sedentary lifestyles are universal. The Active City programme offers tools that can be adapted to the local challenges.

UK PA INITIATIVES AND ORGANISATIONS

Office for Health Improvement and Disparities

OHID (formerly Public Health England) is a government department within the Department for Health and Social Care. OHID focuses on improving the nation's health, reducing health inequalities and helping people to avoid preventable risk factors for ill-health. OHID is responsible for working with the NHS and local government to improve access to services which detect risks to health. They also act on the wider determinants of health, such as work, housing and education, through their partnerships across communities and employers.

Box 19.1 Clinical Considerations: OHID case study

PHYSICAL ACTIVITY CLINICAL CHAMPIONS (PACC)

The OHID PACC programme recruits healthcare professionals such as GPs, nurses and other allied health professionals to a championing role for PA. As part of the role, 'Champions' draw on their local networks and act as advocates for PA, including the provision of training and education to healthcare professionals. This training has increased the knowledge, confidence and regularity of brief interventions between health care professionals and patients. The PACC programme contract may be procured by a new provider in the near future. (Public Health England, 2018).

Within each of the UK's nations, the four national sports councils (Sport England, Sport Northern Ireland, Sport Scotland and Sport Wales) work to provide advice to local governments on sport and physical activity, support national governing bodies and distribute National Lottery Funding (Box 2).

Box 19.2–3 Clinical Considerations: National Governing Body case studies

SPORT ENGLAND STRATEGY

Sport England's mission is to invest in sport and physical activity and to incorporate it into a normal part of life for everyone in England. It receives funding from the National Lottery and the government in order to carry out its projects.

Uniting the Movement is the Sport England ten-year strategy, which runs from 2021–31 and aims to remove existing barriers to physical activity and address many of society's biggest challenges (Sport England, 2021). As England adapts and rebuilds from the disruption caused by the coronavirus pandemic, this strategy aims to use sport and physical activity to support the economy, reconnect communities and rebuild a stronger society. The pandemic has reinforced inequalities in accessing physical activity; Uniting the Movement aims to tackle this by removing barriers to the communities that have traditionally been left behind.

SPORT ENGLAND CAMPAIGNS

Three of Sport England's biggest campaigns include We Are Undefeatable, This Girl Can and Join the Movement.

- We Are Undefeatable was led by a collaboration of 15 health and social care charities and supported by Public Health England (now OHID) and Sport England (We are Undefeatable, 2023). It was designed to motivate people living with long term conditions to become active, in a way that works with each person's condition. By consulting the perspective and experience of those with long term conditions, We Are Undefeatable provides an opportunity to identify and address barriers to physical activity in those with long term conditions. We Are Undefeatable provides practical advice, online resources and community support to those living with long term conditions and empowers them to be physically active. appropriate to their individual circumstances.
- The This Girl Can campaign has been successful in empowering women and girls to be more physically active, regardless of shape, size and ability. Launched in 2015 by Sport England, the campaign celebrates active women and, so far, has inspired three million women to get active (This Girl Can, 2022). This Girl Can recognises there are multiple barriers to physical activity in females, including body image, fear of judgement and a perceived lack of time (due to family, study or work commitments). By using real life examples, This Girl Can empowers women and girls to put aside their fears and to get involved.
- Join the Movement was a campaign to inspire people to become active during the coronavirus pandemic, whilst at home. Since then, it has evolved into a platform to encourage physical activity both at and away from home.

UK PHYSICAL ACTIVITY INITIATIVES

The UK Chief Medical Officer's Guidelines for physical activity have been discussed in the Physical Activity chapter. When updating the guidelines, healthcare professionals have been identified as being important conduits to promoting physical activity (Mutrie et al., 2019) and more generally in the literature (Kime et al., 2020). There are several different projects that aim to support healthcare professionals in helping people become more active.

The Moving Healthcare Professionals is a national programme supporting healthcare professionals to increase their knowledge and ability to incorporate physical activity within routine care. Along with training healthcare professionals, through online modules (on Health Education England's e-learning for healthcare portal) and face-to-face training (by recruiting physical activity champions), Moving Medicine and Active Hospitals have been launched (Brannan et al., 2019).

Moving Medicine

Moving Medicine is an initiative by the Faculty of Sport and Exercise Medicine in partnership with Sport England, the Office for Health Improvement and Disparities, Sport Scotland, NHS Scotland, the British Association of Sport and Exercise Medicine and the Australasian College of Sport and Exercise Medicine (Faculty of Sport and Exercise Medicine, 2023). The initiative has established a collaborative relationship with a broad range of professional bodies and third sector organisations, as well as academic collaborations – with teams at the University of Bristol and Edinburgh.

Moving Medicine was established as part of the former PHE, now OHID. Sport England led the Moving Healthcare Professionals programme in response to the high levels of physical inactivity in the UK.

Physical inactivity is responsible for one in six UK deaths. 40% of long-term conditions could be prevented if everyone met the UK Chief Medical Officer's physical activity recommendations.

Moving Medicine aims to empower people to live active and healthy lifestyles by changing the way healthcare professionals approach physical activity conversations. They aim to integrate physical activity into everyday healthcare by improving the frequency and quality of conversations about physical activity.

Moving Medicine has consolidated the evidence for physical activity in the context of specific clinical conditions and developed a range of time orientated, easy-to-access, online resources for healthcare professionals to use with their patients. The resources were developed, following an extensive development process, to make the huge evidence base around physical activity accessible to all healthcare professionals. Consultation with healthcare professionals identified the most significant barriers to the provision of physical activity advice included lack of time, lack of clinician knowledge and perceived lack of success with changing patient behaviour. This informed the design of resources, structured on a behavioural change framework, to enable time-limited healthcare staff to build continuity through short interactions and provide effective solutions to consultation barriers.

Moving Medicine and the Faculty of Sport and Exercise Medicine aim to create a supportive environment for its contributors, integrating Moving Medicine into Sport and Exercise Medicine training, whilst maintaining and developing resources through evaluation and dissemination of information.

Active Hospitals

Active Hospitals is a Moving Medicine project that aims to change the physical activity culture within hospitals. Integrating movement into routine hospital care is thought to influence subsequent physical activity behaviours (Faculty of Sport and Exercise Medicine, 2023).

The online Active Hospital toolkit provides departments with resources, including staff training, risk management, governance, intervention templates and exercise programmes for patients. The toolkit provides information to support departments and hospital trusts applying to become an Active Hospital.

Box 19.4 Clinical Considerations: Active Hospitals case study

One of the successful Active Hospitals pilot programmes was in the Oxford University Hospital maternity department. Following analysis of clinical pathways and identifying opportunities to influence the capability, opportunity and motivations (see Figure 19.3) of pregnant women, multiple interventions were developed to increase physical activity in maternal care. Successful interventions included: embedding a physical activity calculator, with brief advice, into all booking visits; utilising motivational interviews for women with gestational diabetes; decorating the outpatient environment with posters, a promotional film and distributing new patient information leaflets. The physical activity calculator was successful in identifying women who did not meet the aerobic component of the Chief Medical Officer's physical activity in pregnancy recommendations. This allowed the cause of inactivity to be identified and helped women become more physically active.

SOCIAL AND CULTURAL ISSUES AFFECTING HEALTH IMPROVEMENT AND PHYSICAL ACTIVITY

The determinants of physical activity are widely influenced by environmental, social and cultural issues. Individuals may partake in physical activity because they are in good health and want to reduce stress, meet new people, manage their weight and for enjoyment. However, there may be barriers such as low motivation, perceived lack of time and fear of injury.

Initiatives have focused on addressing these social and cultural issues to design interventions to target key groups. One model frequently used to understand behaviour is the COM-B model, as outlined in Figure 19.3 (West and Michie, 2020). By modifying opportunity, capability or motivation, it may be possible to change behaviour.

Both capability and opportunity influence motivation and, whilst all three influence behaviour change, they are also influenced by the change which occurs. For example, a physically inactive individual may perceive they do not have the skills (capability) to partake in an exercise class. By being offered a free attendance to the class (opportunity), their attendance may allow them to realise they do have the capability required, which may motivate them to change their behaviour.

MULTIPLE CHOICE QUESTION (MCQ) QUESTIONS

1. You attend a lecture on population and public health. According to the World Health Organisation, which one of the following conditions contributes to the highest number of global deaths?

   A. Physical inactivity
   B. Unsafe water, sanitation and hygiene
   C. High cholesterol
   D. Hypertension
   E. Alcohol use

2. A 64-year-old patient comes to discuss her health habits with you following a myocardial infarction. She admits that her physical activity levels are low but is keen to try and improve this. She has been invited on to a hospital pilot scheme that involves a 12-week graded exercise programme to try and reduce the risk of another infarction. Which of the following terms best describes this public health intervention?

   A. Primary Prevention
   B. Secondary Prevention
   C. Tertiary Prevention
   D. Local Prevention
   E. Health Surveillance

3. You are learning more about Public Health in the UK. You try to identify ways to increase physical activity levels and consider a screening programme. The Office of Health Improvement and Disparities (OHID) is currently responsible for which of the following screening programmes?

   A. Prostate cancer
   B. Physical inactivity in Pregnancy
   C. Diabetic eye
   D. Lung cancer
   E. Newborn vision

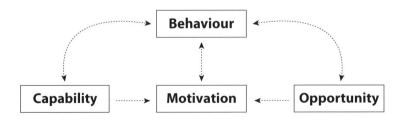

Figure 19.3 COM-B model of behaviour

4. You are trying to promote the importance of physical activity in your clinical practice. Which one of the following programmes or initiatives has been proven to increase knowledge of the UK Chief Medical Officer's physical activity guidelines, increase confidence in discussing physical activity with patients and increase the number of conversations with patients regarding physical activity?

   A. Uniting the Movement, Sport England strategy
   B. World Health Organisation Global Action Plan on Physical Activity (GAPPA)
   C. Physical Activity Clinical Champion (PACC)
   D. The Active Well-being Initiative
   E. The Toronto Charter for Physical Activity: A Global Call for Action

5. At a lecture you attend, you are informed that more people in the South of England meet the recommended physical activity guidelines compared with people living in the North West of England. What is this an example of?

   A. Health inequality
   B. Health commissioning
   C. Social Norm
   D. Screening
   E. Health needs assessment

MULTIPLE CHOICE QUESTION (MCQ) ANSWERS

1. Answer D
   Hypertension is the leading cause of global deaths according to the WHO and is even greater than physical activity (A) and the other suggested causes.

2. Answer B
   This is an example of secondary prevention, with the aim of reducing the impact of a disease that has already occurred. Primary prevention (A) aims to prevent a disease before it occurs e.g. legislation to ban smoking. Tertiary prevention (C) has a focus on softening the impact of an existing disease, such as initial cardiac rehabilitation in this case. Local prevention is action taken on

a community-based level (D) and E is a process of monitoring health.

3. Answer C
   Diabetic eye screening is one of the two adult screening programmes. Newborn hearing is screened, not vision (E). Physical inactivity does not form part of the antenatal programmes (B) and neither Prostate or lung cancer currently have screening programmes.

4. Answer C
   The Physical Activity Clinical Champion (PACC) programme has been independently evaluated by the National Centres' for Sport and Exercise Medicine. This showed that training was successful in the listed outcomes in the question stem.

5. Answer A
   This describes an example of a health inequality: a difference in health experienced by different groups that are avoidable and unacceptable.

FURTHER READING AND REFERENCES

Active Well-being Initiative, 2017. Liverpool: a pioneer city walks the talk. Available from: http://activewellbeing.org/wp-content/uploads/2017/09/OR103-ACTIVE-CITIES-EN.pdf

Active Well-being Initiative, 2018. Global active city label. Available from: http://activewellbeing.org/global-active-city/

Brannan, M., Bernardotto, M., Clarke, N. and Varney, J., 2019. Moving healthcare professionals–a whole system approach to embed physical activity in clinical practice. *BMC medical education*, *19*(1), pp.1-7.

Department of Health (2019) A report from the Chief Medical Officers in the UK on the amount and type of physical activity people should be doing to improve their health. Available from: https://www.gov.uk/government/publications/physical-activity-guidelines-uk-chief-medical-officers-report

Faculty of Sport and Exercise Medicine, 2023. Moving Medicine. Available from: https://movingmedicine.ac.uk

Faculty of Sport and Exercise Medicine, 2023. Moving Medicine – Active Hospitals. Available from: https://movingmedicine.ac.uk/active-hospitals/

Kime, N., Pringle, A., Zwolinsky, S. et al. 2020. How prepared are healthcare professionals for delivering physical activity guidance to those with diabetes? A formative evaluation. *BMC Health Serv Res* 20, 8. https://doi.org/10.1186/s12913-019-4852-0

Moving Medicine—The ultimate resource to help healthcare professionals integrate physical activity conversations into routine clinical care. https://movingmedicine.ac.uk.

Mutrie, N., Standage, M., Pringle, A.R., Laventure, R., Smith, L., Strain, T., Dall, P., Milton, K., Ruane, S., Chalkley, A. and Colledge, N., 2019. Expert Working Group Working Paper Communication and Surveillance UK physical activity guidelines: developing options for future communication and surveillance.

Sport England, 2021. Uniting the Movement. Available from: https://www.sportengland.org/about-us/uniting-movement

The International Society for Physical Activity and Health, 2022. Key Resources. Available from: https://ispah.org/resources/key-resources/

This Girl Can, 2022. This Girl Can. Available from: https://www.thisgirlcan.co.uk

UK Government, 2023. Population Screening programmes: detailed information. [Online]. Available from: https://www.gov.uk/topic/population-screening-programmes

UK Government, 2023. NHS Health Checks: applying All Our Health. [Online]. Available from: https://www.gov.uk/government/publications/nhs-health-checks-applying-all-our-health/nhs-health-checks-applying-all-our-health

We are Undefeatable, 2023. We are Undefeatable. Available from: https://weareundefeatable.co.uk

West, R and Michie, S. 2020. A brief introduction to the COM-B Model of behaviour and the PRIME Theory of motivation. Qeios. doi:10.32388/WW04E6.

World Health Organization, 2018. Global action plan on physical activity 2018-2030: more active people for a healthier world. Geneva: World Health Organization. Available from: https://apps.who.int/iris/bitstream/handle/10665/272722/9789241514187-eng.pdf

World Health Organization, 2022. Physical Activity. Geneva: World Health Organization. Available from: https://www.who.int/news-room/fact-sheets/detail/physical-activity

Psychosocial Aspects of Sport and Exercise Medicine **20**

James W. Burger and Allan Johnston

BEHAVIOUR CHANGE

Helping patients increase their physical activity, and reduce sedentary behaviour, requires finding effective ways to motivate the individual in front of you. Motivation is represented by the direction, origin, intensity, and persistence of behaviours. Finding out *why* patients act in a certain way is central to helping them find power to change. Working collaboratively with the patient, and acknowledging their place in the process of change, may help reduce resistance.

Self-Determination Theory: suggests personal growth and self-actualisation are what motivates people to change. It highlights the importance of intrinsic motivation and that people are driven by competence, autonomy, and social relatedness. Behaviour regulation can occur through external (controlled) regulation or autonomous regulation. External motivation may include punishment or rewards.

Transtheoretical Model of Behaviour Change: behaviour change is a process with many different stages of change. These stages are precontemplation, contemplation, preparation, action, and maintenance, with or without relapse. Identifying the stage of change can allow appropriate engagement in readiness to change.

Social-Cognitive Theory: behaviour is driven by our intentions and beliefs based on our values, expectations, and learnings from our social context. We learn about consequences of behaviours through our experiences and relationships with others.

Dual-Process Theory: behaviour is influenced by both automatic processes and deliberate reflective processes.

Clinical Considerations—Promoting Behaviour Change in the Individual

Using a collaborative, person-centred approach can emphasise autonomy. It is important to understand the context of the behaviour and what motivates the behaviour. Supportive interactions can promote change talk, as well as shifting confidence, knowledge, and attitudes toward physical activity.

- Motivational Interviewing techniques can be useful in eliciting ideas about change and encouraging change talk. Use open-ended questions, affirmations, reflections and summaries (OARS).
- Expressing empathy, supporting self-efficacy and rolling with resistance are important. It may be helpful to include a focus on short-term benefits of affect regulation, rather than only the long-term benefits of physical activity.
- Exploring acceptable and sustainable options for physical activity, using likes and preferences.
- Finding ways to maximise enjoyment and pleasure, which promotes repetition. Prioritise exercise in leisure time and make use of active transport, as these may be more personally meaningful and enjoyable.
- Pre-emptively identifying barriers may help mitigate problems. Help patients prioritise self-care, where they give themselves permission to safeguard time for exercise. Help manage comorbid illnesses or physical ailments that may be barriers. Manage *social physique anxiety* (anxiety about judgement from others). Promoting sport for self-discovery and relationships seems to retain patients in sport more than through performance narratives.

DOI: 10.1201/9781003179979-20

PSYCHOSOCIAL ASPECTS OF SEM

Behaviour change

Transtheoretical model

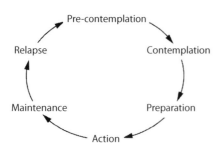

Testing

- SMHAT-1 - IOC sport mental health assessment tool
- SMHRT-1 - IOC sport mental health recognition tool
- BDSA - Baron depression screener for athletes
- POMS - Profile of mood states

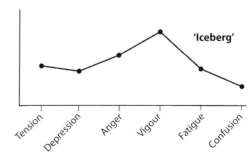

Physical activity

Neurobiological effects
- ↓ Serotonin/noradrenaline reuptake
- ↑ Growth factors
- ↑ Endorphins
- ↑ Endocannabinoid signalling
- ↓ Stress

Psychosocial effects
- Distraction
- Pleasure
- Excitement
- Social connection
- Self-actualisation

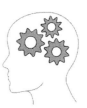

Arousal

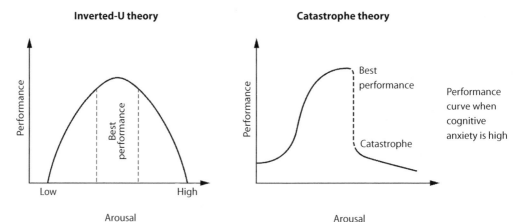

Figure 20.1 Pictorial chapter overview.

Creating an Environment Which Supports Behaviour Change

Occupational, leisure, transport and household contexts should be reviewed for opportunities to include physical activity and reduce sedentary behaviours. Developing prompts and reminders, establishing active workstations, regular breaks and walking meetings can be useful. Ensure adequate equipment and facilities (or safe low-cost alternatives at home) and establish social support and connection with others who are increasing their physical activity, such as through organised sports. Youth may also need a supportive environment and encouragement to be physically active in a developmentally appropriate way.

PSYCHOLOGICAL EFFECTS OF PHYSICAL ACTIVITY

Physical activity has been shown to reduce stress, improve mood, self-esteem, feelings of well-being, cognition and brain plasticity, improve sleep quality and reduce depression and anxiety symptoms. These effects are likely due to multiple mechanisms, which can be grouped broadly as neurobiological effects and psychosocial effects.

Neurobiological Effects

- Neurotransmitter effects—prevent reuptake of serotonin and noradrenaline
- Release of growth factors, e.g. brain-derived neurotrophic factor (BDNF), with neurogenesis in key brain areas, such as the hippocampus
- Endorphin release
- Endocannabinoid signalling
- Reduced inflammation and oxidative stress
- Reduced stress response through Hypothalamic-Pituitary-Adrenal axis
- Epigenetic changes

Psychosocial Effects

- *Cognitive-behavioural effects:* distraction from rumination and from negative affect, with increased positive thoughts and feelings. Exposure to pleasurable experiences, fun, interest, and activities of value. Feelings of physical well-being and improved perceived fitness and body image. Reduced feelings of worthlessness and hopelessness. Excitement of competition.
- *Self-actualising:* feeling challenged, with a sense of achievement, autonomy, and mastery. Physical activity may involve learning new skills or self-improvement.
- *Social connectedness:* enhancing social support, creating social interaction and connection, making friends, having a sense of belonging.

Mood-Enhancing Physical Activity

Physical activity may be particularly beneficial for mood when it is outdoors, involves social connection (e.g. team sport) and is repeatable, with the individual feeling intrinsically motivated and challenged, enjoying the activity, having a sense of achievement and the opportunity to learn new skills.

EXERCISE AS MEDICINE IN PSYCHIATRY

Behavioural Activation

Behavioural activation aims to improve depressive symptoms by increasing engagement with positive stimuli and promoting approach behaviour rather than avoidant behaviour. Together with the patient, activities that increase pleasure or mastery, such as types of physical activity, are identified. Breaking down activities into their components can ease initiation of the activity and progressive completion. This technique involves realistic goal-setting, with routines and scheduled activities.

Prescribing Exercise for Mental Disorders

Exercise is now one of the first-line, evidence-based treatments for people with depression, without the side-effects and stigma of medication (NICE Guidance, 2009). Most of the evidence is for aerobic exercise of at least moderate intensity. Aerobic exercise at the recommended intensity and frequency of public health guidelines has been shown to be effective for treatment of mild to moderate major depressive disorder. There is a moderate effect in reducing anxiety symptoms. Resistance training shows promise. Yoga and tai chi integrate physical activity with meditation and deep breathing, techniques which have their own evidence in mental disorders. Walking also has growing evidence to support its use in mental health management and may be useful for older populations. Supervised exercise interventions under the guidance of exercise professionals have shown larger benefits on symptoms.

Beyond the affective benefits of exercise, there are pro-cognitive effects in dementia and possibly chronic psychotic illnesses. Sustained exercise during the midlife period helps prevent dementia predominantly through lower cardiovascular risk, obesity, and diabetes. Depression and social isolation are also risk factors for dementia, which exercise may minimise.

The exercise programme should include aerobic, resistance, flexibility and neuromotor exercises, with patient readiness assessed using behaviour change principles. Using the frequency, intensity, time and type (FITT) principles as a framework for prescribing exercise may be helpful. The aim is to make the programme accessible to improve confidence and adherence. Patients with mental disorders may benefit from starting slowly, particularly with previous inactivity or if motivation is a challenge. Starting slowly also limits the injuries which may be particularly impactful in the context of a negative cognitive bias.

Managing Physical Health of Patients with Mental Disorders

Those with mental disorders are at higher risk of physical ill-health and higher mortality. This is only in part due to modifiable lifestyle factors, including smoking, diet and physical activity. Psychotropic medications often have significant cardiometabolic, endocrine and neuromotor side effects. Many promote weight gain and the development of metabolic syndrome. Physical activity can help mitigate the predicted weight gain and insulin resistance and promote bone health. Side-effects, such as postural hypotension, may bring potential safety risks, which require tailoring of exercise programmes.

People with severe mental disorders may be less proactive in health-seeking behaviours. Those with mental disorders are also more likely to be stigmatised by healthcare professionals and receive a lower standard of care. This includes less frequent screening for physical conditions, diagnostic overshadowing (attributing their physical symptoms to their mental disorder), hesitancy in providing treatments, as well as these patients being overlooked for health programmes. Providing equitable access to supervised exercise programmes is imperative when they are available.

SPORTS PERFORMANCE: MOTIVATION, AROUSAL AND ATTENTION

Motivation and Goal-Setting

Much of the research into motivation in athletes is based on self-determination theory, placing emphasis on the motivating drive of autonomous goals, competency, and social relatedness. Many athletes may begin sport with high levels of intrinsic motivation (e.g. enjoyment and passion for their sport), although not all will retain this as their core motivation.

Motivation and performance may benefit from clear and appropriate goal-setting. Goal-setting involves identifying and defining explicit targets, priorities and expectations. Setting appropriate goals can improve focus on current tasks and reduce distractions; energise the athlete for the task according to the degree of challenge; organise the efforts of the athlete; keep the athlete accountable; and encourage them to persevere, as well as promote relevant learning and a sense of mastery. Goals should ideally be included in both training and competition.

Outcome goals are targets based on the end results of a task and generally involve external comparisons. These tend to have a binary outcome such as winning or gaining a medal. *Performance goals* are targets based on the end results of an action achieved independently by the athlete, such as scoring a goal or a certain number of points.

Process goals are targets for specific behaviours the athlete will aim to execute during the performance, such as technique, participating in a named number of training sessions in the week, or focusing on a particular attentional cue. Process goals are most effective at promoting better performance and having a multi-goal strategy is usually best. A useful technique for setting goals is using SMART goals (or SMARTER goals).

- *Specific:* clear and precise.
- *Measurable:* able to be quantified, such as comparative to an athlete's previous performance.
- *Accepted:* by all relevant parties.
- *Realistic:* they need to be achievable for the athlete.
- *Time-limited:* explicit time point for achieving the goal.
- *Exciting:* challenging and rewarding goals.
- *Recorded:* need to be documented.

Arousal

Arousal is the level of activation or psychological readiness a person experiences when facing a task. Identifying and maintaining the optimal level of arousal for peak performance can help athletes achieve success. With low arousal, the performance is likely to be suboptimal for sports performance. However, too much arousal can be a barrier. The inverted-U curve visually depicts how levels of arousal that are too low and too high can both be detrimental (Yerkes-Dodson Law). Arousal can then be regulated through arousal reducing and arousal promoting techniques to move up and down the performance curve.

However, the relationship between arousal and performance is more complex, which different theories aim to capture. In the catastrophe model, there is a smooth inverted-U curve for physiological arousal and performance when there is low cognitive anxiety, but this is not the case when there is a high cognitive anxiety. At higher cognitive anxiety, there is a steady increase in performance until a point where there is a catastrophic drop-off, from which it is difficult to down-regulate.

Individual Zone of Optimal Functioning theory suggests moderate arousal and anxiety is not necessarily the ideal for performance. There is an optimum level of pre-competitive state anxiety (or other emotions) for each individual and task, with a zone of optimal functioning where athletes try to place themselves.

Flow state refers to total absorption in an activity with a state of consciousness that results in optimal functioning. It is an autotelic type of experience, where participating in the activity is the purpose in itself. The athlete participates in an intrinsically interesting activity, challenging them at a level matching their ability. Awareness merges with the action, often without an awareness of time. There are clear goals, a sense of control and the athlete receives unambiguous feedback.

Attention

Athletes, like the rest of us, have only limited attentional resources. The ability to attend selectively to stimuli is key to performance, with athletes deciding on which cues to focus. Otherwise, athletes can have their attention overloaded or be unable to shift their attention to relevant cues. Attention can be conceptualised as either having a broad or narrow width, with internal or external direction.

Broad-internal focus involves looking at a wide variety of inward cues, such as using thoughts and feelings to plan for the game ahead.

Broad-external focus places a wide focus external to the athlete, such as paying attention to where teammates and opposition players are on the field.

Narrow-internal focus involves a small number of internal cues, such as when visualising the specific components of an upcoming movement.

Narrow-external focus places focus on a specific external cue or small number of cues, such as returning a serve in tennis.

Learning new skills may require a narrow internal focus on the components of the skill. The skill becomes more automatic with training and experience. However, when under duress or suffering from a loss of confidence, the focus of high-level performers may narrow to the individual motor actions involved in the skill, where flow may be disrupted and external cues missed, negatively affecting performance.

Redirection of attention can help athletes cope with challenging exercise. *Association* focuses attention fully on the activity, whilst *dissociation* focuses attention away from the activity using distraction techniques. Dissociation can potentially reduce unpleasantness with strenuous exercise by distracting from discomfort or pain. However, it could potentially also be less motivating from a mastery and self-actualisation perspective. Using both associative and dissociative strategies may be useful.

STRESS IN ATHLETES

What Is Stress?

Stress is a process where there are physiological and emotional responses to stimuli. Stress can be viewed as a transaction between demands and resources. Stress will naturally occur when these stimuli are interpreted as taking or exceeding personal resources and may affect well-being. The relevance of the stimulus is assessed together with the perceived ability to cope, weighing up the extent of personal control, available coping resources, and perceived probability of effectiveness.

Stressful stimuli occur as one of the four *transactional alternatives*. *Challenge*: athlete perceives that their available resources and extent of control allow for them to cope with demand and they may gain from the situation. *Threat*: athlete perceives that personal resources are outweighed by demand. *Benefit*: athlete perceives that there has already been gain. *Harm*: athlete perceives there has already been harm.

Stressors in Athletes

Although not mutually exclusive, stressors can be personal, competitive, and organisational. Athletes are people first. They may have *personal stressors*, such as daily hassles, relationship conflict, financial difficulties, or dealing with bereavement or trauma. Athletes may also display personality traits like perfectionism, which can become maladaptive when combined with high levels of self-criticism. *Competitive stressors* include demands directly from performance, such as injury, underperformance, retirement, chronic joint pain, and major competition. Both failure and success can place strain on available resources. Athletes may struggle with managing pressure, feelings of emptiness, uncertainty about future goals, and post-competition dysphoria even when achieving. *Organisational stressors* are system demands from functioning within a larger organisation, such as team dynamics, psychological climate, bullying and harassment, leadership issues, or logistic issues.

Overtraining

Functional overreaching requires a balance between training and recovery to prevent Overtraining Syndrome (OTS), where the athlete experiences chronic maladaptation to stressors and performance decline. This burnout process results in symptoms of fatigue, apathy, depressed mood, anxiety, insomnia, poor concentration, appetite changes and weight loss. Depression in athletes shares many features with OTS and is found commonly in athletes with OTS.

Injury and Rehabilitation

Injury is often highly significant for athletes and is a risk factor for increased stress, mental health symptoms and disorders. Stress can also, itself, result in higher risk of injury. Stress causes physiological changes (e.g. increased muscle tension) and can affect attention, with attentional narrowing and distractibility. Emotional responses to injury can be varied and may fluctuate. Adherence to rehabilitation programmes requires sustained effort and motivation. Athletes may have a smoother return to play if they use available social support and psychological coping skills rather than avoidant coping and risky behaviour. The injury event may be personally traumatic and lead to acute stress disorder or post-traumatic stress disorder, which reinforce avoidance. There may be the emergence or relapse of substance misuse or eating disorders. Depression may also affect rehabilitation if not identified. At times, the secondary gains of being injured can be a barrier to recovery. Social support should be provided through the different phases of rehabilitation, from injury onset through to return to play. It can take the form of emotional support, self-esteem support, information and guidance, and tangible or physical support. SEM clinicians play a key role.

Sport-related concussion is an injury that requires particular attention from a mental health perspective. Concussion may present with various cognitive, affective, sleep, and physical symptoms. There can be persistent symptoms, difficulties with functional return to work or study, mental health symptoms, and long-term complications of concussion. Repeated concussions have been linked with depression, cognitive impairment, and suicide in later life.

Trauma, Harassment and Abuse

Trauma is the response to a highly stressful event that causes harm and overwhelms the ability to cope. Traumatic events can include accidents and injuries, sexual harassment and abuse, acts of violence, or natural disasters. Sexual exploitation by coaches and health practitioners can take advantage of power imbalances and trust. Organisations need to safeguard athletes, with clear channels for dealing with incidents when they occur.

Career Transitions

Any change can be a stressor, but career termination and transitions are peak times for stress. Sudden retirement due to injury or being cut from the team can be particularly challenging. Organisations and athlete entourage should educate athletes about career transitions and help manage these challenges proactively. Athletes with adequate coping skills, social support and planning for retirement may transition more easily. Developing personal management skills throughout their career can assist with maintaining a daily structure, financial management, and decision making after retirement. Adaptation to their next life phase depends on the extent of their athletic identity and whether they have developed other aspects of their identity. Organisations should aim to develop rounded athletes and encourage them to broaden their social identity. Collegiate athletes may also have difficulties in transition out of college sport. Exploring aspirations and discussing life beyond sport early may help athletes cope.

Athletes with Disabilities

Paralympians may find career transitions particularly challenging due to a more significant change in their social identity and perceived value by others, from celebrated elite athlete to a person with a disability. These athletes also have the additional pressure to be inspirational for others. Although shifting other stereotypes, the 'Supercrip' narrative may reinforce that these athletes have tragedies to overcome and imply that they can only be viewed as valuable if they achieve extraordinary goals.

SPORT PERFORMANCE: COPING STRATEGIES

Coping strategies can be *problem-focused* or *emotion-focused*. Encourage athletes to check the facts about the situation so they can challenge their automatic judgements. When an athlete's emotions are appropriate for the facts, the situation is the problem. *Problem-focused coping strategies* aim to remove or adjust the environmental stimulus causing the stress, by selecting the situations in which they place themselves or modifying them. If the emotion does not fit the situation, *emotion-focused coping strategies* may help regulate intense emotions and reduce stress. Various techniques can help redirect attention, reframe cognitive interpretations of the situation, or regulate responses. Coping through an *avoidant coping style* (e.g. distraction, removing oneself for a period) may provide temporary relief from distress. However, an *approach coping style* may be necessary for longer term solutions.

There are psychological skills which can be taught, to manage athletes' thoughts, emotions, or physiological arousal. Psychological skills training requires skills education, acquisition, and practice. Skills do not easily transfer to different situations and generalising skills may require explicit encouragement and practice.

Reflective Practice

Identifying the best strategies and skills for managing stress and performance requires purposeful reflection. This can identify benefits and barriers to performance (such as negative automatic thoughts, hyperarousal, or being fixated on mistakes). Recording thoughts, feelings and the effects of behaviours in a journal can be useful for identifying patterns and the best way forward.

Useful Psychological Skills

Self-talk: the inner dialogue of a person, which can be in the form of thoughts or spoken words. Self-talk happens organically but can also be performed strategically to reframe negative thoughts, focus attention, or adjust arousal levels. Positive, instructional and motivational self-talk may be particularly useful for performance.

Imagery/visualisation: purposefully creating an experience in the mind using memories, thoughts, mental images, senses and emotions. These could be visual (seeing the images) or kinaesthetic (feeling the movement). Some athletes may be better at imagining their internal experience rather than the external experience, or vice versa.

Breathing exercises: deep, slow breathing can aid relaxation and reduce arousal, such as through diaphragmatic breathing exercises.

Progressive muscle relaxation: progressively shifting focus between muscle groups as the athlete tenses, then relaxes, each group. This aids relaxation and a better sense of control over muscle tension.

Biofeedback: measurements of physiological variables, such as heart rate, give feedback on the body's response to breathing and relaxation techniques. This helps athletes learn more about their body and better control of their physiological variables.

Meditation: meditation is a practice of awareness and focusing the mind. Mindfulness is the awareness that arises by bringing attention to the present experience, on purpose and without attachment or judgement. Mindfulness has similarities with other performance concepts in athletes like flow state. Mindfulness training may help athletes to develop their selective attention and be fully present in their activity.

Routines and Rituals: may help focus attention on the task. Routines may be easier to implement during the performance in self-paced sports (e.g. golf), or at specific times in other sports (e.g. penalties in football).

Music: pre-task music can be used as part of a ritual or to adjust arousal. Music can aid as a dissociative strategy and can be comforting.

Sleep hygiene: sleep has a role in performance, recovery, training adaptations, and quality of life. General advice includes: trying to create a routine for sleep with consistent bed times; winding down; creating a suitable environment (e.g. cool, dark and quiet); using the bed only for sleep (or sex); avoiding lying in bed if not sleepy; exercising regularly (ideally, not just before bed); exposure to morning natural light; switching off electronic devices at night; limiting caffeine, alcohol, and heavy meals close to bed time; and limiting naps if struggling with sleep. However, athletes may need to supplement their limited opportunity for sleep through naps to improve their mood, alertness, and cognition prior to performance. If athletes choose to nap, it is best to limit the duration to under 30 minutes, at an appropriate time. Athletes may also need to plan for predicted shortages of sleep and consider 'banking' sleep. Sleep monitors may aggravate sleep anxiety in some athletes, so they should be used with caution.

SPORT PERFORMANCE: TEAM DYNAMICS

Teams interact with each other and depend on each other to reach shared goals. They identify as their own separate entity, with a social structure of norms and roles. When conflict and divisions are managed, heterogeneous and culturally diverse groups may outperform more homogenous groups as they can draw on more varied resources. Groups tend to progress through various stages: *forming* (independent participants with superficial engagement), *storming* (conflict arises), *norming* (resolving conflict), *performing* (established roles and norms, clear leadership, autonomy in decisions) and *adjourning* (separation or ending of team/season). Teamwork involves preparation, execution, evaluation and adjustment phases.

Team cohesion is the tendency of a team to continue to operate as a unit to pursue their goals. It is a dynamic process made of two independent components: *task cohesion* and *social cohesion*. Task cohesion is the extent to which teammates work together to reach a goal. Social cohesion is the extent to which teammates enjoy being teammates. Team cohesion can be influenced by team size, individual player satisfaction and leadership. Team cohesion may be developed by promoting mastery orientation, creating spaces where teammates get to know each other personally, developing an awareness of the roles of other players, promoting pride within subgroups of large teams, avoiding social cliques, focusing on self-comparisons and avoiding jealousy, encouraging cooperation through team drills, encouraging ownership, setting goals and celebrating areas of success—even in loss. Positive perception of a player's or coach's role in a team depends on the role clarity, beliefs about self-efficacy, role satisfaction and role acceptance.

Coaching aims to help players develop and perform. Psychosocial coaching highlights the importance of psychological and social factors driving the technical, tactical and physical aspects of coaching. Coaches' behaviours and interpersonal style can impact a team's psychological climate. The TARGET framework aims to reduce social comparison and encourage a mastery-oriented climate, which may help foster a positive psychological climate.

- *Task:* The tasks should be challenging, varied, and promote self-referenced goals.
- *Authority:* Players should play an active role in their development and make meaningful autonomous decisions.

- *Recognition*: Appropriate individual feedback on progress and effort.
- *Grouping*: Breaking into heterogeneous groups for tasks.
- *Evaluation*: Feedback is mastery-oriented and self-referenced.
- *Time*: Allow flexibility so all ability levels can master the task.

MENTAL HEALTH SYMPTOMS AND DISORDERS

The World Health Organisation defines *mental health* as 'a state of well-being in which an individual realises his or her own abilities, can cope with the normal stresses of life, can work productively and is able to make a contribution to his or her community' (WHO, 2022). It makes up a core part of health—there is no health without mental health. Mental health lies across a spectrum from being mentally healthy to having a mental disorder.

Mental health symptoms are self-reported negative thoughts, feelings, or behaviours that may cause distress and impact on functioning.

Mental disorders are clinically diagnosed according to diagnostic criteria and cause significant distress or functional impairment.

Untreated mental disorders, like depression, can have a performance impact, injury risk, morbidity through suffering and functional impairment, and mortality risk—such as through suicide.

Common Mental Disorders in Athletes

Elite athletes have similar prevalence rates to the general population for most mental disorders. In addition to general risk factors like adverse life events, there are unique demands on elite athletes. There may be periods which present a higher risk for mental health symptoms, such as following injury or concussion, high profile losses, career transitions, and with overtraining.

Athletes can commonly have depression, anxiety, sleep problems, alcohol use, and eating disorders. Athletes may present atypically when it comes to depression, with more prominent irritability, apathy toward training, loss in pleasure of competing, or substance use. Eating disorders may occur more commonly in sports with weight classes or when being lean may be an advantage. ADHD may be more common in athletes because of the attraction to fast-paced physical activity.

Athletes may use substances for performance benefits, recreational use or due to substance use disorders. SEM clinicians can identify these issues to assist athletes before they suffer long-term consequences. Other forms of behavioural addictions are also reported in athletes, such as gambling disorder and exercise dependence.

Barriers to Help-Seeking

Athletes may not access help for their mental health problems for many reasons. Low mental health literacy can result in athletes not being aware of symptoms, having limited insight into the benefits of seeking help, or not knowing how to access help (Gorczynski et al., 2021). Stigma is still common, both in terms of self-stigma and public stigma. Athletes may have concerns over the consequences of seeking help, such as confidentiality or impact on team selection.

Organisations and coaches can encourage help-seeking through education and normalising emotional expression and mental health conversations. Mobilising social support and role modelling behaviour, through player leadership, may assist help-seeking. Clear channels to access familiar mental health professionals confidentially can reduce potential barriers.

Identifying Athletes Who May Need Help

Mental health symptoms may be recognised by the athlete themselves or any of the athlete family or entourage. The International Olympic Committee has developed the *IOC Sport Mental Health Recognition Tool-1 (SMHRT-1)* (Gouttebarge et al., 2021) to identify experiences that may suggest mental health problems. The *IOC Sport Mental Health Assessment Tool-1 (SMHAT-1)* was developed for use by health professionals and is validated for elite athletes. The SMHAT-1 triages athletes by screening for psychological distress using the Athlete Psychological Strain Questionnaire. If screening positively, this is followed by disorder-specific screening tools and clinical assessment. Diagnosis of mental disorders requires clinical assessment by a trained health professional.

Management Principles

Assessment should be confidential. Performing an adequate risk assessment is imperative, including explicit enquiry of suicidal ideation and warning signs. Managing acute risk is a priority. SEM clinicians who have sufficient experience in managing mental disorders may be the primary practitioner. However, appropriate referral to a specialist in athlete mental health may be required.

Psychoeducation may help the athlete make autonomous decisions about treatment options. First-line management of mental disorders in athletes is generally non-pharmacological with counselling or psychotherapy, unless the athlete has a moderate to severe disorder. Return-to-play decisions require balancing the benefits of participation, exercise and social support, with athlete safety (Reardon et al., 2019).

When prescribing medication, the choice is particularly important in athletes. Prior to initiating medication, prescribers must carefully consider the physiological effects. Medications that cause sedation, weight gain, tremors, and cardiac effects can have deleterious effects on performance. Practitioners need to be ethical, ensuring there are no unfair ergogenic effects from medication, beyond return to normal functioning. Applying for a Therapeutic Use Exemption through the World Anti-Doping Agency should be done if there are no appropriate choices with fewer performance effects.

Mental Health Emergency Action Plans

To safeguard the mental health of their athletes and act in accordance with their duty of care, sports organisations should develop a formal, documented Mental Health Emergency Action Plan (MHEAP). This policy document would include definitions of mental health emergencies, emergency contact details, and a comprehensive outline of the procedures with named role-players. There must be adequate training of stakeholders and rehearsal of the MHEAP implementation.

PSYCHOLOGICAL AND PSYCHOMETRIC TESTING

Psychometrics broadly refers to the measurement of psychological constructs. In sports, these measures have been used to try to predict performance. However, they can be controversial in their application. There are numerous athlete-specific and general population tools that are used to measure psychological constructs in athletes.

Psychometric testing can include screening tools for mental health symptoms, such as the SMHART-1 and Baron Depression Screener for Athletes (BDSA). The Profile of Mood States (POMS) assesses the transient mood states, namely tension, depression, anger, vigour, fatigue and confusion. A typical 'iceberg' profile has been described in athletes. The iceberg profile shows athletes being low in the negative mood states and high in vigour.

Psychometric testing can be used to describe personality traits of athletes, using personality inventories. Personality can be defined as individual differences in characteristics of thoughts, feelings, and behaviours, which endure and are relatively stable over a person's life. Theories of personality development include psychodynamic theory and trait theory. The Five Factor Model of Personality describes the 'Big Five' traits: Extraversion, Neuroticism, Conscientiousness, Openness, and Agreeableness. Within each trait, there is a spectrum. Psychometrics of personality may be assessed through projective measures and structured questionnaires. The NEO—Five Factor Personality Inventory measures the 'Big Five' traits. Athletes often differ from other populations in their personality profiles on these measures, but there is variation among athletes and across different sports. Athletes tend to be higher in extraversion and conscientiousness and lower in neuroticism. Perfectionism is another trait that is common in athlete populations, which can be positive or maladaptive. Data are conflicting about the ability to separate skill levels of athletes according to personality traits.

CLINICAL CONSIDERATIONS

Medical support staff are in a unique position to destigmatise mental health support, make initial assessments and management plans, and determine when specialist input is advisable. While it may be tempting to shy away from discussing mental health with athletes, perhaps due to inexperience or uncertainty, the only way to become more comfortable is through experience and training. Consider accessing further training in mental health, as managing athletes holistically is essential in SEM. Become acquainted with the local sports psychiatrists and sport psychologists for complex cases, advice, and referrals.

Clinicians must equip themselves with the knowledge and skills to motivate at-risk and general populations to exercise. Behaviour change is a process. Be curious about the experience of your patient and trust the process.

With exercise having a primary role in the management of patients with common mental disorders, a robust understanding of mental health is required to be able to prescribe exercise appropriately in this cohort. There is no health without mental health.

MULTIPLE CHOICE QUESTION (MCQ) QUESTIONS

1. A 34-year-old male with newly diagnosed diabetes has come to see you on request of their partner. He is interested in incorporating more physical activity into his leisure time. According to Self-Determination Theory, one of the most powerful motivators for him to become more physically active would include:

   A. Text message reminders of the potential negative effects of physical inactivity
   B. Monetary rewards for physical activity goals completed
   C. Regular praise and approval by the doctor
   D. Goals identified by the patient
   E. Competition with a neighbour

2. A 28-year-old archer became shaky and restless in the gold medal match at the Olympics. They tried their usual routines and breathing techniques. However, they found these to be ineffective on this occasion, leading to underperformance. Which best represents the relationship depicted in the Catastrophe model?

   A. An inverted U-shape depicts the relationship between arousal and performance
   B. An autotelic experience results in optimal functioning
   C. The relationship between arousal and performance is unpredictable
   D. Each individual has a zone of optimal functioning

   E. High cognitive anxiety changes the relationship between arousal and performance

3. A 32-year-old reserve goalkeeper needed to be substituted on for a penalty. During the penalty taker's approach, he watches their body language and takes note of their eyes being locked to his left. How would his selective attention be best described?

   A. Narrow-external focus
   B. Narrow-internal focus
   C. Broad-external focus
   D. Dissociation
   E. Association

4. A 26-year-old wrestler has recently suffered a groin injury. They were administered a Profile of Mood States (POMS), which showed depression above the population norm. What describes the usual 'iceberg' profile for athletes?

   A. High anger
   B. High vigour
   C. Low across all mood states
   D. Low depression and high across all other mood states
   E. High tension

5. An 18-year-old football player plays professionally for her premier club. Her coach is a 32-year-old male who has coached her for three years. They have had an on-and-off sexual relationship for the last two years. He often praises her in front of teammates and gives her special treatment. There are times when she feels he is inappropriate in front of others but has not been able to bring herself to confront him. She reports feeling pressured to continue being intimate with him as he may influence her career. What is the most appropriate next step for the SEM clinician?

   A. Inform her that you have limited ability to intervene as she is a consenting adult
   B. Ask her the details of the sexual acts to evaluate further
   C. Encourage her to return to you if he is hostile or violent
   D. Follow the organisation's sexual harassment protocol
   E. Discuss your concern with the team captain for more information

MULTIPLE CHOICE QUESTION (MCQ) ANSWERS

1. **Answer D**
    Self-Determination theory highlights the relative importance of intrinsic motivation and autonomy.
2. **Answer E**
    When there is high cognitive anxiety, increasing arousal past a threshold will cause a catastrophic drop-off in performance. Once crossed, it may be difficult to return to the performance level of lower arousal levels. At low cognitive anxiety, there is a smoother inverted-U curve.
3. **Answer A**
    Although association involves focusing on the task at hand, this case describes the cues the goalkeeper is using. They are focusing on a small number of external cues and excluding other information.
4. **Answer B**
    The iceberg profile describes how athletes report high vigour, and lower than average negative mood states.
5. **Answer D**
    The player is uncomfortable and reaching out for help. Agency may be limited by distinct power imbalances and extensive personal repercussions. The behaviour does not need to be hostile or violent to be considered harassment. Organisations have a duty to create clear channels for reporting abuse.

REFERENCES AND FURTHER READING

Articles and Guidelines

English Institute of Sport. *Sports Performance Resources*. Available at: https://eis2win.co.uk/all-resources/

Gorczynski, P., et al. (2021). Developing mental health literacy and cultural competence in elite sport. *Journal of Applied Sport Psychology*, 33(4), pp. 387–401.

Gouttebarge, V., et al. (2021). International Olympic Committee (IOC) Sport Mental Health Assessment Tool 1 (SMHAT-1) and Sport Mental Health Recognition Tool 1 (SMHRT-1): Towards better support of athletes' mental health. *BJSM*, 55(1), pp. 30–37.

International Olympic Committee. (2021). *IOC Mental Health in Elite Athletes Toolkit*. Available at: https://stillmed.olympics.com/media/Document%20Library/IOC/Athletes/Safe-Sport-Initiatives/IOC-Mental-Health-In-Elite-Athletes-Toolkit-2021.pdf

NICE Guidance. 2009. *Depression in Adults: Recognition and Management*. Available at: www.nice.org.uk/guidance/cg90 (Predicted to be updated 2022).

Reardon, C.L., Hainline, B., Aron, C.M., et al. (2019). Mental health in elite athletes: International Olympic Committee consensus statement (2019). *BJSM*, 53, pp. 667–699.

World Health Organization. (2022). *Health and Wellbeing*. Available at: https://www.who.int/data/gho/data/major-themes/health-and-well-being

Textbooks

American Psychiatric Association. (2013). *Diagnostic and Statistical Manual of Mental Disorders*. 5th ed. Arlington, VA: American Psychiatric Publishing.

Cox, R.H. (2012). *Sport Psychology: Concepts and Applications*. 7th ed. New York, NY: McGraw-Hill.

Currie, A., Owen, B. (2016). *Sports Psychiatry*. Oxford, UK: Oxford University Press.

FSEM UK Recommended Reading List.

Glick, I., Kamis, D., Skull, T. (2018). *The ISSP Manual of Sports Psychiatry*. International Society for Sports Psychiatry. New York, NY: Routledge.

Lam, L.C.W., Riba, M. (2016). *Physical Exercise Interventions for Mental Health*. Cambridge, UK: Cambridge University Press.

Mistry, A., McCabe, T., Currie, A. (2020). *Case Studies in Sports Psychiatry*. Cambridge, UK: Cambridge University Press.

Rollnick, S., Fader, J., Breckon, J., Moyers, T. B. (2020). *Coaching Athletes to Be Their Best: Motivational Interviewing in Sports*. New York, NY: The Guilford Press.

Tod, D., Thatcher, J., Rahman, R. (2010). *Sport Psychology*. London, UK: Red Globe Press.

Zenko, Z., Jones, L. (2021). *Essentials of Exercise and Sport Psychology: An Open Access Textbook*. Minneapolis: Society for Transparency, Openness, and Replication in Kinesiology. https://doi.org/10.51224/B1000

Radiology 21

James Hamilton, Dane Vishnubala, Brook Adams, Richard Collins and Carles Pedret

BASIC PRINCIPLES

The development of imaging technology has revolutionised many aspects of modern medicine. Sports and exercise medicine clinicians often find themselves working in environments with easy access to imaging, but referrers must be aware of its limitations. Developing a good relationship with radiologists can optimise the use of imaging. The basic principles will provide a simple introduction to the key terms in radiology reports and on how to use different modalities in diagnosis.

Ultrasound

Ultrasound is commonly performed, ideal for the imaging of many superficial and soft tissue structures. It is cheap, safe, well tolerated and readily accessible (Table 21.1).

Ultrasound uses high frequency sound waves that are both emitted and received via a transducer. Two different tissues will attenuate (absorb) sound to different degrees, creating an acoustic boundary from which some sound reflects. This leads to production of an image by the transformation of sound waves to electrical impulses. A water-based gel is applied to the transducer to facilitate transmission of ultrasound waves between the transducer and patient's skin.

Various ultrasound probes are available with characteristics appropriate to the type of examination; a combination of probe choice and machine setting determines the type of image produced, relevant to the clinical application. High frequency probes are best suited to MSK imaging, allowing a high-resolution image of superficial structures to be generated.

An image is produced in real time, allowing dynamic assessment of structures, which is a useful adjunct to clinical examination or even cross-sectional imaging (Figure 21.2). A well optimised ultrasound image can provide great detail of superficial structures such as tendons, ligaments or superficial joints and can also differentiate between a joint effusion or synovitis. The Doppler feature highlights flow within blood vessels, thereby demonstrating hyperaemia, and this can be used to characterise soft tissue lesions or inflammatory pathology.

Ultrasound is highly vulnerable to artefacts. An example is anisotropy, whereby a structure not imaged perpendicularly falsely appears darker, due to fewer sound waves reflected back to the transducer.

Magnetic Resonance Imaging (MRI)

MRI makes use of highly complex physics, but at its most basic level uses a magnet with the transmission and reception of radio waves to generate cross sectional images. These are presented in groups called 'sequences', that are modified to enhance particular tissue characteristics relevant to the potential diagnoses of a given area. In general, most pathological processes increase the amount of fluid (oedema) in an area, so the design of a protocol for an MRI study will often be a combination of sequences to delineate anatomy (T1 sequences) and fluid-sensitive sequences to highlight areas of pathology (T2 sequences). See Table 21.2.

DOI: 10.1201/9781003179979-21

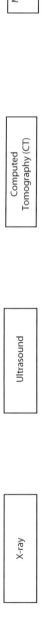

Radiology

X-ray
- Common first line modality
- Accessible and cost effective
- Detects acute bony injury and joint abnormalities, very specific
- Can detect calcification
- Low radiation compared to CT
- Not sensitive
- Generally poor for soft tissue pathology

Ultrasound
- Real time information, low acquisition time
- Cost effective
- No radiation
- Dynamic, multi-plane imaging
- Power-doppler can help detect inflammatory pathology
- Can compare sides
- Great for superficial soft tissue structures
- Cannot image whole body or deeper structures
- User dependent

Computed Tomography (CT)
- Unlimited tissue depth penetration
- Good for bony injury/trauma
- Good for complex joints, intraarticular and axial structures
- 3D reconstructions may be helpful
- High radiation dose
- Poor soft tissue contrast

Magnetic Resonance Imaging (MRI)
- No radiation
- Great for soft tissue injuries
- High spatial resolution
- Can help differentiate between degenerative, inflammatory and traumatic pathology
- Expensive, high acquisition time
- Patients can be claustrophobic and contraindicated with certain metal implants

Figure 21.1 Overview.

Table 21.1 Key terms in your report

Echogenicity	Highly echogenic structures such as soft tissue return a brighter or 'hyperechogenic' image. Low echogenic structures, such as fluid, allow more sound waves to pass through, giving a darker image on the screen.
Acoustic Enhancement	Effect that occurs at the interface beyond a fluid filled structure, due to a large difference in sound transmissibility; this is useful for characterising cystic lesions
Acoustic Shadowing	Solid tissues block the transmission of sound waves, causing areas of void or shadowing on the image. For example, bone or calcified structures will lead to acoustic shadowing beyond them.
Doppler flow	Blood flow in a region can be measured in many ways and with great sensitivity. This tissue characterisation demonstrates areas of higher blood flow.

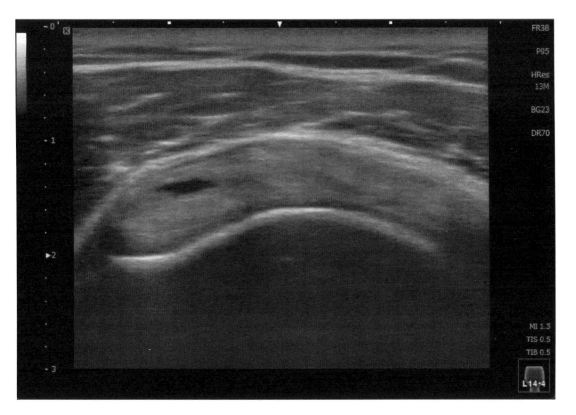

Figure 21.2 Ultrasound image of an intrasubstance supraspinatus tear of the shoulder. Note the hypoechoic defect with echogenic boundaries.

The resolution of MRI is enhanced using different magnetic field strengths measured in 'Tesla' units. A greater field strength allows more of the protons within the body to be polarised. In clinical practice, the commonly used field strengths are 1.5T and 3T. In addition to these, the image quality is highly dependent on the calibration of sequence parameters, and radiographers will often adjust these depending on patient characteristics.

Table 21.2 MRI Sequences

T1 weighted	Commonly used sequence weighting to demonstrate anatomical characteristics. At the most basic level, fluid appears dark and fat appears bright. T1 sequences are required when using gadolinium contrast agents, as gadolinium will increase T1 signal.
T2 weighted	Purely T2 weighted sequences tend to show fat and fluid as bright areas of the image. Looking at areas of fluid that are known, such as the bladder or cerebrospinal fluid, can help identify a sequence.
Fluid weighted (STIR)	Sequences that are described as fluid weighted will highlight areas of fluid likely to represent oedema. All pathology is wet so this highlights possible areas of abnormality. This technique uses fat saturation (see below).
Signal dropout	These are areas that return no signal, such as calcifications or gas.
Fat saturation	These sequences use various techniques to remove fat signal from the image. In MSK imaging, this is used to show bone marrow oedema—the fat signal from normal bone marrow is suppressed in the image, highlighting any oedema. Fat signal will appear dark on these images.

Contrast can be used to enhance for assessment of neoplastic or inflammatory pathology, and intra-articular contrast is used in arthrogram studies to delineate fine intra-articular structures within a joint such as the labrum in the shoulder or the hips.

Contrast

Although this could refer to the inherent difference in brightness between adjacent tissues, in radiology this often refers to the administration of a substance that enhances the contrast between tissues to demonstrate pathology. Contrast media can be used in all imaging modalities in order to distinguish tissue characteristics. In MSK imaging, this could be intravenous contrast in CT/MRI, which allows assessment of the vascularity of a region; or intra-articular contrast, which increases the contrast around fine structures such as joint labra or ligaments, to allow for characterisation of tears or soft tissue tumours. A study using intraarticular contrast is called an arthrogram.

X-ray, Fluoroscopy and CT

The basic principle of plain radiographs is the generation of X-rays (essentially Gamma rays) from bombardment of a tungsten electrode across a large voltage gap. X-ray, Fluoroscopy and CT all use ionising

radiation, and the safety of these medical exposures are a particular concern for Radiologists. In the UK, medical radiation exposure is regulated by both health and safety law and Ionising Radiation (Medical Exposure) Regulations (IRMER). Clinicians should apply the principle that radiation dose should be 'As Low as Reasonably Practical' (ALARP) when requesting and protocolling studies. All exposures to medical radiation should be justified; this means that the risk of the radiation exposure is outweighed by the diagnostic or therapeutic benefit.

A plain X-ray image can broadly demonstrate five densities; air, fat, fluid/soft tissue, bone and metal, and this guides the types of pathology that are well demonstrated. X-ray is first line for investigation of most fractures, a useful starting point to evaluate joint pathology and commonly used for post-operative follow up of metalwork.

A CT scanner is essentially a more advanced form of X-ray, that mounts an X-ray tube in a gantry that spins around a patient allowing formation of a cross-sectional image. These thin slices can be scrolled through and often reconstructed to create images in different planes for precise anatomical definition of pathology. Each area of the image (voxel) is assigned a radiographic density measured in Hounsfield Units. Images are displayed in grey scales with voxels above the selected range displayed in negative colours (black or white) and this allows each tissue to be assessed using optimal parameters for detection of pathology.

Fluoroscopy uses similar principles to X-ray to generate continuous images. Historically, this was used extensively in investigation of joint pathology, although is now more commonly used for interventions such as joint and spinal injections. Radiologists often favour fluoroscopic injections for joint interventions, as an intraarticular injection of radiopaque contrast is an accurate indicator of intra-articular needle placement.

Nuclear Medicine

Nuclear medicine has less use in the sport radiology context. This modality involves injection of a radioactive tracer, which is specifically absorbed by the tissue of interest, before radioactive isotopes are emitted from the patient and detected by a gamma camera.

This can be fused with CT images to enhance sensitivity and provide anatomical information. Metalwork complications are a common use of nuclear medicine studies in this way. Some institutions still assess for occult or stress fractures (e.g. scaphoid fractures) but MRI availability has largely superseded this, without the drawback of ionising radiation.

Guided Injections and Targeted Therapy

All radiological modalities can be used to guide targeted therapy (Table 21.3). Ultrasound allows direct visualisation of a needle and can be used to access soft tissue and intra-articular structures. Many radiologists use fluoroscopy for intra-articular injections, which, in conjunction with contrast, confirms intra-articular needle placement. More complex intervention can be provided under CT guidance, giving enhanced anatomical information for needle placement, but with increased radiation exposure and procedure time.

Ultrasound assessment allows diagnosis and therapy in the same appointment, which is an important consideration when designing a service. Fusion ultrasound is a relatively new technology, that combines ultrasound images with CT or MRI, potentially allowing more complex interventions with greater accuracy than could be performed under ultrasound alone.

Spinal Imaging

In acute spinal trauma, CT is the preferred method of imaging in the Emergency Department; plain film is rarely used.

Table 21.3 Key Image-Guided Interventions	
Steroid injection	These injections are used where there is localised inflammatory pathology. Important considerations include post-injection flare, risk of infection, systemic effects of steroid medication and local tissue damage.
Platelet Rich Plasma (PRP)/ autologous blood	Platelet rich plasma uses a patient's blood, which is spun in a centrifuge, to separate the constituents. Autologous blood is injected directly. Both therapies are intended to place blood products that promote healing into damaged tissue. Evidence for some applications is poor.
Hyaluronic acid injection	Synthetic hyaluronate injection is primarily used to ameliorate symptoms of arthritis, although use has been reported in other synovial lined structures.
Shoulder Hydrodilation	Treatment for adhesive capsulitis involves intra-articular injection of steroid and saline in order to distend the joint capsule.
Barbotage	Using a needle to agitate a region. This can be used for calcific tendinopathy, and calcium deposits can also be aspirated in the acute phase. Some use of dry needling has been documented in insertional tendinopathies.
Nerve root block/ Transforaminal epidural	Targeted intervention to spinal nerve roots using injection of steroid and local anaesthetic. This can be therapeutic to relieve pain but also diagnostic to confirm irritation of a nerve root prior to surgery.
Ablation	Use of radiofrequency, microwave or extreme cold to destroy a focal area of tissue. This can be used to relieve pain, if targeted at nerve roots, or to treat some tumours.

The need for cervical spine imaging is predicted by the Ottawa or Nexus C-spine rules. Clinicians should be familiar with the features predicting the need for spinal imaging to allow clinical clearance, particularly when managing players with head injuries.

MRI of the spine allows for assessment of the bone marrow signal. The discs, ligaments, cord and nerve roots can be assessed, and imaging of the spine in trauma is often performed when evaluating potentially unstable spinal injuries, or where there are neurological signs.

Bone marrow is a metabolically active tissue that responds to insults in many ways. Radiology reports regularly discuss bone marrow oedema, which is a non-specific response of bone marrow to multifactorial insult. In spinal imaging in sports medicine, this is usually a result of trauma: either acute, or as a result of overuse injuries (e.g. pars interarticularis defects). Malignancy is another important cause of bone marrow signal change to consider.

KNEE

Knee injuries are common in sports medicine. In the emergency department, the acutely swollen post-traumatic knee is usually initially investigated with X-ray, which allows exclusion of severely displaced fractures and assessment for joint effusion or lipohaemarthrosis. The results of this, in conjunction with clinical impression, guide the use of further, more advanced imaging and different institutions may vary in their approach.

Classic Injury Patterns

When imaging the knee, there are classic patterns of bone marrow oedema that are associated with common injuries, and this can provide a useful indicator of the structures likely to be injured (Table 21.4). It can also direct 'review areas' for particularly detailed examination, especially if these appear normal initially.

Fractures Around the Knee

Many fracture types occur in contact sports and these usually occur in conjunction with other injuries. An important plain film sign to appreciate in an acute

setting is lipohaemarthrosis. In the knee, this is seen in the suprapatellar region, where there is extensive joint swelling secondary to haemarthrosis with a layer of fat sitting on top. The fat is of lower density (think back to the five radiographic densities) and gives a characteristic appearance. As the fat comes from bone marrow, following disruption of the cortex, there must be a fracture. Further investigation is mandated if this is occult on initial imaging.

Ligaments and Menisci

Plain X-ray is often the first line investigation for an acutely painful knee; though for accurate visualisation, MRI is the first line modality for imaging the cruciate ligaments, collateral ligaments and menisci. The menisci are well demonstrated, and various types of meniscal tear can be delineated. The X-ray can still be useful for the appreciation of small fractures, such as the sometimes subtle 'Segond' fracture at the lateral tibial plateau (indicative of an ACL rupture). Joint swelling caused by an effusion can be seen, and should prompt consideration of more significant pathology.

On MRI, the ACL should be examined in all planes. Rupture of the ACL is well demonstrated with secondary signs such as the 'lateral notch sign' and anterior tibial translocation (Figure 21.3). Similarly, the menisci are well demonstrated on standard MRI and should be evaluated in all planes.

Meniscal tears are generally categorised as horizontal, vertical, radial or complex—meaning a combination or multiple morphologies. Further characterisation includes whether a tear extends to the meniscal root (the meniscal peripheries are more vascular and small tears may heal); the degree of displacement; and special types of tear—such as the Wrisberg rip or 'ramp' lesions—involving the meniscal attachments and having important implications for surgery.

Thickening of the MCL is commonly seen in the context of a low grade or chronic injury, with oedema around the collateral ligaments suggesting a grade 2 injury. Ligamentous rupture will demonstrate redundancy of the split ligament ends, with extensive surrounding soft tissue swelling. Similar principles apply to the assessment of the lateral collateral ligaments. Although the posterolateral corner structures are variable and often poorly seen on MRI, this region should be examined carefully—especially in the context of ACL rupture.

Table 21.4 Knee Injury Patterns Seen on MRI

Pivot Shift	Marrow oedema (contusion) is seen on the posterolateral tibial plateau and mid-lateral femoral condyle, indicating there has been valgus stress on an externally rotated knee. This can be associated with ACL injury.
Hyperextension	Contusion is seen on the anterior tibial plateau and anterior femoral condyle. It suggests hyperextension, often with the foot planted, and may be associated with ACL, PCL, meniscal and even dislocation injuries.
Patellar dislocation	Contusion is seen on the anterolateral lateral femoral condyle and medial patella. It suggests dislocation, often from a twist to a flexed knee, and may be associated with medial patellofemoral ligament or patellar retinaculum injury.

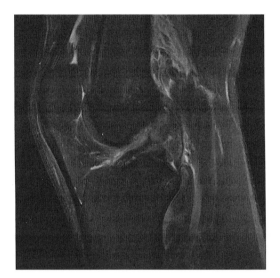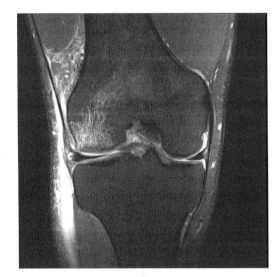

Figure 21.3 MRI knee showing a complete ACL tear. Note the pattern of bone bruising consistent with a pivot shift mechanism.

The Articular Cartilage

Articular cartilage has a fairly high-water content, which allows for optimised sequences to show cartilage pathology (proton density imaging). Various terms describe articular cartilage pathology and types of chondral surface defect in MRI. These can be confined to the chondral surface or extend to the subarticular bone, where they are termed an osteochondral defect. These are commonly seen in sports injuries.

The stability of an osteochondral defect can be predicted from MRI: if fluid is seen beneath a defect, this is likely to be unstable and orthopaedic referral is indicated.

Patellofemoral Instability

The patellofemoral joint is a highly variable joint with a range of variance that can predispose to instability or early degeneration. The patella is a sesamoid bone, and patellar instability is a common presentation in sports medicine. As with most presentations, plain film is beneficial in acute dislocation, even if reduced. The skyline view can be useful, as it permits assessment of subtle avulsion fractures, the retinacular insertions and is a useful adjunct to MRI. The retinaculum, articular surface damage and associated intra-articular fragments can be assessed on MRI, as can factors predisposing to patellar instability:

such as patella alta, increased TT-TG (tibial tuberosity to trochlear groove) distance and trochlear facet asymmetry.

Patella maltracking refers to signs associated with suboptimal motion of the patella across the femoral trochlea. Defects of the articular surface of the patella—particularly when the degree of degeneration at the patellofemoral joint is out of proportion to the degeneration in the medial and lateral compartments—are signs of chronic issues with patellar tracking. The infrapatellar and quadriceps fat pads are often oedematous with mechanical issues at the patellofemoral joint, and fat pad impingement often presents in the paediatric age group. The infrapatellar fat pad is an important pain generator around the knee joint in all ages.

The Extensor Mechanism

The quadriceps tendon is developed from all the quadriceps muscles and it attaches to the superior pole of the patella. The part coming from the rectus femoris crosses over the patella and has continuity with the patellar tendon. The patellar tendon origin is in the inferior pole of the patella bone and attaches to the tibial tuberosity. These tendons can undergo tendinopathic change and severely tendinopathic tendons can rupture. From a radiological point of view, the patellar and quadriceps tendons are superficial structures, well visualised on ultrasound. Tendinopathic features, such as fusiform thickening, hypervascularity, calcifications and hypoechoic clefts, can be readily identified and can be graded. In cases of complete rupture, an ultrasound examination can completely characterise the injury.

FOOT AND ANKLE

Fractures of the metatarsals are common in athletes, both as a result of trauma and stress response. Simple metatarsal fractures are well demonstrated on X-ray but injuries to the base of the metatarsals, involving the Lisfranc ligament complex, should always prompt further imaging, usually with CT. Ongoing suspicion of an injury in this area following a normal appearing X-ray also warrants CT to exclude the possibility of an occult Lisfranc fracture—which can have devastating consequences for mobility if left untreated.

An insidious onset of pain in the metatarsals (or at the base of the 5th metatarsal) raises suspicion of a stress fracture, more accurately described in imaging terms as a stress response. As with many presentations in sports medicine, an initial plain X-ray is advised. This can show not only an advanced stress fracture, but also subtle early periosteal reaction. It is worth noting stress fractures can sometimes be seen on ultrasound, and this is an important review area. Stress fractures can occur at other locations in the foot, such as the calcaneus. If clinical suspicion remains, then MRI allows detection of occult fractures or an early stress response—changes in the marrow are apparent before a cortical break occurs. MRI also allows to diagnose the bone oedema which could be a source of pain itself, as well as a precursor of a stress fracture or a stress reaction.

Complex fractures of the foot and ankle are usually imaged with CT to aid planning. In initial assessment of injuries in the Emergency Department, plain X-ray can identify signs of ankle instability, such as widening of the medial clear space. It is also important to assess for associated injuries, e.g. a posterior malleolar fracture.

Joint Pathology

With many ankle injuries, plain film imaging remains the first line for exclusion of fractures and assessment of the joint space. Osteochondral defects of the talar dome can be appreciated on plain film. Appreciation of ankle joint swelling and radiological signs of instability are all important when assessing the plain X-ray. MRI can be a useful adjunct to characterise joint pain with assessment of subchondral oedema and articular cartilage.

Ligamentous injury can be assessed with ultrasound, which can rapidly aid the grading of injuries in a point-of-care scenario. High grade ankle injuries will often be supplemented by MRI imaging, allowing excellent visualisation of the ligamentous structures and assessment of associated injuries. Note that MRI tends to underestimate the grading of ankle ligament injuries.

Ultrasound can visualise the major tendinous structures of the ankle and can be used to evaluate chronic tendinopathy and rupture of major tendons. Ultrasound is the first line test in acute Achilles tendon rupture and allows for assessment of extent of rupture, size of defect and a functional test of the Achilles tendon under direct imaging.

Table 21.5 Pelvic Tendinous Insertions

Anterior Superior Iliac Spine	Sartorius, Tensor Fascia Lata
Anterior Inferior Iliac Spine	Rectus Femoris (direct head)
Ischial tuberosity	Hamstrings
Greater Tuberosity	Gluteal tendons
Lesser tuberosity	Iliopsoas tendon

Tendinopathy is commonly observed on MRI of the foot and ankle, and tears can be visualised and graded.

When imaging the foot and ankle, functional factors should be considered—MRI can show minor changes in soft tissues simply due to footwear.

HIP AND GROIN

Pelvic fractures are rare, even in contact sports. Additional injuries are probable due to the high impact involved. CT is usually appropriate in these cases, often with a dedicated trauma CT protocol. More chronic stress fractures can be subtle on plain film, so MRI should be considered if there is a high index of suspicion.

More common fractures in younger athletes are avulsions of the major pelvic tendinous insertions (Table 21.5).

Groin pain in athletes is complex. From an imaging point of view, clinical history is crucial, as some findings can be seen both in healthy controls and symptomatic individuals. This is due to the complexity of the pelvic tendinous attachments and the complex function of all muscle groups in the pelvis that can create functional disbalances as they act in an agonist/antagonist fashion. Intervention (targeted injection or surgical) must be in conjunction with a bespoke rehabilitation programme.

Hip pathology can manifest as groin pain. X-ray of the hip is the first line study for assessment of hip morphology (Figure 21.4), possibly followed by advanced imaging such as MRI or MR arthrograms.

Debate exists as to whether MRI at 3T or arthrography at 1.5T optimises diagnosis. MRI of the pelvis allows assessment of the hip joint morphology, effusions, synovitis and cartilaginous injuries. MRI arthrogram is good for labral tears, which are often highly symptomatic due to the rich labral blood supply. If there is a suspicion for labral pathology, liaison with a Radiologist is important to ensure optimal imaging protocols.

The process of true femoral acetabular impingement involves rapid degeneration of the hip joint when an anatomical disposition occurs. Femoroacetabular impingement (FAI) is broadly split into two types: Pincer and Cam type deformity, with a mixed picture also seen. Abnormal morphology of the femoral head causes increased wear of the cartilage and acetabular labrum, which can progress to early severe degenerative OA. A substantial number of healthy control subjects have a similar hip morphology, leaving clinicians to determine which patients will benefit from intervention balanced against the risk of harm.

Other common diagnoses demonstrable on pelvic MRI are muscle injuries of the adductor group, gluteal injuries and imaging features supporting a diagnosis of greater trochanteric pain syndrome.

SHOULDER

The shoulder is a complex functional unit and imaging should be interpreted with this in mind. Fractures of the shoulder girdle are imaged with plain film in the first instance, and this allows assessment of the congruency of the glenohumeral joint. Some non-displaced fractures such as greater tuberosity fractures are often misdiagnosed by X-ray and ultrasound scan can be more sensible in these cases. The acromioclavicular joint is a common area of injury, particularly in contact sports, and the Rookwood classification is used to delineate these injuries. MRI is sometimes useful for surgical planning or where there is concern for other intra-articular injury.

When considering soft tissue injuries around the shoulder, these can be categorised into rotator cuff injuries (commonly seen in older adults as a result

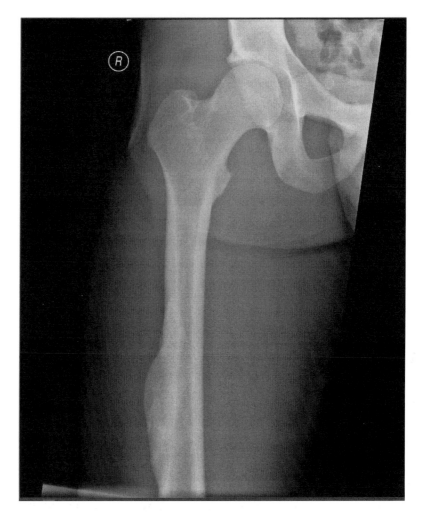

Figure 21.4 X-ray of the right femur of a rugby player following subacute trauma. Further imaging confirmed Myositis ossificans.

of degeneration) and non-rotator cuff injuries—incorporating the ligamentous and intra-articular structures around the shoulder girdle. When interpreting radiology reports, there are several normal adaptations in elite sports players, which are useful to be aware of.

Biceps and Pectoral Rupture

The biceps muscle has two tendinous attachments, the long head attaches to the glenoid labrum and the short head to the coracoid process. Ultrasound can diagnose ruptures of both the biceps tendon origins,

but delineation of the distal biceps insertion can be difficult. MRI remains the gold standard, especially using the FABS view (elbow flexed, shoulder abducted, forearm supinated). These cases should be imaged promptly if surgical repair is possible.

Pectoral rupture can be diagnosed on ultrasound but, again, MRI is the most appropriate examination. This is an injury commonly seen among patients undertaking heavy weightlifting. It is important to make the suspicion of pectoral rupture clear on radiological requests, as the field of view required extends more inferiorly compared to a standard shoulder MRI protocol.

Dislocation and Instability

Anterior dislocation of the shoulder is frequently seen in the context of contact sports, such as rugby. Plain film will diagnose this, and a follow-up film is required to confirm relocation and exclude fracture. The associated Hill Sachs lesion (humeral head depression fracture) and Bankart lesion (inferior glenoid fracture) can sometimes be seen on plain film and are useful review areas in the acute setting.

The glenoid forms part of a complex with the glenoid labrum and associated capsular ligaments, which are important stabilisers of the shoulder joint. MRI or MRI arthrography is the imaging modality of choice for assessment of the glenoid labrum and the bicipital-labral complex.

Anterior inferior dislocation often causes injury to the inferior glenohumeral ligament and, as a result, trauma to the closely attached glenoid labrum occurs. There are several variants of soft tissue Bankart lesions, with varying combinations of injury to the labrum and middle or inferior glenohumeral ligaments. Humeral avulsion of the glenohumeral ligament is another variation of this pattern.

Whilst SLAP (superior labral anterior-to-posterior) tears can be difficult to diagnose (with a great deal of normal variants around the bicipital-labral complex), these lesions can be of little clinical significance and should be put into context.

Rotator Cuff

The rotator cuff can be effectively examined using ultrasound, which has equal sensitivity to MRI as it has a very standard examination routine. Tendinopathic changes are easily demonstrated and both partial and full thickness tears can be characterised. Examination includes the acromioclavicular joint, to determine morphology and predisposing factors to subacromial impingement, and there should be a dynamic assessment for subacromial and subscapular impingement. The degree of fatty atrophy of the rotator cuff musculature should be judged, as this has important surgical implications.

ELBOW

Lateral epicondylopathy is an overuse injury of the common extensor tendon, usually seen in racquet sports and in those whose occupation requires gripping heavy objects. Diagnostic features can be seen on both ultrasound and MRI. Similar imaging features are seen at the medial epicondyle, which, although termed 'golfers' elbow', is also seen in tennis players. This involves the common flexor tendon insertion.

MRI is generally the best modality for imaging the medial and ulnar collateral ligaments.

The paediatric elbow is predisposed to a different pattern of injury. Awareness of the order of ossification centres is essential for assessment of paediatric elbow films. Little Leaguer's Elbow is a medial epicondyle apophysitis associated with baseball pitching, secondary to repetitive valgus stress. As with other forms of apophyseal injury, the fragmented appearances of the apophysis can be seen on X-ray. These appearances are variable and MRI remains the optimal modality to evaluate the physis and for pathological marrow oedema.

MRI can detect osteochondral defects, whether secondary to osteochondritis dissecans or degenerative disease.

A commonly seen pathology around the elbow are nerve entrapments. This can be secondary to entrapments of the ulnar (most common), median or radial nerves and their branches. Medial epicondylopathy is closely associated with ulnar neuropathy, caused by entrapment in the cubital tunnel. Both MRI and ultrasound have a role: signs of nerve thickening or oedema can be seen on both. Ultrasound can give real-time information about ulnar nerve subluxation.

The distal biceps tendon attaches at the radial tuberosity, with a complex attachment at the lacertus fibrosus. As with long head of biceps rupture, urgent MRI remains the best test to characterise distal biceps tendon injury, given a relatively short timescale for successful surgical repair.

HAND AND WRIST

Scaphoid fractures are usually seen following a fall on an outstretched hand. The importance of these injuries is that the scaphoid has a retrograde blood supply, so a more proximal fracture is at high risk of avascular necrosis. Subsequent effects on carpal stability have an impact on function in these (often young) patients. Specific radiographic scaphoid views improve sensitivity. Follow-up films are usually performed 10 days following splint applications and, if clinical concern remains, the most appropriate investigation is MRI. This could be performed at an earlier stage following initial plain film in the setting of professional sport. Injuries with a similar clinical presentation include base of thumb metacarpal fractures or distal radius fractures, which can be significant if there is intra-articular involvement.

Hamate fractures can be difficult to appreciate on plain film. These are often seen in contact or combat sports, and can be associated with dislocation of the ring and little finger metacarpals. When assessing this area, make sure the ring and little finger CMC joints are congruent and that the hook of the hamate can be seen. Isolated hook of hamate fractures are more commonly associated with impaction, e.g. in racquet sports. A chronic stress response injury is also possible.

Many fractures of the hand and wrist have been given eponymous names, some of which are associated with certain sports.

The scapholunate ligament (SLL) connects the scaphoid to the lunate and has a volar, intraosseous and dorsal component. Established high grade scapholunate rupture can be appreciated on a plain film, with widening of the scapholunate interval beyond 4 mm. SLL injuries may occur following a fall on an outstretched, extended and pronated hand, or be a more chronic presentation of carpal instability. More subtle injuries are usually detected on MRI, although dynamic ultrasound testing is also possible in expert hands.

If available, 3T MRI provides excellent imaging quality; otherwise, the best imaging choice is either an arthrogram or standard MRI, depending on clinical suspicion. MRI of the wrist allows for excellent assessment of pathology involving the bones, tendons and nerves. The smaller ligaments and triangular fibrocartilaginous complex (TFCC) are optimally assessed with a 3T scan and/or MR arthrography.

Both 'Gamekeeper's' and Skiers thumb refer to injuries of the ulnar collateral ligament of the thumb—either chronic or acute, respectively. An avulsion fracture at the ulnar corner of the first metacarpal head or base of the proximal phalanx may be seen on X-ray. However, to assess the ligament, ultrasound is often used, which can assess the position of a bony fragment. If this becomes trapped beneath the adductor pollicis muscle, this is termed a Stener lesion and should be fixed surgically. MRI can be used for grading.

MUSCLE INJURY AND GRADING

Muscle injuries are the most common injuries in elite sport and they occur due to the high demands of this environment. Imaging is mainly performed to have an early and accurate diagnosis, but also to guide rehabilitation. The availability of ultrasound lends itself to initial assessment of muscle injury and functional assessment can be undertaken simultaneously. In well built, muscular individuals, ultrasound may not be able to delineate deep structures, so MRI is used.

Several grading systems have been proposed to categorise the area and location of muscle injuries, with the most commonly used system being BAMIC (British Athletics Muscle Injury Classification). This was initially used in hamstring injuries in track and field athletes with an MRI diagnosis (Table 21.6).

Table 21.6 BAMIC Muscle Injury Classification	
Grade 0	0a focal injury with normal MRI 0b features of DOMS (Delayed Onset Muscle Soreness)
Grade 1 a: myofascial (peripheral)	STIR signal <10% cross sectional area or longitudinal length and <1 cm fibre disruption
Grade 2 b: myotendinous junction/ muscular	STIR signal 10–50% cross section; length <15 cm and <5 cm fibre disruption 2c means that there is a moderate intramuscular tendon tear
Grade 3 c: tendinous	STIR signal >50% cross sectional area, longitudinal length >15 cm and >5 cm fibre disruption 3c means that there is an extensive intramuscular tendon tear
Grade 4 Complete Tear	4a Myofascial, muscular or myotendinous 4b Tendinous

MRI characterises injuries according to the amount of muscle oedema measured on a STIR sequence, fibre disorganisation, the location of the tear and especially if there is an affection of the dense connective tissue. Grades 1–3 can be classified as a) myofascial, b) myotendinous junction/muscular or c) tendinous.

CLINICAL CONSIDERATIONS

Other commonly used muscle injury classification systems include Pedret et al., (2020) for the ultrasound classification of gastrocnemius injuries and Prakash et al., (2018) for the MRI classification of calf injuries. Classification systems can be limited and do not take into account factors such as injury history, limb dominance, age and playing position when trying to predict return to sport times.

MULTIPLE CHOICE QUESTION (MCQ) QUESTIONS

1. A 13-year-old county level athlete has recently been training for a 110-metre hurdle event. He presents to your clinic following an acute popping sensation around his leading right hip. X-ray demonstrates a small bony fleck adjacent to the anterior inferior iliac spine.
   Which of the following statements is correct?

   A. Findings are suggestive of acute sartorius tendon avulsion.
   B. This is a commonly seen normal variant and a low-grade quadriceps injury is more likely.
   C. This is a typical finding of rectus femoris tendon avulsion.
   D. MRI arthrogram is indicated to assess the acetabular labrum.
   E. Findings are suggestive of hamstring tendon avulsion.

2. A 35-year-old male patient presents to your clinic with a 4-week history of worsening pain within the metatarsals of his right foot following the introduction of a new training programme. There is no history of trauma. On examination, there is point tenderness over the midshaft of the second metatarsal but no other significant findings. Which of the following statements is correct?

   A. A normal plain film would exclude a stress fracture and a biomechanical cause for pain should be sought.
   B. Ultrasound performed in clinic will exclude a stress response in this case.
   C. Bone marrow oedema on MRI is indicative of a stress response in this case.
   D. Bone scintigraphy demonstrates areas of bone marrow oedema typical of a stress response.
   E. CT should always be performed in assessment of foot fracture.

3. A 65-year-old former professional golfer attends your clinic with recurrent right hip pain. X-ray has demonstrated features of moderate osteoarthritis, with moderate degenerative change in the lumbar spine. A shared decision is made to proceed with a corticosteroid and local anaesthetic injection into the right hip as both a diagnostic and therapeutic procedure. Which of the following statements is correct?

   A. Ultrasound cannot be used to guide injections into the hip joints as the needle cannot be visualised at lower frequencies.
   B. MRI must be performed prior to injection to exclude alternative causes for the presentation.
   C. Contrast injection should be used when performing an ultrasound guided injection to confirm needle placement.
   D. Ultrasound and fluoroscopic techniques can both be used for intra-articular injection in this circumstance.
   E. A labral tear is a contraindication to corticosteroid injection.

4. A 23-year-old male footballer presents to the outpatient clinic with a 4-month history of right sided groin pain of insidious onset. The pain is difficult to localise but clinically there is no suspicion of a hernia. Plain film of the pelvis demonstrates small bilateral CAM morphologies with no other abnormality. With regard to the following statements regarding contextualising the subsequent MRI findings, which is correct?

   A. A standard MRI protocol, without intra-articular contrast, at 1.5T can usually exclude a labral tear.

B. Symmetrical marrow oedema at the symphysis pubis is indicative of a clinically significant stress response that explains this presentation.

C. A small area of anterior acetabular marrow oedema in this context is strongly suggestive of clinically significant FAI.

D. The stability of a small osteochondral defect of the articular surface of the femoral head cannot be predicted on MRI.

E. A 'sportsman's hernia' is a small abdominal wall defect easily seen on MRI.

5. Whilst on a team training camp abroad, a 28-year-old female footballer complains of sudden onset pain in the hamstring region whilst sprinting. Clinically, you suspect a hamstring strain with no loss of power and a local MRI is performed. The report describes a region of oedema within the biceps femoris muscle measuring 30% of the cross-sectional area of the muscle, extending into the distal myotendinous junction over an approximate length of 10 cm. Which BAMIC grade injury does this represent?

A. 2b
B. 3a
C. 3b
D. 2c
E. 2a

MULTIPLE CHOICE QUESTION (MCQ) ANSWERS

1. Answer C
Pelvic tendon insertions are common exam questions.

2. Answer C
Bone marrow oedema on MRI is a key sign of stress response. This cannot be excluded on plain film and, whilst ultrasound can demonstrate periosteal swelling or a cortical breach, the test is not sensitive enough to exclude a stress fracture. Scintigraphy demonstrates tracer uptake secondary to osteoblastic process rather

than marrow oedema and was previously used to detect stress fractures. CT should be performed in assessment of complex fractures such as a Lisfranc fracture.

3. Answer D
Both ultrasound and fluoroscopic techniques can be used. In cases of osteoarthritis evident on plain film, in an appropriate age group, MRI imaging is not required. A labral tear is not a contraindication to a steroid injection and may be an expected finding in this case.

4. Answer C
Congruent findings of a Cam defect and focal articular surface wear would be suggestive of Cam impingement. A labral tear is difficult to exclude at 1.5T without intra-articular contrast. Marrow oedema at the symphysis pubis is often seen in normal subjects and is variable according to skeletal maturation. Osteochondral defect stability can be graded according to surrounding oedema. A 'sportsman's hernia' is a non-specific term relating to athletic groin pain and no abdominal wall defect is visible on MRI.

5. Answer A
The BAMIC grading system is a useful means of grading muscle injuries on MRI.

FURTHER READING AND REFERENCES

Pedret, C., Balius, R., Blasi, M., Dávila, F., Aramendi, J.F., Masci, L and de la Fuente, J. 2020. Ultrasound classification of medial gastrocnemious injuries. *Scand J Med Sci Sports.* 30(12), pp. 2456–2465. doi: 10.1111/sms.13812. Epub 2020 Sep 16. PMID: 32854168.

Pollock, N., James, S.L.J., Lee, J.C and Chakraverty, R. 2014. British athletics muscle injury classification: a new grading system. *British Journal of Sports Medicine 2014*; 48, pp. 1347–1351.

Prakash, A., Entwisle, T., Schneider, M., Brukner, P and Connell, D. 2018. Connective tissue injury in calf muscle tears and return to play: MRI correlation. *Br J Sports Med.* Jul; 52(14), pp. 929–933. doi: 10.1136/bjsports-2017-098362. Epub 2017 Oct 26. PMID: 29074478.

Index

Note: Page numbers in *italic* indicate a figure and page numbers in **bold** indicate a table on the corresponding page.

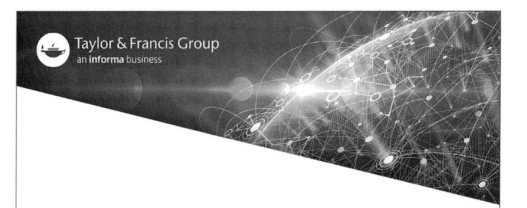
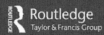
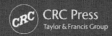

Printed in the United States
by Baker & Taylor Publisher Services